COMPREHENSIVE WELLNESS FOR FIREFIGHTERS

Fitness and Health Guide For Fire and Rescue Workers

Jon Pearson

John Hayford, M.S.

Wendi Royer, M.S.

Summit Fitness Services

JOHN WILEY & SONS, INC.
New York • Chichester • Weinheim • Brisbane • Singapore • Toronto

Comprehensive Wellness for Fighters (CW-F) is an innovative training program designed specifically for use by fire and emergency medical services departments in promoting the fitness and health of their members. The program provides detailed instructor materials, including videotape and slide support, for teaching the information contained in this book. To order or learn more about the CW-F program, please contact Summit Fitness Services, PO Box 478, Blue Ridge Summit, PA 17214, 717-794-2269.

This book is not intended as a substitute for medical advice. Readers who suspect that they may have specific medical problems should consult a physician about any suggestions made in this book.

Originally published as ISBN 0-442-02068-6

For ordering and customer service, call 1-800-CALL-WILEY.

Library of Congress Cataloging-in-Publication Data

Pearson, Jon

Comprehensive wellness for firefighters : fitness and health guide for fire safety workers/ Jon Pearson, John Hayford, Wendi Royer

p. cm.

Includes bibliographical references and index.

ISBN 0-471-28709-1 (pbk.)

1. Fire Fighters —Health and hygiene. I. Hayford, John. II. Royer, Wendi III. Title.

RC965.F48P43 1995 95-4598

613'.08'83633—dc20 CIP

To all our nation's fire and rescue workers,

whose fitness and health benefit us all.

And to Pat.

CONTENTS

DEVELOPMENT TEAM

This book is based on the **Comprehensive Wellness For Firefighters** training program developed by Summit Fitness Services. Key members of the instructional design team are:

David Barillo, M.D., is Clinical Assistant Professor of Surgery at a large southwestern university, specializing in the transport and critical care of severely burned patients. He has served as Medical Director for the Hazardous Materials Team and Fire Surgeon for the Newark (NJ) Fire Department, Deputy Chief of the Newark (NJ) Auxiliary Fire Department, and consultant to the United States Fire Administration and National Fire Academy.

Dan Fabyan provides management consulting and teaching services to fire organizations. Previously, he was Deputy Chief of Operations for the Miami Fire Department with responsibility for fire suppression, rescue, training, and physical fitness. He has served as the City of Miami Fire Marshal, Chief of the Department's Fire Prevention Bureau, and Adjunct Faculty member for the National Fire Academy.

John Hayford, M.S., is Exercise Physiology Coordinator for the National Hospital for Orthopaedics and Rehabilitation. He directs programs for health and fitness promotion involving a comprehensive series of medical and physical fitness examinations and assessments. Mr. Hayford's clients include fire and rescue departments, law enforcement agencies, corporations, athletic teams/clubs, and members of the general public.

Jon Pearson, President of Summit Fitness Services, has served as instructional designer and developer on many National Fire Academy and Emergency Management Institute courses and videotapes. As a management consult, he has directed major projects in training development, curriculum planning, target audience analysis, application of instructional technologies, organizational analysis, and management information system design.

Dade Royer is President of American Fitness Inc. and co-owner of Family Fitness, Inc., which manages fitness and aerobic centers and programs. He directs an on-site corporate fitness center, and has co-authored training manuals for fitness consultants, fitness instructors, aerobic instructors, and clerical management. Previously, he owned and managed a health food and nutritional supplies outlet and two health food cafes.

Wendi Royer, M.S., is a certified Professional Aerobics Instructor, co-owner, aerobics director, and instructor for fitness clubs, and aerobics director for the Citicorp Fitness Center. She develops and conducts training for aerobics instructors, and participates in training development projects for the National Fire Academy and Emergency Management Institute. She has also served as manager and nutritional consultant to local weight loss centers.

Ellen Ternes is a television, radio, and videotape script writer and producer for a broad range of clients. She has developed education, information, and entertainment programs, including projects for the National Fire Academy, a public health information series, nutrition videotapes for athletes, and an information video on the U.S. Army's fitness program.

ACKNOWLEDGMENTS

Special thanks to Chief Gary Hawbaker and members of the Hagerstown (MD) Fire Department, IAFF Local 1605, for their help and good spirits throughout this project. Also, our gratitude to Tom Healy, Murray Loflin, Dennis Rubin, and Gordon Sachs for reviewing early drafts of the manual and providing valuable insight and support. Finally, thanks to Andrew Sussman and Tracy Holliday for their talent, hard work, and faith in the outcome.

Photographs by Pictures Plus, Waynesboro, Pennsylvania.

INTRODUCTION

Studies have repeatedly shown that firefighters and rescue workers need high levels of strength, endurance, aerobic capacity, and flexibility to do their jobs. But just being fit isn't enough for this dangerous occupation. To minimize risks, each member of the department also needs to take an active role in managing his or her own health in areas as diverse as nutrition, weight control, stress management, substance abuse prevention, and personal safety. In other words, every worker needs to think of fitness as part of **comprehensive wellness**, a philosophy that emphasizes the total health and well-being of each individual through the active prevention of illness and injury.

Comprehensive Wellness for Firefighters (CW-F) has been prepared to help the fire service community address this critical health and safety issue. In the following chapters, you will learn about the health risks faced by firefighters, and why you need higher levels of fitness than most other professions. You will examine basic concepts and techniques for building your physical capabilities, and design exercise routines that meet your own needs and interests. You will receive up-to-date information on related health issues, and develop personal action plans that serve as a "road map" to improved vitality and well-being.

The rest is up to you—no long-term gain will occur unless you want it to. But if you make a commitment to health and fitness, the benefits can be tremendous! They include:

- Greater strength and stamina
- Weight reduction and/or control (maintenance)
- Lower cholesterol and blood pressure levels
- Decreased risk of death, injury, or disability from disease
- Heightened job performance and enjoyment from work
- Improved performance in sports and other physical activities
- Better posture, joint functioning, and appearance
- Reduction of anxiety, stress, tension, and depression
- Increased energy, general vitality, and mental sharpness
- Enhanced self-esteem and self-image
- More restful and refreshing sleep

In short, ***increasing your level of physical fitness and taking better care of your health can greatly improve your life***. This is not just a grand statement—it's a fact! Therefore, you are encouraged to accept responsibility for your own fitness and health by incorporating wellness into your daily routine. Like other good things, it may take some effort, but the results will be worth it. **Do it for yourself!**

WHAT YOU WILL LEARN

This book is designed as a resource and practical guide to help you get in shape and stay in shape throughout your entire career. The information is divided into two areas: 1) developing and maintaining high levels of physical fitness needed for fire and rescue work, and 2) establishing lifestyle patterns and behaviors that contribute to long-term health and enjoyment.

To develop and maintain fitness, you need to participate in a regular program of appropriate exercise activities. Chapters 1-5 provide in-depth information on exercise principles and options, including simple self-assessment methods, sample workout routines, and tools to help you prepare your own exercise plan. Material on related topics—human physiology, disease risk factors, back problems, etc.—is integrated throughout. Since everyone is different, a major focus is placed on identifying activities that are right for <u>you</u>. Remember, research shows that people usually don't stick with an exercise program unless they enjoy it and it produces results.

Although physical fitness is critical to health and performance, it's only one component of wellness. Chapters 6-10 contain information and guidelines on related subject areas, including nutrition, weight control, substance abuse prevention, stress management, and personal safety. This material is designed to provide a framework for thinking through your own lifestyle—what you're doing right and what might be improved. Building on this knowledge, you establish simple action plans that reflect your own interests and priorities. The book concludes with material that emphasizes the comprehensive nature of wellness and the skills needed to <u>maintain</u> a healthy lifestyle.

The material in this book is appropriate for all fire and rescue department members who have current medical approval to participate in vigorous exercise and fitness assessment activities. After completing the book, you should be able to:

- Explain key fitness terms and concepts.
- Describe major health risk factors associated with common lifestyles and fire service activities.
- Assess your own current levels of physical fitness.
- Select exercise activities and programs that are right for you.
- Evaluate your own lifestyle in each major component of wellness.
- Develop strategies and a personal action plan to promote your own wellness.
- Adopt a long-term commitment to physical fitness and a healthy lifestyle.

CHAPTER OVERVIEW

Chapter 1—Physical Fitness and the Fire Service begins the book by examining why high levels of fitness are needed for fire and rescue work. A special emphasis is placed on risk factors for coronary heart disease. General fitness terminology and concepts are introduced, and you are given an opportunity to think about your own attitudes concerning fitness and health. Fire department fitness programs are discussed, and the relationships among fitness, health, and job performance are analyzed.

Chapter 2—Fitness Assessment: Finding Your Starting Point explains the purpose and benefits of conducting a personal fitness evaluation as part of your exercise program. You are guided through a series of simple procedures designed to help you assess your current capabilities in each of four areas: flexibility, cardiovascular fitness, muscular fitness, and body composition. You will use these results in later chapters to develop individualized exercise plans.

Chapter 3—Physiology and Flexibility: The Science of Stretching first identifies the major muscle groups and connecting tissues in the human body. The components of an effective fitness workout (warm-up, exercise, and cool-down) are described. You learn the basic principles of flexibility training, and review effective stretches for a comprehensive workout. Then you apply this information to develop a personal flexibility training plan that takes into account your own abilities and goals. Finally, tips for promoting exercise adherence—the ability to stick with your fitness program—are discussed.

Chapter 4—Cardiovascular Fitness: Run (or Walk) for Your Life explains the principles of cardiovascular conditioning and the requirements of an effective aerobic exercise program. Guidelines for a productive and practical walking and running program are presented, addressing such factors as clothing, weather conditions, and exercise intensity. Then you review a range of exercise options as a basis for preparing a personal cardiovascular workout plan.

Chapter 5—Muscular Fitness: Building Strength Safely and Effectively defines the nature and components of strength, and explains basic principles for effective muscular conditioning. Proper technique for various exercises for all the major muscle groups is described. You learn about back injuries and preventive measures for avoiding future problems. Finally, you develop your own strength training routine and comprehensive exercise plan based on guidelines for an effective workout.

Chapter 6—Nutrition: Practical Guidelines for Good Health explains the importance of nutrition for health and performance. First, basic concepts and terminology are reviewed. You then learn a series of simple yet comprehensive guidelines for healthful eating based on current research. Suggestions and tools for examining your own diet and applying the guidelines to your unique situation are presented. The chapter concludes with a simple nutrition action plan format and related reference materials.

Chapter 7—Body Composition and Weight Control examines the statistics and health risks associated with excess weight and obesity in this country. The principles of effective weight management—what works and what doesn't—are examined, with a special emphasis on the benefits of proper nutrition and physical activity. You identify common eating problems, analyze your own eating behaviors, identify areas for improvement, and establish short-term weight management goals for your daily life.

Chapter 8—Substance Abuse: Alcohol, Drugs, and Tobacco focuses on the health impacts of the three most important preventable risk factors in this country. First, the nature of substance abuse is discussed, and its impact on society and the fire service is examined. Information describing the usage and effects of alcohol, illicit drugs, and tobacco in the United States is presented. You review common causes and symptoms of the problem, and assess your own potential for chemical dependency. Finally, you learn about some possible sources of assistance, and think about your own role and responsibilities.

Chapter 9—Managing Stress On and Off the Job defines the nature and impacts of stress on health and performance. Chronic and traumatic stress in the fire service is discussed. You identify common causes and symptoms of stress, assessing your own potential for problems. Coping techniques for dealing with personal and occupational stress—relaxation, exercise, time management, role clarification, support groups, and departmental employee assistance programs—are examined. You then have an opportunity to identify various sources of stress in your own life, and to develop a personal stress management action plan.

Chapter 10—Maintaining Wellness Through Lifestyle Management reinforces and summarizes the information in preceding chapters by placing fitness and health issues within the context of total wellness. You learn about health trends in the United States, and evaluate your own behaviors in five major wellness categories. You think about ways to make and maintain long-term lifestyle changes, and review guidelines for personal growth. Finally, you prepare a long-term wellness plan that serves as a road map on your journey to a lifetime of fitness and good health.

Chapter 1

Physical Fitness and the Fire Service

CHAPTER INTRODUCTION

Physical fitness is a critical component of health and performance. Without high levels of fitness, fire and rescue workers can't do their jobs either safely or well. Being fit also contributes to overall health by helping to minimize problems associated with heart disease, excess weight, stress, and other risk factors.

For these reasons, every fire and rescue service member should conduct a regular program of physical exercise that promotes general health and develops the levels of fitness required for his or her assigned responsibilities. This goal is best accomplished through a gradual and progressive exercise program based on workouts that are tailored to the individual's own abilities, needs, and interests.

Chapter 1—Physical Fitness and the Fire Service is an introduction to the book and to some important physical fitness terms and concepts. You will learn why physical fitness is particularly important to fire and rescue workers, both for personal health and for job performance. The dangers and primary risk factors of heart disease, the nation's number one killer, are reviewed. You will examine the relationship between physical fitness and overall wellness, especially the need to manage your **lifestyle** to promote good health.

LEARNING OBJECTIVES

After learning the information in this chapter, you will be able to:

- Explain the need for high levels of physical fitness in the fire and rescue services.
- Identify the primary risk factors for coronary heart disease.
- Discuss your own attitudes about physical fitness and fire department fitness programs.
- Define the four components of physical fitness and related terms.
- Describe important benefits of physical fitness for personal health and wellness.
- Determine the need for medical screening before starting an exercise program.

THE IMPORTANCE OF FIREFIGHTER FITNESS

FIREFIGHTERS AND PHYSICAL FITNESS

The U.S. Fire Administration (USFA) states that "Firefighting is known to be one of the most physically and mentally demanding occupations today. Each year, over 50% of the firefighters who die in the line of duty succumb to heart failure and other stress-related problems. Studies have shown that an increased level of fitness for firefighters can reduce the risk of these deaths; thus, physical fitness is a critical aspect of firefighter health and safety." (USFA 1990)

A large body of scientific research supports this position. Well-designed physical fitness programs have been proven to reduce the incidence and severity of on-the-job injuries, which result in lost time and unnecessary medical costs. More importantly, improved fitness helps counteract risk factors associated with heart disease, responsible for a major portion of firefighter fatalities, disabilities, and early retirements. Other recognized benefits include improvements in member work performance, morale, and well-being.

"Fire departments shall provide and require the structured participation of all members in a program to develop and maintain appropriate levels of physical fitness."

NFPA 1500, 8-5.1

As a result, a National Fire Protection Association standard (NFPA 1500), *Standard on Fire Department Occupational Safety and Health Program*, mandates that all fire departments have a physical fitness program. This requirement is generally supported by both fire service management and labor organizations. For example, the International Association of Fire Chiefs Foundation concluded in a study that "a combination of benefits can be realized by implementing physical fitness programs in the fire service....These benefits justify inclusion of a mandatory physical fitness program in the daily activities of fire fighters." (IAFCF 1977)

The International Association of Fire Fighters (IAFF), as a matter of policy, also supports physical fitness for all its members. A position paper by the organization states that "a program of physical fitness should be the objective of every fire department."

RESEARCH ON FIREFIGHTING AND FITNESS

It has been said that firefighters expend as much energy during a major emergency as the players in a rigorous handball match. This assertion is supported by many studies that demonstrate the need for and benefits of high levels of physical fitness in the fire service. Other research proves that well-designed and managed fire service fitness programs result in improved job performance for participants, reduced incidence and severity of on-the-job injuries, and lower costs. Key findings of some of these studies can be summarized as follows:

- Available data indicates that firefighters have increased risk for injuries, pulmonary disease, heart disease, cancer, and noise-induced hearing loss. Strenuous work demands, exposures to carbon monoxide and other toxic substances, and acute respiratory changes may particularly stress the cardiovascular system.

- Although the total number of deaths is decreasing, the fatality rate for career firefighters is one of the highest in all industries. Heart attacks are responsible for about 50 percent of firefighter deaths. In 1990, 760 firefighters suffered a heart attack or stroke on the job. (Karter and LeBlanc 1991)

- According to a National Fire Protection Association (NFPA) survey, strains, sprains, and muscular pain accounted for over 40 percent of the 100,000 firefighter injuries in 1990. Over one fifth of all injuries were caused by overexertion or strain. (Karter and LeBlanc 1991)

- Statistics from the Seattle Fire Department showed that roughly 21-26 percent of firefighters reported injuries each year. About 50 percent or more involved sprains or strains, including muscles, joints, pinched nerves, and "slipped" discs.

- Studies have shown that firefighting requires working at near maximal heart rates for prolonged periods of time, often after limited warm-up. Heavy protective equipment and heat from the fire contribute to this physical load. Wearing protective gear can decrease work efficiency by as much as one-third.

- Firefighting requires a physical performance profile reflecting high aerobic capacity, high muscular strength and endurance, above average lean body weight, and minimal body fat. A USFA-funded study showed that fit fire-fighters took half the time to complete simulated fire ground tasks as did their less fit counterparts.

- In spite of the physical requirements of firefighting, studies have shown that male firefighters often score only average to slightly above average when compared with other adult males. The most serious shortcoming noted is excess body fat, considered particularly significant because of the burden placed on the cardiovascular system and the negative effect on muscular performance. Another study concluded that as many as two-thirds of firefighters do not meet the required physical performance profile.

- Several fire departments have documented that improved fitness results in significant cost savings through reduced incidence and severity of on-the-job injuries. Of particular note are reductions in back injuries and improvement in heart disease risk factors. Organizational costs include paying for disabilities and premature retirements.

In short, firefighting imposes significant physical demands, requiring high levels of fitness to minimize the risk of injury or even death. Unfit firefighters are not only a danger to themselves, but they pose an added risk to their co-workers and the community they serve. They also contribute to higher costs and are a factor in reduced performance.

Unfortunately, too many firefighters are not fit enough for the job—over 25 percent by some estimates. For this reason, the USFA stated as follows in a recent publication:

> **"You have the responsibility of servicing the public with a level of physical fitness that enables you to respond to a host of unforeseen emergencies....Regular participation in a physical fitness program is essential" to meet this requirement.**

HEART DISEASE: THE NUMBER ONE KILLER

Despite a dramatic 39 percent decline in death rates over the past twenty years, heart disease is still the leading cause of death for both men and women. About 7 million Americans are affected by coronary artery disease, and more than 1.5 million suffer a heart attack each year. In 1989, 733,867 people died from diseases of the heart. That translates to one life every 43 seconds. Another 145,551 died from stroke. (NCHS 1992)

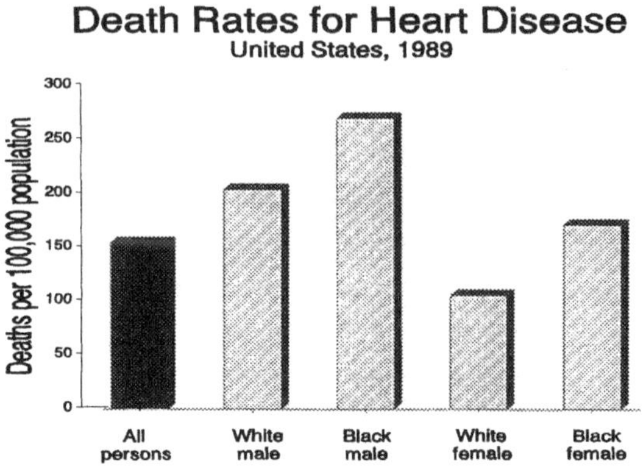

In 1985, coronary heart disease (CHD) was the leading cause of early retirement among firefighters, second only to cancer as a cause of death. According to the New England Research Institute, studies seem to suggest that firefighters have from 2 to 10 times the risk of CHD as the general population. Unfortunately, there is some uncertainty over this data because of the limitations of existing research. However, "it is not unreasonable to expect elevated risk for heart disease, since firefighters are faced with high carbon monoxide exposures and extreme physical demands (with no warm-up period)." (NERI 1989)

WHAT IS CORONARY HEART DISEASE?

The cardiovascular system—heart and blood vessels—functions as the body's "plumbing system" by carrying oxygen and nutrients to the muscles and other tissues. The heart, through its pumping action, provides the pressure needed for moving blood throughout the system.

Like other muscles, the heart needs energy to function. The harder the heart works, the more oxygen and nourishment it needs. Most heart disease is due to a progressive narrowing of the **coronary arteries** that supply blood, and thus energy, to the heart muscle. This happens when cholesterol and fat, circulating in the blood, build up on artery walls, forming a raised "plaque." The partial restriction of blood flow due to plaque, called **atherosclerosis**, can cause chest pain during exercise; complete blockage can cause a heart attack. Most heart attacks occur when a clot forms at a narrow part of an artery.

RISK FACTORS FOR HEART DISEASE

Clinical studies show that certain characteristics and lifestyles are statistically linked with heart disease. These "danger signs," called **risk factors**, can help identify people who are more likely to develop problems. Think of these risk factors as "germs" of heart disease. If they are not controlled, the odds increase that heart disease may develop. As the number of risk factors goes up, so does the chance of developing a serious problem.

High blood pressure, high blood cholesterol, and **cigarette smoking** have long been recognized as major risk factors for coronary heart disease. More recently, **physical inactivity**, known to contribute to heart disease and stroke, has been elevated to the status of a "primary risk factor." Remember: the likelihood of developing heart problems increases with the number of risk factors you have. A person with any two risk factors can have four times the risk of someone without any; three risk factors can indicate eight times the risk.

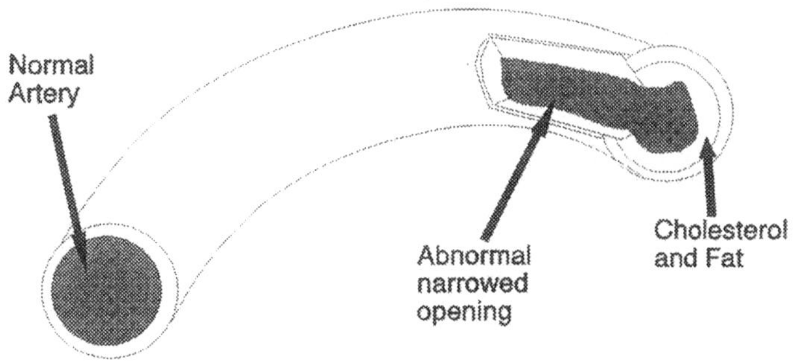

High Blood Pressure

When the heart beats, it forces blood into the arteries, which act like a network of pipes to carry oxygen and food throughout the body. Blood pressure is the force exerted against the artery walls as blood moves through them. Think how a hose nozzle works: when open, it takes little pressure to force water through the hose; when the opening is restricted, pressure in the hose increases.

Blood pressure is measured using a "blood pressure cuff," or sphygmomanometer. Two readings are taken: the higher (systolic) measures the maximum pressure on the arteries caused by the heart's contraction; the lower (diastolic) represents the pressure between beats. A reading of 120/80 (millimeters of mercury) is considered "normal." Although acceptable levels may vary somewhat, systolic readings above 140 and/or diastolic readings above 90 typically indicate high blood pressure, or **hypertension**.

High blood pressure can eventually damage arteries in various parts of the body, possibly leading to stroke, kidney failure, and blindness. It also increases the risk of heart disease and heart attack by contributing to the build-up of fatty deposits in the arteries.

> **"Individuals with uncontrolled high blood pressure are three times as likely to develop coronary heart disease, six times as likely to develop congestive heart failure, and seven times as likely to have a stroke as individuals with controlled high blood pressure."**
> **American Heart Association**

About 30 percent of American adults have high blood pressure, which is about one-third more common among blacks than among whites. Approximately half of all heart attack victims and two-thirds of all stroke victims have high blood pressure. Although the cause of most cases is unknown, persons more likely to develop hypertension include:

- Older adults
- Overweight persons
- Alcohol abusers
- Oral contraceptives users (women)
- Individuals who are sensitive to sodium (salt)
- Members of families with a history of hypertension
- Physically inactive persons

Unfortunately, the 1976-80 National Health and Nutrition Examination Survey found that only 11 percent of people with a blood pressure equal to or greater than 140/90 had it under control. About 20 percent of Americans with hypertension didn't even know they had the condition. This is why high blood pressure is often described as "the silent killer."

High Blood Cholesterol

Cholesterol, a fat-like substance transported in the blood, is one of the major components of plaques that form on artery walls. Although your body needs cholesterol to function normally, high levels in the blood have been shown to contribute to atherosclerosis, heart attack, and stroke. Therefore, many experts believe that cholesterol levels should be maintained below 200 milligrams per deciliter (mg/dl) of blood.

Studies show that the risk of heart attack for persons with blood cholesterol levels at 240 mg/dl is about twice that at 200 mg/dl; it increases to at least four times as high at 300 mg/dl. Even moderately elevated blood cholesterol levels increase the risk of heart disease. Unfortunately, **more than half of all adults have total blood cholesterol readings above recommended levels, and about one in four has a level considered "high" (i.e., 240 mg/dl or above).**

There are several types of cholesterol. The two most important are LDL (Low-Density Lipoprotein) and HDL (High-Density Lipoprotein) cholesterol. LDL cholesterol can be thought of as "***l***ethal" or "bad" since elevated levels contribute to the build-up of plaque on artery walls. HDL cholesterol is "***h***elpful" or "good," since it acts to prevent plaques by removing cholesterol from the bloodstream. The ratio of total cholesterol to HDL cholesterol should be less than 5.0. For example, if total cholesterol is 200 mg/dl, HDL cholesterol should not be less than 40 mg/dl (200/40 = 5.0).

The most important factor affecting cholesterol levels is diet. Large amounts of cholesterol are found in egg yolks, red meats, organ meats, dairy products (whole milk and cheeses), butter, and shellfish. Foods high in saturated (hydrogenated) fats also tend to raise the level of cholesterol in the blood. Conversely, unsaturated fats (such as canola, olive, peanut, sunflower, and corn oils) tend to lower cholesterol levels. Other possible contributing factors include obesity, genetic disorders, thyroid problems, diabetes, and diseases of the liver and kidney.

Smoking

Most people are aware of the relationship between smoking and lung disease. However, according to the AHA, smoking also doubles the risk of heart attack and increases the risk of sudden cardiac death two to four times. Smoking contributes to high blood pressure by constricting blood vessels and increasing the heart rate. Carbon monoxide in cigarette smoke also reduces the oxygen-carrying capacity of the blood, adding an additional burden on the heart. Smoking acts to lower HDL (helpful) cholesterol levels and appears to promote the formation of plaques on artery walls.

About 26 percent of the American population 25 years of age and older smoked in 1990. Among men, about 28 percent smoked; among women, the percentage was about 23. Fortunately, the proportion of the adult population that is aware that smoking is one of the major risk factors for heart disease has increased dramatically over the last 15 years. As a result, the percentage of adults who smoke has steadily declined (down 8 percent since 1979).

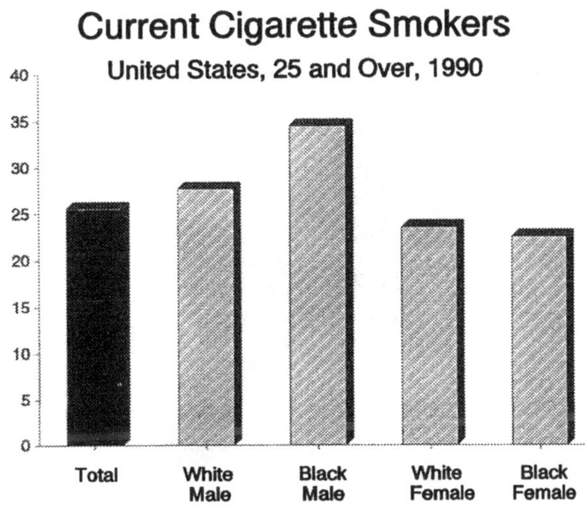

Smoking may pose a particular problem for firefighters since it contributes to elevated levels of carbon monoxide on the fireground. The additional cardiovascular stress may also trigger a heart attack due to a sudden clot or arrythmia. Fortunately, research shows that people who stop smoking decrease their risk of heart attack by 50 percent after two years. After 10 years, a former pack-a-day smoker has about the same risk as someone who never smoked a single cigarette.

Physical Inactivity

Studies indicate that inactive people have a higher risk of heart attack and a lower chance of post-heart-attack survival. A sedentary lifestyle contributes to total blood cholesterol and excess weight. Moreover, a regular program of exercise has been shown to increase HDL cholesterol levels in the blood while decreasing LDL levels.

In 1990, a National Health Interview Survey indicated that 41 percent of adults 18-64 years of age "exercised regularly." However, only about 5 percent of the respondents were aware how often and how long exercise must be performed to promote cardiovascular fitness. In another survey conducted by the Centers for Disease Control, roughly 60 percent of adults reported that they maintained a "sedentary lifestyle," defined as fewer than three 20-minute sessions of leisure-time physical activity per week. Almost 30 percent did not engage in **any** physical activities (other than regular job duties) during the previous month.

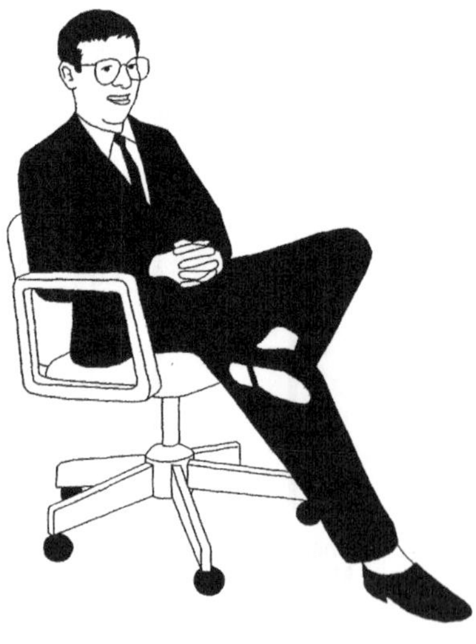

Studies of Los Angeles County firefighters have shown that physical activity and work capacity seem to be related to heart disease and insurance claims for heart injury. **Unfortunately, typical job activities performed by firefighters do <u>not</u> provide adequate levels of activity to promote fitness.** According to materials published by the National Fire Protection Association, "firefighting has many periods of inactivity, followed by sudden demands for physical strength and endurance. In view of the proportion of working hours spent firefighting, we would classify firefighting as a sedentary activity. Therefore, you are more likely to develop cardiovascular disease because of the relative **lack** of physical activity." (Davis and Curtis)

Other Factors Related to Coronary Heart Disease

In addition to the primary risk factors, other traits have been statistically linked to coronary heart disease. Some of these secondary risk factors are controllable through lifestyle changes; others are not. Persons with one or more of the following characteristics should pay even closer attention to their health risk profile:

- **Excess Weight.** Being overweight puts a strain on your heart and may lead to other cardiac risk conditions, such as high blood pressure, high blood cholesterol, and adult diabetes.

- **Diabetes.** One form of diabetes (inability to regulate blood sugar) develops most often in overweight adults. It produces abnormalities in lipoproteins that may accelerate atherosclerosis, and may raise the risk for heart attack in other ways not well understood.

- **Age.** Atherosclerosis often worsens progressively over time, leading to increased heart disease in older persons.

- **Race.** Black Americans have a greater risk of heart disease than white Americans, in large part due to higher average blood pressure levels.

- **Hormonal Factors.** Men have more heart attacks than women and have them earlier in life, but women narrow the gap after menopause.

- **Family History of Early Heart Attack.** There is a significant genetic component to heart disease. Someone with family members (parents, siblings, cousins, aunts, uncles, grandparents) who have had a heart attack should strongly consider avoiding all other controllable risk factors.

- **Alcohol.** Excess consumption of alcohol promotes weight gain, increases blood pressure, raises blood fat levels, and produces heartbeat irregularities. (Although some researchers suggest that moderate intakes of alcohol may actually reduce heart attacks, most experts stress that this potential benefit does not justify drinking alcohol because of other inherent health risks.)

- **Stresses of Modern Society.** Personal and occupational stress may provoke other risk factors and lead to excessive smoking, drinking, and eating. Furthermore, some personality types may be at increased risk for heart disease.

Activity 1-1

ATTITUDES ABOUT FITNESS

Why do some individuals enjoy physical fitness activities and others find them boring or unpleasant? Why do some fire and rescue workers stick with their exercise routine and others quit after a short period of time? The answer seems to lie in the "psychology of fitness." In other words, your beliefs and attitudes about fitness strongly influence your response to any fitness program (and to the information in this book).

Before going further, it might be useful to examine what you really think and feel about physical fitness and exercise programs:

- How important is physical fitness to your health and well-being? How fit do you need to be? How fit do you want to be?
- Do you have any responsibilities to others about your physical fitness? To your department and co-workers? To your family and loved ones?
- What are your personal fitness goals? What are you willing to do to achieve them?

Take this opportunity to think about your own beliefs and attitudes by completing the simple activity on the next page (Figure 1-1). Remember: **there are no right or wrong answers**. Everyone is different. Like other values, your beliefs and attitudes about fitness are an individual matter that reflect your own personality and a lifetime of experience. However, keep in mind that making any lifestyle change, like starting a new exercise program, is easier when your values support what you plan to do. Lower scores on this activity might indicate the opposite.

PHYSICAL FITNESS: WHAT DO YOU BELIEVE?

Each of the pairs of statements below can be seen as different ends of a continuum defining a range of values about some aspect of physical fitness. For each pair of statements, circle the number that best reflects your beliefs: 1 if you strongly agree with the statement on the left, 3 if you strongly agree with the statement on the right, or 2 if you fall somewhere in between.

Figure 1-1

Statement 1	Score	Statement 2
1a. Exercise has to be hard work—no pain, no gain.	1 2 3	1b. Exercise can be a pleasant and rewarding activity.
2a. Many people who don't exercise live as long and well as those who do.	1 2 3	2b. The odds are that my level of fitness will affect my future health and happiness.
3a. People care about me for who I am, not my physical abilities or how I look.	1 2 3	3b. My fitness and appearance affect my attitude about myself and how others feel about me.
4a. My health and fitness are my own business, not the department's or anyone else's.	1 2 3	4b. My health and fitness are a real concern to the department and to those who care about me.
5a. My performance on the job is not affected by my level of physical fitness.	1 2 3	5b. If I was in better physical condition, I could do my job even better.
6a. Physical fitness isn't a high priority for me—other aspects of my life are more important.	1 2 3	6b. When it comes to fitness, I want to be the best that I can be.

FIRE SERVICE PHYSICAL FITNESS PROGRAMS

Formal data on fire service physical fitness programs currently in place around the country is limited. A 1977 survey of over 1,000 departments by the International Association of Fire Chiefs (IAFC) Foundation found that 18% had some type of active program at that time. The scope and content of these programs varied considerably, with about half using some type of organized or "packaged" materials, generally available commercially. The vast majority, however, had no physical fitness program, and a significant number (11%) had discontinued programs due to lack of support, injuries, or other problems. (IAFCF 1977)

Since that time, many more departments have recognized the benefits of providing their members with opportunities to exercise. As noted in the National Fire Academy course *Firefighter Safety and Survival: The Company Officer's Responsibility*, "there are literally thousands of physical fitness programs in operation today. Although many of these programs are good, some are lacking, and thousands of firefighters, both paid and volunteer, have no physical fitness programs at all." (NFA 1988)

FIRE SERVICE FITNESS PROGRAMS

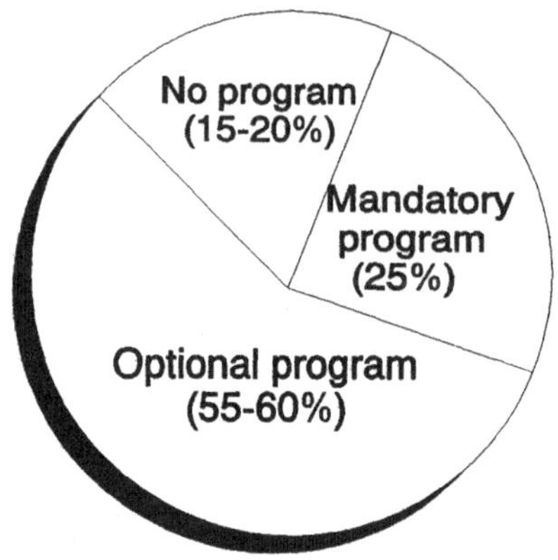

An informal survey of 123 fire departments conducted by a candidate for the National Fire Academy's Executive Fire Officer (EFO) Program determined that about 25 percent had a mandatory fitness program, 55-60 percent had optional programs, and 15-20 percent had no program at all. (Skinner, 1991) However, few small and volunteer departments—those which have the most difficulty implementing a comprehensive physical fitness program—participated in the survey.

The bottom line is that each department is different, just like each person. You need to understand and follow your own department's unique policies and procedures. Remember: since fitness is a critical component of firefighter health and safety, it's part of the job.

FEATURES OF SUCCESSFUL PROGRAMS

The IAFC Foundation study identified factors which appear to contribute to a successful physical fitness program. To be fully effective, physical fitness programs should include:

- Efforts to reduce other risk factors that affect the health and performance of firefighters. The most important are excess weight and cigarette smoking.

- Evaluation of each member's condition prior to beginning a physical fitness program. Departments should have early and continuing medical advice.

- Adequate training of all department members. In particular, members must learn why physical fitness is so important to their health and well-being.

- Exercises designed to develop and maintain the cardiovascular and muscular skelctal systems. An exercise schedule that does not meet both these essentials is unsatisfactory.

- Cooperation of fire department management, members, and the community's elected and appointed officials.

OBSTACLES TO PROGRAM DEVELOPMENT

A survey of 76 fire departments conducted by the Institute of Human Performance identified the most frequently cited factors involved in the failure to develop an effective departmental physical fitness program. (USFA 1990) These are listed below.

- √ Lack of funding
- √ Lack of equipment or facility
- √ No standards or adequate tests
- √ No appreciation for program benefits
- √ No support from employee organization
- √ Legal liabilities
- √ No support from department officials

"You, the individual firefighter, are the one who will benefit most by attainment of optimal fitness. It's a benefit that can't be taken away but, rather, one that you take away. Fitness goes with you wherever you are. In the final analysis, the firefighter who wishes to maintain optimal health and fitness will find the time needed for regular exercise, whether time is provided on duty or off."

U.S. Fire Administration

FITNESS AND WELLNESS

Before beginning any type of program, it's important to understand some of the terminology and basic concepts used in the field. Much information about physical fitness is fairly new. Ongoing research and experimentation has produced a dynamic area of study that continues to undergo constant change and to yield exciting new developments.

THE COMPONENTS OF PHYSICAL FITNESS

Fitness professionals divide fitness into four separate components: **flexibility, cardiovascular fitness, muscular fitness, and body composition**. Muscular fitness is further divided into muscular strength, endurance, and power.

Each component is equally important, and one component should not be emphasized over the others. Furthermore, each component is measured separately, and there are specific methods to improve fitness in each area. **For individuals to be considered "physically fit," they must possess acceptable levels of fitness in all four fitness components.** The four components are described below briefly; more detail is presented in later chapters.

Flexibility

Flexibility is the ability to move the joints of the body through their normal range of motion. An adequate degree of flexibility is important to prevent injury and to maintain body mobility.

Cardiovascular Fitness

Cardiovascular fitness, also known as aerobic fitness, is the capacity of the heart-lung system to supply the working muscles with oxygen, and the ability of muscle tissues to use that oxygen to produce energy. Since stamina is built through this component, cardiovascular fitness measures your ability to participate in sustained vigorous physical activity for long periods of time. Aerobic fitness also plays a major role in preventing artery disease, high blood pressure, diabetes, and obesity.

Muscular Fitness

Muscles are bundles of tissues that shorten, or contract, when stimulated. Through their connection to bones and joints, they provide a system of levers which permit movement. Muscles also contribute to the maintenance of body heat, since a by-product of contraction is heat production.

Subcomponents of this dimension of fitness include:

- **Muscular strength**—the force a muscle or muscle group can generate with maximum effort, measured by how much weight can be pushed or pulled. This is sometimes known as absolute strength.

- **Muscular endurance**—the ability of a muscle or group of muscles to generate force without fatiguing, measured by the length of time or number of times the action can be repeated (multiple or sustained contractions).

- **Muscular power**—the speed with which muscular strength can be applied.

Body Composition

Body composition is defined as the ratio of the body's lean and fat tissues. Lean body mass—consisting of muscles, bones, nervous tissue, skin, and organs—represents the metabolically active part of the body that makes a direct and positive contribution during exercise. Body fat is tissue that stores energy for use during some forms of exercise, but otherwise does not contribute directly to performance. Although some body fat is essential, excess body fat acts as a dead weight, contributing to injuries and a number of health-related problems.

FITNESS AND HEALTH

Fitness is best defined as a state of optimal physical well-being. Fitness means having the energy and physical ability to maintain a desirable quality of life—enthusiasm for living, without fatigue or exhaustion from routine required activities. Persons with high levels of fitness are, on average, healthier and more able to participate in activities for personal enjoyment. Persons with low fitness levels may have difficulty completing daily requirements, and usually have little or no energy left for other activities.

Health may simply be described as the absence of illness. A person with excellent health is usually considered to be someone who is not sick, not requiring medical attention, and not dependent upon medications on a daily basis. Many healthy individuals are also physically fit. However, it's important to realize that health and fitness are not always the same—you can be one and not the other.

FITNESS AND PERFORMANCE

What is the relationship between fitness and performance, i.e., how well you do on the job, in sports, or on some other task? Simply stated, it depends on the task—fitness is more important for some activities than it is for others.

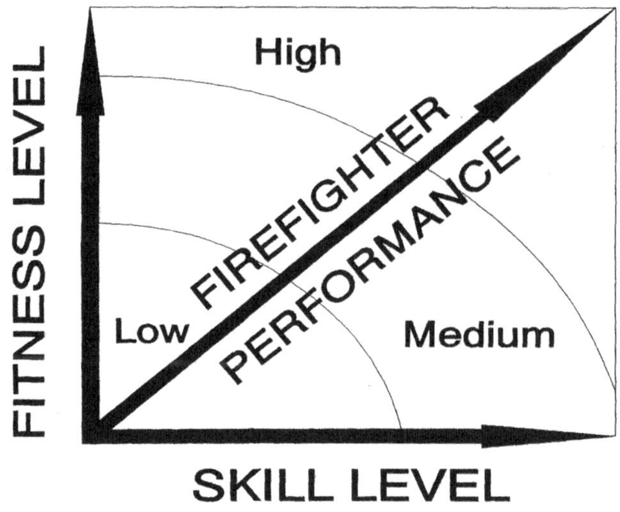

Performance is generally defined in terms of athletics and skill. However, high athletic ability and skill may or may not be related to physical fitness. It is possible for a highly skilled individual to have a low level of fitness. It is also just as possible for a physically fit individual to have little or no athletic skills.

Good performance requires that you have at least the levels of fitness required to accomplish the task at hand. Some activities involve high levels of overall fitness. Others demand exceptional levels of one or more of the four components of fitness (e.g., runners require high levels of cardiovascular fitness, while football players may need more strength). For still other activities, such as playing pool, fitness is relatively unrelated to performance.

For fire and rescue work, studies have shown that fitness is directly related to performance. Fit personnel are able to perform tasks more quickly and with fewer injuries than non-fit personnel. As shown in the graphic, performance generally improves as fitness and skills increase, but <u>both</u> are necessary. Neither a high level of fitness combined with a low level of skill, nor a high level of skill combined with a low level of fitness, will result in outstanding performance.

Therefore, the levels of fitness you need depend on 1) the requirements of general health, 2) daily needs at home and work, and 3) your personal goals and interests. Obviously, everyone should strive at least to stay healthy.

Emergency services personnel, in addition, must maintain levels of fitness above those of most other workers because of their physically demanding occupation. Research indicates that the most important component of fitness for fire suppression tasks is muscular strength, followed by muscular endurance. Aerobic capacity is also important, especially in longer duration incidents. Flexibility and body composition affect performance, but less directly than the other components, by reducing the efficiency of movement or contributing to injuries. (O'Connor 1994)

FITNESS AND WELLNESS

Wellness is any activity, behavior, or attitude that improves the quality of life and enables daily functions to be performed with energy and interest. Physical fitness is obviously an important component of wellness. Other areas include:

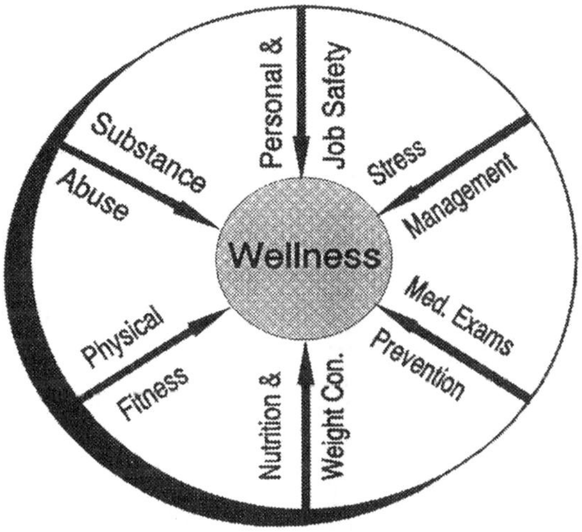

- Nutrition and weight control
- Stress management
- Personal and occupational safety
- Substance abuse prevention
- Medical examinations and disease prevention

Fitness is developed and maintained through a regular program of vigorous physical activity which addresses all four components—flexibility, cardiovascular fitness, muscular fitness, and body composition. Such a program contributes to personal health, performance, and overall wellness. Some of the most important benefits of regular exercise are described below.

Heart Disease

Heart disease is the leading cause of death in the United States for both men and women. Recent medical findings report that by age 55, 33 percent of all men will show symptoms of coronary artery disease. By age 60, men have a 20 percent chance of heart attack—that's one man in every five!

Cardiovascular disease is often referred to as the "disease by choice." It is estimated that 70 percent of all deaths from this disease could be prevented by lifestyle changes. Regular aerobic exercise is one of these changes.

Aerobic exercise slows the buildup of plaque in the arteries of the heart, helps prevent obstructive blood clots from forming in the arteries, improves the levels of cholesterol in the bloodstream, and contributes to normal blood pressure. Aerobic exercise also makes the heart a stronger and a more efficient pump. Resting heart rates usually decrease after exercise training because the heart can pump more blood per beat. Therefore, it needs to beat fewer times to circulate the same amount of blood.

Cancer

Studies have found that men and women who exercise are less likely to get colon cancer. Research also suggests that women who do not exercise have more than two and a half times the risk of developing cancer of the reproductive system, and almost twice the chance of getting breast cancer.

> The Journal of the American Medical Association in November 1989 reported that those who exercise moderately, compared to those who do not exercise at all, reduce their risk of early death from cancer and heart disease by **50 percent**.

Exercise and Weight

According to the National Center for Health Statistics, "half the adult population of the United States (70 million) is considered overweight." Other sources report even higher figures of 83 percent of the population as overweight (on average, 17 pounds for women and 18.5 pounds for men).

Exercise is essential in any successful weight reduction program. Exercise burns calories, so weight lost through an appropriate diet accompanied by exercise is more likely to be fat rather than water or valuable muscle tissue.

Weight loss is also more likely to be maintained with regular exercise. Repeated weight loss and weight gain, known as the yo-yo dieting syndrome, causes a drop in the metabolic rate. By preventing the loss of active muscle tissue, regular exercise helps maintain a healthy metabolism that will assist in weight maintenance.

Studies of weight loss participants reported that those who tried to maintain weight loss through diet alone were not successful, regaining an average of seven pounds. However, those participating in an exercise program regained an average of only two pounds.

Exercise and Aging

Although aging is inevitable, there is great variability in the aging process. Research has shown a direct relationship between physical fitness and the physiological changes that occur in the body due to aging. The rate of deterioration can be slowed by the maintenance of adequate fitness levels through regular physical activity.

Exercise strengthens muscles, joints, tendons, and ligaments. This may prevent, improve, or correct certain ailments such as lower back problems, tendinitis, bursitis, and some types of arthritis. Weight-bearing exercise also prevents the loss of bone minerals which can lead to osteoporosis.

In fact, exercise may actually counteract the effects of aging. Exercise slows the loss of stamina, strength, flexibility, bone density, metabolic rate, and general enthusiasm for being active. Exercise may counterbalance the age-related decrease in work capacity and physical performance, and contribute to the ability to maintain and sustain an independent lifestyle. This benefit increases the likelihood that you'll enjoy the years of retirement you've worked so hard for.

Exercise and Mental Health

Exercise has been shown to contribute to psychological health and well-being in a number of ways:

- **Fatigue**—Exercisers go to sleep more quickly, sleep more soundly, and are more refreshed than those who do not exercise. Physically fit individuals are also more resistant to fatigue, and tend to have more energy to participate in activities typical of high-quality, productive lifestyles.

- **Stress**—Exercise dissipates hormones and other chemicals that build up during periods of high stress. Exercise also generates a period of substantial emotional and physical relaxation that sets in approximately an hour and a half after an intense workout.

- **Depression**—In her book Mental Skills for Physical People, Dr. Dorothy V. Harris wrote, "exercise is nature's best tranquilizer." Researchers have found that mildly to moderately depressed individuals who engage in aerobic exercise 15 to 30 minutes per day at least every other day typically experience a positive mental adjustment in two to three weeks.

- **Self-Esteem**—Research has documented the assertion that individuals who exercise regularly feel better about themselves than sedentary individuals.

- **Mental Sharpness**—Individuals who exercise regularly appear to have better memory capability, reaction times, and levels of concentration than non-exercisers.

Exercise and Other Lifestyle Choices

Individuals who make a fitness commitment and strive to maintain and improve the quality of their lives through physical fitness tend to extend these pursuits into other lifestyle choices. Related health-promoting habits—like avoiding tobacco, alcohol, and other harmful substances—often accompany the decision to exercise regularly.

STAYING PHYSICALLY ACTIVE

Our bodies are designed for physical activity. Unfortunately, many people in today's technological society are not as active as our ancestors, who often worked hard as part of their daily routine. Even firefighters, on average, don't get enough physical activity on the job to improve their level of fitness or positively affect their health.

Our sedentary lifestyles have resulted in a category of diseases that are actually caused by or made worse by a lack of physical activity. These include coronary heart disease, high blood pressure, obesity, anxiety, depression, and lower back problems. For some of these problems, fire and rescue workers face an even greater risk than the general population.

In addition to health considerations, physical fitness is necessary for a balanced and quality lifestyle. It contributes to performance on the job, in sports, and in many other areas of life. Emergency services personnel, in particular, need levels of fitness above those of most other workers because of their physically demanding profession.

Therefore, fire and rescue workers need to plan a program of ongoing and relatively intense physical activity into their daily lives. The studies overwhelmingly suggest that individuals who exercise regularly tend to be healthier at any given age. Although the process takes time and commitment, the physiological (body) and psychological (mind) improvements are well worth the effort.

MEDICAL SCREENING

Although exercise is safe and beneficial for the vast majority of people, you cannot automatically assume you're one of them. Some people—especially those who have been sedentary for a long period, are older, use certain medications, or have particular medical conditions—should consult with a doctor before beginning any exercise program.

The American Heart Association advises that "most people do not need to see a doctor before they start, since a gradual, sensible exercise program will have minimal health risks." Medical screening is recommended for those over age 40 and for anyone with cardiac, orthopedic, or other risk factors as determined by a simple questionnaire. (Figure 1-2)

The American College of Sports Medicine suggests that you consult with your doctor if:

- You are 45 or older.
- You are 35 or older and have any risk factors for heart disease.
- You have a diagnosis or any symptoms of cardiovascular or lung disease.

Your doctor may recommend that you take a treadmill or stress test (exercise electrocardiography), the best available screening test for coronary disease. During this procedure, heart activity is monitored while you exercise until fatigue or warning signs appear. The procedure, which usually takes 10-15 minutes, can be administered in a suitably equipped doctor's office, hospital, health club, or other facility.

The American College of Sports Medicine recommends stress testing for anyone over 45 years of age before starting an exercise program. Other experts recommend stress testing for men between 40 and 45 and women older than 55. Exercise electrocardiography should also be performed in younger individuals with cardiac risk factors. (Barillo 1993)

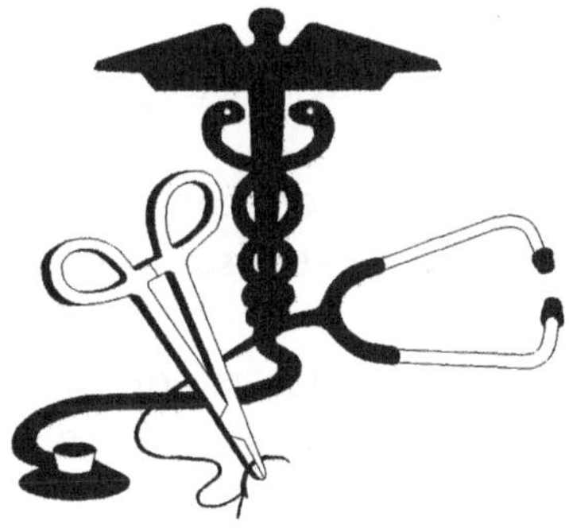

Figure 1-2

AMERICAN HEART ASSOCIATION GUIDELINES

Most people do not need to see a doctor before they start since a gradual, sensible exercise program will have minimal health risks. However, there are some people who should seek medical advice. To find out if you should consult a doctor before you start, use the following checklist:

- ☐ Your doctor said you have heart trouble or a heart murmur, or you have had a heart attack.
- ☐ You frequently have pains or pressure in the left or mid-chest area, left neck, shoulder, or arm during exercise or right after you exercise.
- ☐ You often feel faint or have spells of lightheadedness.
- ☐ You experience extreme breathlessness after mild exertion.
- ☐ Your doctor said your blood pressure was too high and is not under control. Or you don't know whether or not your blood pressure is normal.
- ☐ Your doctor said you have bone or joint problems such as arthritis.
- ☐ You are over 40 and not accustomed to regular exercise.
- ☐ You have a family history of premature coronary artery disease.
- ☐ You have a medical condition not mentioned here which might need special attention in an exercise program. (For example, insulin-dependent diabetes.)

If you've checked one or more items, talk to your doctor before you start. If you've checked no items, you can start on a gradual, sensible exercise program tailored to your needs.

CHAPTER SUMMARY

Physical Fitness and the Fire Service introduced the personal philosophies of fitness and wellness, including some important terms and concepts. You learned why physical fitness is particularly important for fire and rescue workers because of their demanding occupations. In particular, the nature of heart disease and related risk factors were examined.

You also examined your own attitudes about fitness and the state of fire department fitness programs. You read about the relationships among fitness, wellness, and job performance, and the many benefits of exercise for your health and well-being. Finally, you reviewed guidelines for medical screening before exercise programs.

Having completed this chapter, you should now be able to:

- Explain the need for high levels of physical fitness in the fire and rescue services.
- Identify the primary risk factors for coronary heart disease.
- Discuss your own attitudes about physical fitness and fire department fitness programs.
- Define the four components of physical fitness and related terms.
- Describe important benefits of physical fitness for personal health and wellness.
- Determine the need for medical screening before starting an exercise program.

BIBLIOGRAPHY

American Heart Association, *Exercise and Your Heart*, Pamphlet.

Barillo, David, M.D., *Medical Aspects of a Fire Department Exercise Program*, Summit Fitness Services, 1993.

Davis, Paul O., Ph.D., and Arthur V. Curtis, Ph.D., *The Firefighters Survival Manual: A Guide to Physical Fitness*, National Fire Protection Association.

International Association of Fire Chiefs Foundation, *Fire Service Physical Fitness Programs*, September 1977.

Karter, Michael J., and Paul R. LeBlanc, "U.S. Fire Fighter Injuries - 1990," *NFPA Journal*, November/December 1991.

National Center for Health Statistics, *Health, United States, 1991*, Hyattsville, MD: Public Health Service, 1992.

National Fire Academy, "Unit II: Firefighter Health and Physical Fitness," *Firefighter Safety and Survival: The Company Officer's Responsibility*, NFA-SO-FSCO, 1988.

National Fire Protection Association, *Standard on Fire Department Occupational Safety and Health Program* (NFPA 1500), 1992 Edition.

New England Research Institute, Inc., *Development and Evaluation of a Computer Driven Health Risk Tool for Fire Fighters*, February 1989.

O'Connor, Jack, Ph.D., "Components of Fitness," *Firefighter's News*, August-September 1994.

Pollock, Michael L., Jack H. Wilmore, and Samuel M. Fox III, *Health and Fitness Through Physical Activity*, New York: John Wiley & Sons, 1978.

Skinner, Paul A., *Current Trends in Fire Service Fitness - 1991*, National Fire Academy Executive Fire Officer Program Report, August 1991.

Sothmann, M.S., Ph.D., F. Landy, Ph.D., and K. Saupe, M.S., "Age as a Bona Fide Occupational Qualification for Firefighting," *Journal of Occupational Medicine*, Vol. 34, No. 1, January 1992.

United States Fire Administration, *Physical Fitness Coordinator's Manual for Fire Departments*, FA-95, September 1990.

COMPREHENSIVE WELLNESS FOR FIREFIGHTERS

Chapter 2

Fitness Assessment: Finding Your Starting Point

Chapter Introduction

The CW-F Assessment Process

Body Composition Assessment

Flexibility Assessment

Muscular Fitness Assessment

Cardiovascular Fitness Assessment

Evaluating the Results

Chapter Summary

CHAPTER INTRODUCTION

PHYSICAL FITNESS ASSESSMENT

Before starting any exercise program, it's a good idea to evaluate your current level of fitness. This evaluation, called a fitness assessment, measures your capabilities in each of the four components of fitness: flexibility, cardiovascular fitness, muscular fitness, and body composition.

A fitness assessment is an important part of your exercise program because it helps you to:

- Plan exercise that is appropriate for your needs and abilities.
- Establish a baseline for evaluating future progress.
- Establish realistic expectations for your exercise program.
- Stay motivated to stick with the program (exercise adherence).

LEARNING OBJECTIVES

Simple physical fitness assessment techniques are described in this chapter. The procedures will give you a general measure and understanding of your own level of physical fitness. The results will also be used in later chapters to help you develop your own individualized exercise plan in each area of fitness.

After learning the information in this chapter, you will be able to:

- Define the purpose and nature of a physical fitness assessment.
- Describe the benefits and limitations of the CW-F fitness assessment process.
- Identify various techniques and methodologies for evaluating fitness.
- Assess your current level of flexibility, cardiovascular fitness, muscular fitness, and body composition.

THE CW-F ASSESSMENT PROCESS

This chapter introduces a series of simple techniques you can use to assess your current level of flexibility, cardiovascular fitness, muscular fitness, and body composition. Based on your score, you are classified into one of three general **fitness levels** for each component of fitness. These levels are defined as follows:

Level 1—Basic Conditioning. Persons at this level need to gradually improve their conditioning in order to participate in a more rigorous physical fitness program. Non-exercisers, and those who don't exercise enough to have a lasting fitness effect, fall into this category.

Level 2—General Fitness. Persons at this level demonstrate some positive fitness and health effects from exercise. Maintaining at least this level of fitness is considered the **minimum** requirement for any fitness program. However, higher levels of fitness may be appropriate for fire and rescue workers.

Level 3—Performance Fitness. Persons at this level experience the full health benefits associated with good physical fitness. They demonstrate levels of fitness more appropriate for the strenuous requirements of firefighting and rescue tasks.

Scores for the separate components are totaled to give you an overall measure of fitness. The components are weighted differently in the scoring process, reflecting their relative importance in firefighting and rescue work. The highest possible score is 100 points.

CW-F PROTOCOLS

The CW-F Program uses the following procedures, or protocols, to measure fitness in each of the component areas.

1. Body composition—body mass index
2. Flexibility
   - Sit and reach
   - Back of thigh
   - Front of thigh
   - Shoulder
   - Chest
3. Muscular fitness
   - Push-ups
   - Sit-ups
   - Jump and reach
   - Wall-sit
4. Cardiovascular fitness—15 minute walk/run test

LIMITATIONS OF THE MODEL

The assessment techniques described here correlate well with the components of physical fitness, and are particularly useful for demonstrating progress and improvements over time. Another advantage is that they do not require special equipment, supplies, and facilities to administer.

However, keep in mind that more sophisticated and accurate means are available for assessing physical fitness. These services can be found through local health care facilities or sports medicine clinics. Some methods are costly and time-consuming, requiring highly trained technicians and expensive equipment.

Also, remember that the fitness assessment process described here is not specifically designed to measure your ability to perform firefighting or rescue tasks. That process, usually called a **physical performance assessment (PPA)**, typically involves the simulation of essential job tasks (victim rescue, hose advance, etc.) and the establishment of minimum standards for gauging individual capabilities.

Although the process described here doesn't directly measure firefighting ability, it does assess physical fitness, which is essential for satisfactory job performance and for passing the PPA. Thus, your results on this assessment can be considered a valuable indicator of your ability to do well on the job and on the PPA. Furthermore, a well-designed fitness assessment like this will help you develop and maintain the abilities you need to pass the performance test year after year.

Another point to keep in mind: most fitness assessment processes are designed to compare men and women of the same age in the general population. However, **all fire and rescue workers, regardless of age or sex, need to maintain levels of physical fitness that are adequate for the job.** Therefore, such comparisons are less useful in this situation, and are de-emphasized in the CW-F assessment process.

PREPARING FOR THE ASSESSMENT

The same medical screening guidelines discussed in Chapter 1 for starting an exercise program apply here. You should consult with your physician if you have any concerns or special conditions (diseases, injuries, etc.) which could affect your ability to undergo the assessment. This is particularly true for women over age 50, men over age 40, and persons with musculoskeletal problems or risk factors for heart disease.

Otherwise, use common sense in preparing for the assessment. Wear appropriate clothing for exercise, especially if some activities will be conducted out of doors. Wait at least two hours after eating a heavy meal. Warm up thoroughly before all activities, followed by some gentle stretching. And don't overexert yourself beyond your abilities—pushing too hard or too fast is an excellent way to get injured.

You will need the following common equipment and supplies: a weight scale, yardstick or ruler, stopwatch or watch with a second hand, and a piece of chalk or chalk dust. You may also want to bring a towel. You will need a partner for some activities, so recruit a friend who can help out for an hour or so. Finally, you will need access to a smooth wall 10-12 feet high and a level, measured running track, perhaps at a local school or YMCA.

COMPLETING THE ASSESSMENT

Follow the procedures described in the next four sections to conduct the physical fitness assessment. Record your results on a copy of Exhibit 2-1, the **Firefighter Fitness Assessment Tally Sheet**, which appears on the next page. The Tally Sheet is divided into two sections so your can compare your results now with those at some future date, perhaps three to six months down the road.

When you have finished all four parts of the assessment, use the procedures described at the end of the chapter to total your scores and determine your fitness category (Level 1, 2, or 3) in each of the four areas of fitness.

Keep in mind as you complete the process that a fitness assessment is not a test or a competition. There is no expected grade or minimum score required. Each person is different, so you shouldn't become either discouraged or overconfident. Whether your scores are high or low, <u>everyone</u> has room to improve. The results are merely a tool to help you plan a personal exercise program and to monitor your progress over time.

Exhibit 2-1

FIREFIGHTER FITNESS ASSESSMENT TALLY SHEET

Name________________________ **Age**____ **Sex**____ **Height**____

Date________ Wt________

BODY COMPOSITION ASSESSMENT

Body Mass Index ______ Score _____/25

LEVEL **1** **2** **3**

FLEXIBILITY ASSESSMENT

Sitting

Sit and Reach _____ in.	0	1	2	3		
Lying on Back						
Back of Thigh	T	F			1	3
Shoulders	T	F			1	3
Chest	T	F			1	3
Lying on Stomach						
Front of Thigh	T	F			1	3

Score _____/15

LEVEL **1** **2** **3**

MUSCULAR FITNESS ASSESSMENT

Pushups					
# in 2 minutes ______	1	2	4	6	8
Situps					
# in 2 minutes ______	1	2	3	4	5
Jump and Reach					
Best jump (in.) ______	1	2	4	6	8
Wall Sit					
Time (min/sec) ___/___	1	2	4	6	8

Score _____/29

LEVEL **1** **2** **3**

CARDIOVASCULAR FITNESS ASSESSMENT

Miles in 15 min. ______ VO2 Max ______

Score _____/31

LEVEL **1** **2** **3**

TOTAL SCORE ________/100

Date________ Wt________

BODY COMPOSITION ASSESSMENT

Body Mass Index ______ Score _____/25

LEVEL **1** **2** **3**

FLEXIBILITY ASSESSMENT

Sitting

Sit and Reach _____ in.	0	1	2	3		
Lying on Back						
Back of Thigh	T	F			1	3
Shoulders	T	F			1	3
Chest	T	F			1	3
Lying on Stomach						
Front of Thigh	T	F			1	3

Score _____/15

LEVEL **1** **2** **3**

MUSCULAR FITNESS ASSESSMENT

Pushups					
# in 2 minutes ______	1	2	4	6	8
Situps					
# in 2 minutes ______	1	2	3	4	5
Jump and Reach					
Best jump (in.) ______	1	2	4	6	8
Wall Sit					
Time (min/sec) ___/___	1	2	4	6	8

Score _____/29

LEVEL **1** **2** **3**

CARDIOVASCULAR FITNESS ASSESSMENT

Miles in 15 min. ______ VO2 Max ______

Score _____/31

LEVEL **1** **2** **3**

TOTAL SCORE ________/100

BODY COMPOSITION ASSESSMENT

Body composition describes the relationship between the body's lean and fat tissues. Measuring your percentage of body fat—the amount of fat weight you have in comparison to total body weight—is more meaningful than using height/weight tables, which fail to take into account skeletal frame size and muscle development. Genetic and age factors affect body composition, but diet and activity patterns are mostly responsible for individual differences.

Different methods can be used to measure body composition, and these are discussed further in Chapter 7. This assessment uses your **body mass index**, calculated by dividing your weight in kilograms by the square of your height in meters. Desirable totals range from 20 to 25 for men and 19 to 24 for women.

DETERMINING BODY MASS INDEX (BMI)

1. Weigh yourself in shorts or underwear, and record the result on the Tally Sheet.

2. Refer to Table 2-1 on the next page. Find your height in inches along the left side of the table, and your weight (to the nearest five pounds) along the top. The intersection of the two is your body mass index. For example, a person six feet tall (72 inches) and weighing 180 pounds has a body mass index of 24.5.

3. Your score for the assessment is found on the chart below. The highest possible score is 25. Enter this score on the Tally Sheet.

FEMALES		MALES	
BMI	SCORE	BMI	SCORE
Under 24	25	Under 25	25
24-25	15	25-27	15
26-27	8	28-29	9
Over 27	0	Over 29	0

Table 2-1
BODY MASS INDEX CALCULATIONS

HEIGHT IN INCHES	WEIGHT IN POUNDS																			
	100	**105**	**110**	**115**	**120**	**125**	**130**	**135**	**140**	**145**	**150**	**155**	**160**	**165**	**170**	**175**	**180**	**185**	**190**	**195**
60	19.6	20.6	21.6	22.5	23.5	24.5	25.5	26.5	27.4	28.4	29.4	30.4	31.4	32.3	33.3	34.3	35.3	36.3	37.2	38.2
61	19.0	19.9	20.9	21.8	22.8	23.7	24.7	25.6	26.5	27.5	28.4	29.4	30.3	31.3	32.2	33.2	34.1	35.1	36.0	37.0
62	18.4	19.3	20.2	21.1	22.0	22.9	23.9	24.8	25.7	26.6	27.5	28.5	29.4	30.3	31.2	32.1	33.0	34.0	34.9	35.8
63	17.8	18.7	19.6	20.4	21.3	22.2	23.1	24.0	24.9	25.8	26.7	27.6	28.4	29.3	30.2	31.1	32.0	32.9	33.8	34.7
64	17.2	18.1	18.9	19.8	20.7	21.5	22.4	23.3	24.1	25.0	25.8	26.7	27.6	28.4	29.3	30.1	31.0	31.9	32.7	33.6
65	16.7	17.5	18.4	19.2	20.0	20.9	21.7	22.5	23.4	24.2	25.1	25.9	26.7	27.6	28.4	29.2	30.1	30.9	31.7	32.6
66	16.2	17.0	17.8	18.6	19.4	20.2	21.1	21.9	22.7	23.5	24.3	25.1	25.9	26.7	27.5	28.3	29.2	30.0	30.8	31.6
67	15.7	16.5	17.3	18.1	18.9	19.6	20.4	21.2	22.0	22.8	23.6	24.4	25.2	25.9	26.7	27.5	28.3	29.1	29.9	30.7
68	15.3	16.0	16.8	17.5	18.3	19.1	19.8	20.6	21.4	22.1	22.9	23.7	24.4	25.2	25.9	26.7	27.5	28.2	29.0	29.8
69		15.6	16.3	17.0	17.8	18.5	19.3	20.0	20.7	21.5	22.2	23.0	23.7	24.5	25.2	25.9	26.7	27.4	28.2	28.9
70		15.1	15.8	16.6	17.3	18.0	18.7	19.4	20.2	20.9	21.6	22.3	23.0	23.8	24.5	25.2	25.9	26.6	27.4	28.1
71			15.4	16.1	16.8	17.5	18.2	18.9	19.6	20.3	21.0	21.7	22.4	23.1	23.8	24.5	25.2	25.9	26.6	27.3
72			15.0	15.7	16.3	17.0	17.7	18.4	19.1	19.7	20.4	21.1	21.8	22.5	23.1	23.8	24.5	25.2	25.9	26.5
73				15.2	15.9	16.6	17.2	17.9	18.5	19.2	19.9	20.5	21.2	21.8	22.5	23.2	23.8	24.5	25.2	25.8
74					15.5	16.1	16.8	17.4	18.0	18.7	19.3	20.0	20.6	21.3	21.9	22.5	23.2	23.8	24.5	25.1
75					15.1	15.7	16.3	16.9	17.6	18.2	18.8	19.4	20.1	20.7	21.3	22.0	22.6	23.2	23.8	24.5
76						15.3	15.9	16.5	17.1	17.7	18.3	18.9	19.5	20.2	20.8	21.4	22.0	22.6	23.2	23.8
77							15.5	16.1	16.7	17.3	17.9	18.4	19.0	19.6	20.2	20.8	21.4	22.0	22.6	23.2
78							15.1	15.7	16.2	16.8	17.4	18.0	18.6	19.1	19.7	20.3	20.9	21.5	22.0	22.6
79								15.3	15.8	16.4	17.0	17.5	18.1	18.7	19.2	19.8	20.4	20.9	21.5	22.0
80									15.4	16.0	16.5	17.1	17.6	18.2	18.7	19.3	19.8	20.4	20.9	21.5

HEIGHT IN INCHES	WEIGHT IN POUNDS																			
	200	**205**	**210**	**215**	**220**	**225**	**230**	**235**	**240**	**245**	**250**	**255**	**260**	**265**	**270**	**275**	**280**	**285**	**290**	**295**
60	39.2	40.2	41.2	42.1	43.1	44.1	45.1	46.1	47.0	48.0	49.0									
61	37.9	38.9	39.8	40.8	41.7	42.7	43.6	44.6	45.5	46.5	47.4	48.4	49.3							
62	36.7	37.6	38.5	39.5	40.4	41.3	42.2	43.1	44.1	45.0	45.9	46.8	47.7	48.6	49.6					
63	35.6	36.4	37.3	38.2	39.1	40.0	40.9	41.8	42.7	43.6	44.4	45.3	46.2	47.1	48.0	48.9	49.8			
64	34.5	35.3	36.2	37.0	37.9	38.8	39.6	40.5	41.3	42.2	43.1	43.9	44.8	45.6	46.5	47.4	48.2	49.1		
65	33.4	34.2	35.1	35.9	36.7	37.6	38.4	39.2	40.1	40.9	41.8	42.6	43.4	44.3	45.1	45.9	46.8	47.6	48.4	49.3
66	32.4	33.2	34.0	34.8	35.6	36.4	37.3	38.1	38.9	39.7	40.5	41.3	42.1	42.9	43.7	44.5	45.4	46.2	47.0	47.8
67	31.4	32.2	33.0	33.8	34.6	35.4	36.2	36.9	37.7	38.5	39.3	40.1	40.9	41.7	42.4	43.2	44.0	44.8	45.6	46.4
68	30.5	31.3	32.0	32.8	33.6	34.3	35.1	35.9	36.6	37.4	38.1	38.9	39.7	40.4	41.2	42.0	42.7	43.5	44.3	45.0
69	29.6	30.4	31.1	31.9	32.6	33.3	34.1	34.8	35.6	36.3	37.1	37.8	38.5	39.3	40.0	40.8	41.5	42.2	43.0	43.7
70	28.8	29.5	30.2	31.0	31.7	32.4	33.1	33.8	34.6	35.3	36.0	36.7	37.4	38.2	38.9	39.6	40.3	41.0	41.8	42.5
71	28.0	28.7	29.4	30.1	30.8	31.5	32.2	32.9	33.6	34.3	35.0	35.7	36.4	37.1	37.8	38.5	39.2	39.9	40.6	41.3
72	27.2	27.9	28.6	29.3	29.9	30.6	31.3	32.0	32.7	33.3	34.0	34.7	35.4	36.1	36.8	37.4	38.1	38.8	39.5	40.2
73	26.5	27.1	27.8	28.5	29.1	29.8	30.5	31.1	31.8	32.4	33.1	33.8	34.4	35.1	35.8	36.4	37.1	37.7	38.4	39.1
74	25.8	26.4	27.1	27.7	28.3	29.0	29.6	30.3	30.9	31.6	32.2	32.9	33.5	34.1	34.8	35.4	36.1	36.7	37.4	38.0
75	25.1	25.7	26.3	27.0	27.6	28.2	28.9	29.5	30.1	30.7	31.4	32.0	32.6	33.2	33.9	34.5	35.1	35.7	36.4	37.0
76	24.4	25.0	25.7	26.3	26.9	27.5	28.1	28.7	29.3	29.9	30.5	31.2	31.8	32.4	33.0	33.6	34.2	34.8	35.4	36.0
77	23.8	24.4	25.0	25.6	26.2	26.8	27.4	28.0	28.6	29.2	29.8	30.3	30.9	31.5	32.1	32.7	33.3	33.9	34.5	35.1
78	23.2	23.8	24.4	24.9	25.5	26.1	26.7	27.3	27.8	28.4	29.0	29.6	30.2	30.7	31.3	31.9	32.5	33.1	33.6	34.2
79	22.6	23.2	23.7	24.3	24.9	25.4	26.0	26.6	27.1	27.7	28.3	28.8	29.4	30.0	30.5	31.1	31.7	32.2	32.8	33.4
80	22.0	22.6	23.2	23.7	24.3	24.8	25.4	25.9	26.5	27.0	27.6	28.1	28.7	29.2	29.8	30.3	30.9	31.4	32.0	32.5

FLEXIBILITY ASSESSMENT

Flexibility is defined as the range of movement in a joint or group of joints. Normal muscle flexibility allows a full range of movement, while reduced flexibility results in tighter muscles and a restricted range of movement. People with limited flexibility are more susceptible to injuries of the muscles and tendons. (Flexibility is discussed further in Chapter 3.)

Since flexibility is specific to each joint, no single assessment procedure can be used to measure overall flexibility. Therefore, a score for total flexibility is obtained by combining the scores from several separate flexibility measures, each of which focuses on different areas of the body. High scores are indicative of "normal" flexibility; lower scores suggest "tight" muscles or joints.

This Flexibility Assessment procedure consists of **five** individual protocols:

- Sit and Reach
- Back of Thigh
- Shoulder
- Chest
- Front of Thigh

The procedure for each assessment is found on the following pages. Scores for each protocol should be recorded on the Tally Sheet. The highest possible total score for the Flexibility Assessment is **15 points**.

Remember to warm up for at least five minutes before taking the assessment to increase circulation and muscle pliability. Marching or running in place, brisk walking, or other gentle movements can be used for this purpose.

1. Sit and Reach

This procedure assesses the flexibility of your back, buttocks, hamstrings, and calves.

Sit with your legs straight (back of knees against the floor) and the soles of your feet flat against a wall, step, or box. Attempt to reach slowly forward toward your toes. **Do not lunge or bounce forward.** Your legs must stay straight, with the back of both knees against the floor at all times.

Using a yardstick or ruler, have your partner measure, to the nearest half inch, the distance from your toes to your closest finger tip. Record the best of three trials on the Tally Sheet.

SCORE

0	More than 9 inches
1	More than 6, up to 9 inches
2	More than 3, up to 6 inches
3	Less than 3 inches

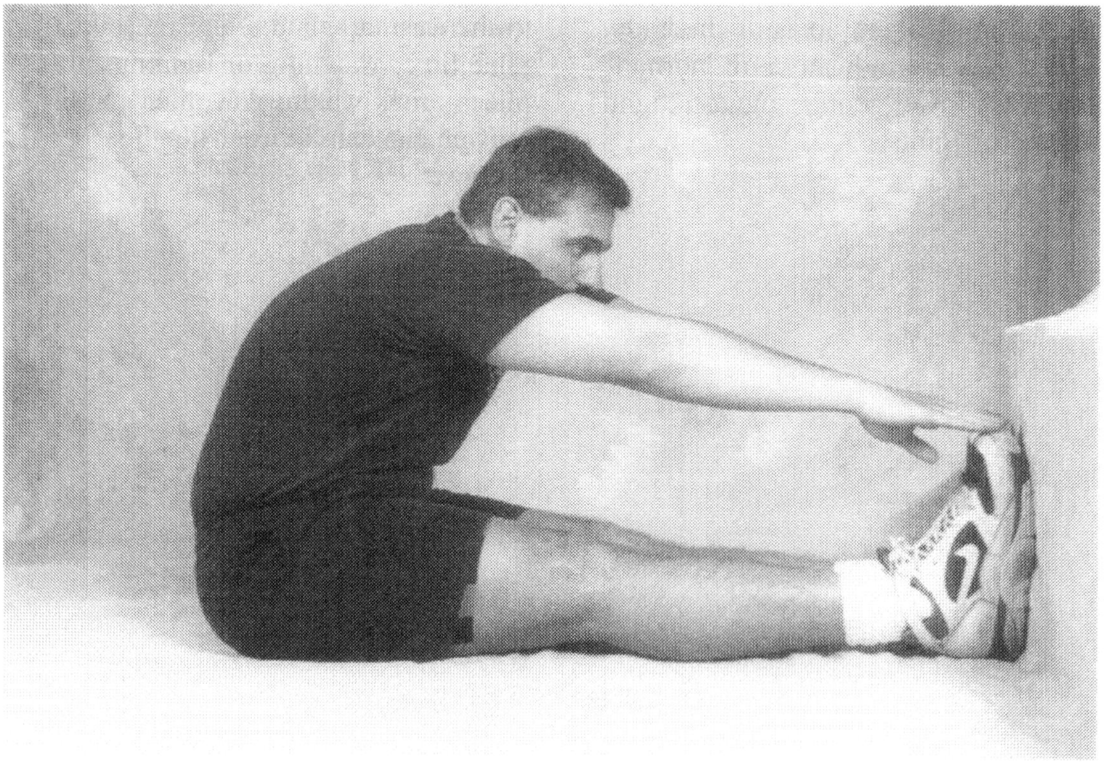

2. Back of Thigh

This protocol is used to assess the flexibility of your hamstring muscles, which run along the back of your upper leg.

For this procedure, use your dominant leg (the one you would normally use for kicking). Lie on your back and bend your leg at the knee with the thigh at a 90 degree angle to your body. The other leg should be straight and flat on the floor; if this can't be performed, the muscle is already "Tight."

Keeping your head down, grasp the bent leg behind the knee and attempt to **slowly** straighten it, pointing your heel towards the ceiling. Anything less than a completely straight leg is "Tight." The other leg must stay flat on the floor throughout.

SCORE

1	Tight
3	Flexible

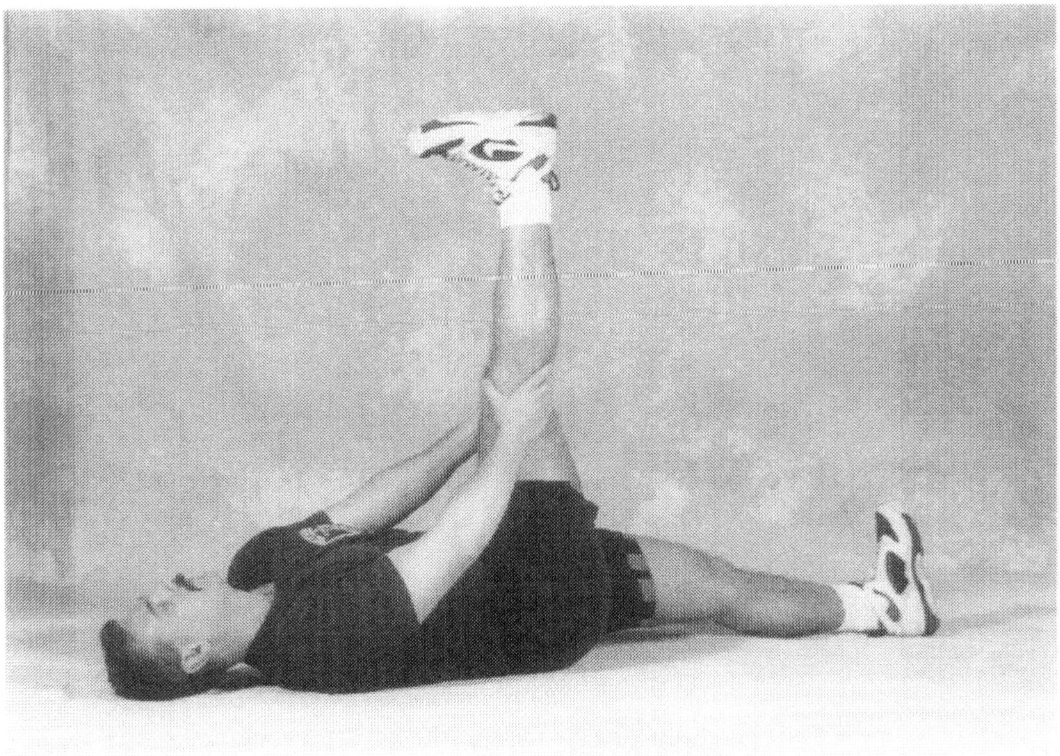

3. Shoulder

This procedure can be used to test the flexibility of your shoulder flexors.

Use your dominant arm during this assessment. Lie down on your back. Keeping your back flat against the floor, try to bring your arm straight back overhead to touch your wrist on the floor over your head. Do not arch your back during this movement; have your partner place his/her hand beneath your lower back to make sure you don't lift your lower back off the floor.

If you can touch the floor over your head with your arm straight, your shoulders are considered "Flexible." The inability to do this is considered "Tight."

SCORE

1	Tight
3	Flexible

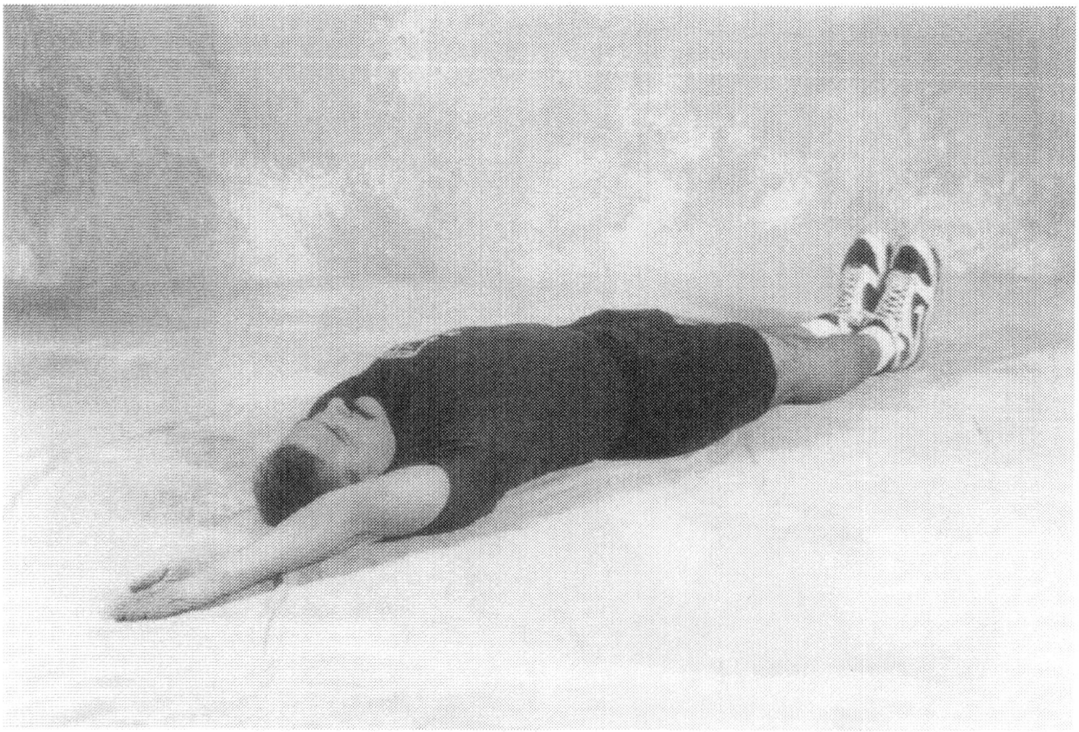

4. Chest

This protocol assesses the flexibility of your pectoralis (chest) muscles.

Lie on your back, with your arms at your side, palms facing in towards your body. Try to relax and not tense any of the muscles in your upper body.

Have your partner view you from a position at the top of your head. The posterior (back) portion of both your shoulders should be lying flat against the floor, i.e., your shoulders should not be rounded forward, with space between the floor and the back of your shoulder.

If your partner can run his/her fingers between your shoulders and the floor, your chest is considered "Tight." Otherwise, list yourself on the Tally Sheet as "Flexible" for this procedure.

SCORE

1	Tight
3	Flexible

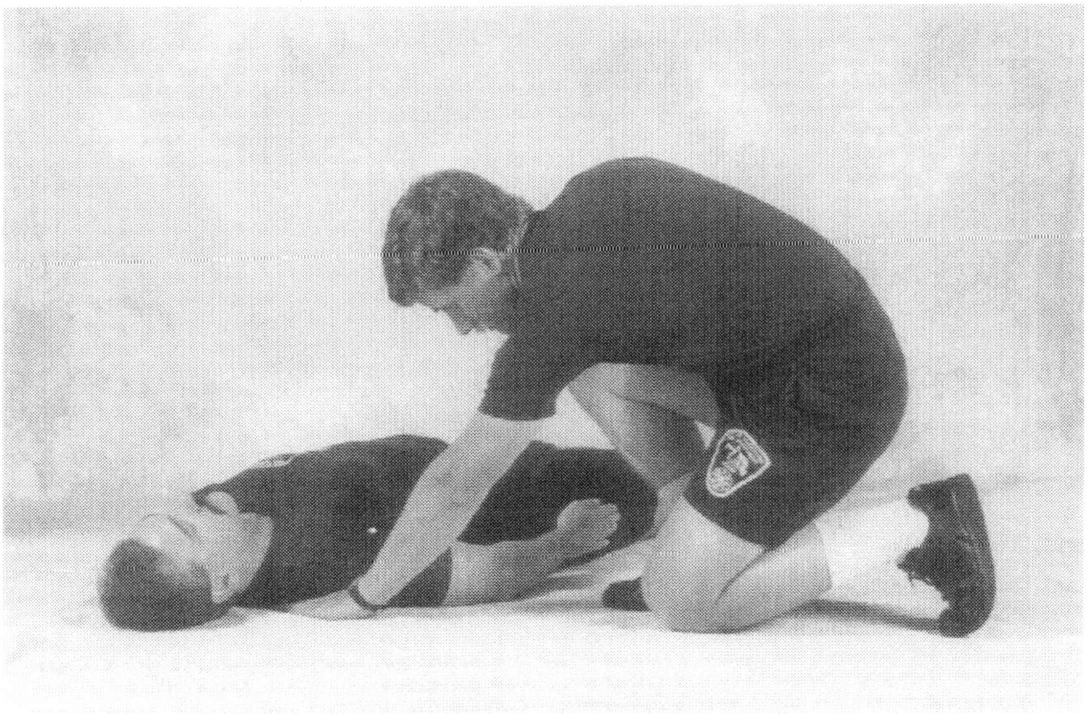

5. Front of Thigh

This procedure is used to assess the flexibility of your quadriceps (thigh) muscle, which runs along the front of your upper leg.

Again, use your dominant leg during this assessment. Lie on your stomach on the floor. Relax your leg muscles and allow your partner to bend your leg for you. Your knees should remain together, not deviating out to the side.

Have your partner bring the heel of your foot gently up towards your buttocks. He/she should be instructed to stop as soon as resistance to this movement is encountered. **Do not try to force the leg further.** If your partner is unable to easily bring your heel all the way to your buttocks, your quadriceps is considered "Tight."

SCORE

1	Tight
3	Flexible

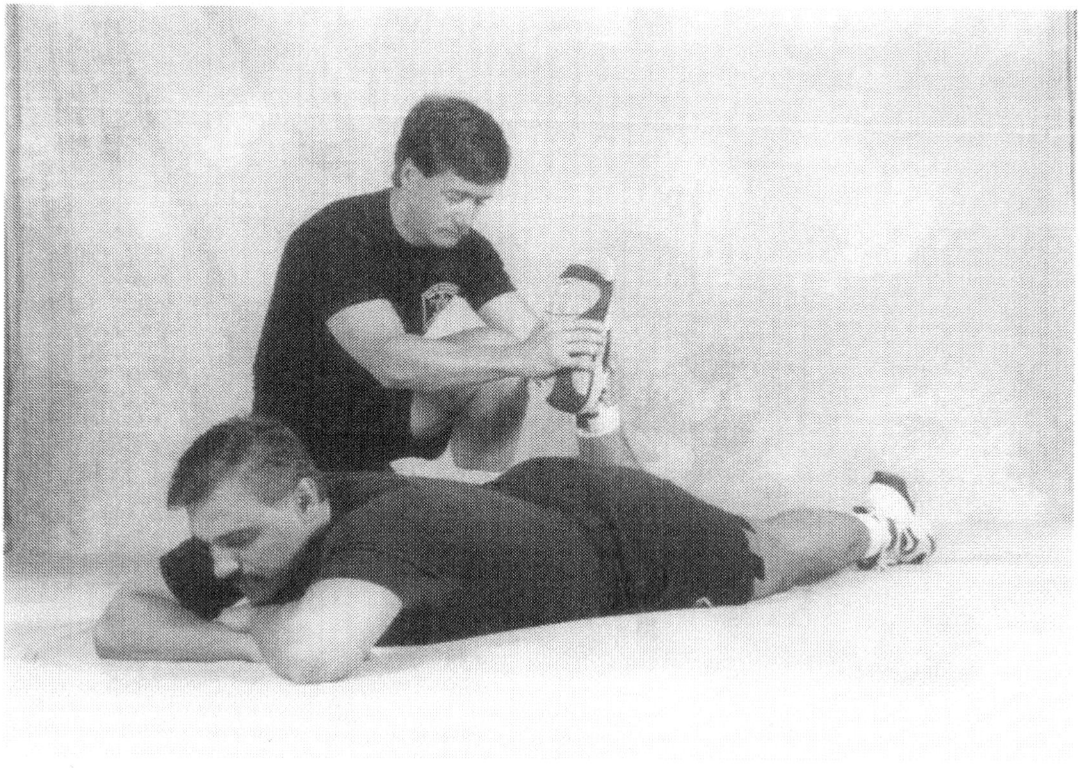

MUSCULAR FITNESS ASSESSMENT

Higher levels of strength, endurance, and power increase your ability to repeat and sustain muscular contractions, and to perform faster and more forceful movements. Studies show that muscular fitness helps reduce the chance of strains and injuries resulting from physical activity. Stronger muscles also help absorb shock and protect the body's structures. (More on muscular fitness is presented in Chapter 5.)

Overall muscular fitness is usually estimated by combining several separate measures, each of which focuses on different areas of the body. Although genetics, sex, and age have an effect upon abilities in this area, participation in a strength training program can improve performance for almost everyone.

This muscular fitness assessment procedure consists of **four** separate protocols:

- Pushups
- Situps
- Jump and Reach
- Wall Sit

Before beginning, make sure you warm-up thoroughly with gentle stretching and other light activities (e.g., brisk walking or marching in place). This reduces the chance of injury and ensures that your body is fully prepared to perform the various strength exercises.

The procedure for each assessment is found on the following pages. The highest possible total score for the Muscular Fitness Assessment is **29 points**. Scores for each protocol should be recorded on the Tally Sheet.

1. Pushups

This procedure tests the strength and endurance of your chest, shoulders, and arms.

During this assessment, you will perform as many pushups as possible, without pausing, in a two-minute time period, or until muscular fatigue occurs. The inability to exercise continuously or to maintain proper form, as described below, indicates the end of the protocol.

Begin the pushup in the "up" position. Keep your body straight and rigid with your arms straight, hands beneath your shoulders. Lower yourself until your chest touches the floor, then return to the starting position. Do not "bounce" your chest off the floor, and maintain straight body posture at all times.

Have your partner keep time for two minutes and count the number of pushups you perform. Your partner should also place his/her hand flat on the floor beneath your chest. You must contact this hand with your chest in order for the pushup to be counted.

SCORE	**# of Pushups**
1	Under 10
2	10 - 20
4	21 - 30
6	31 - 40
8	Over 40

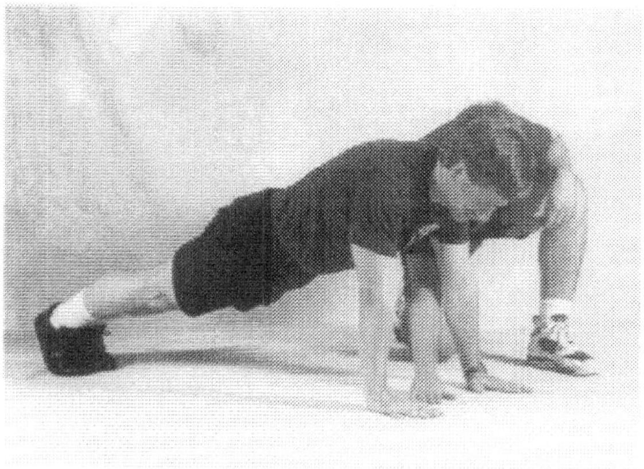

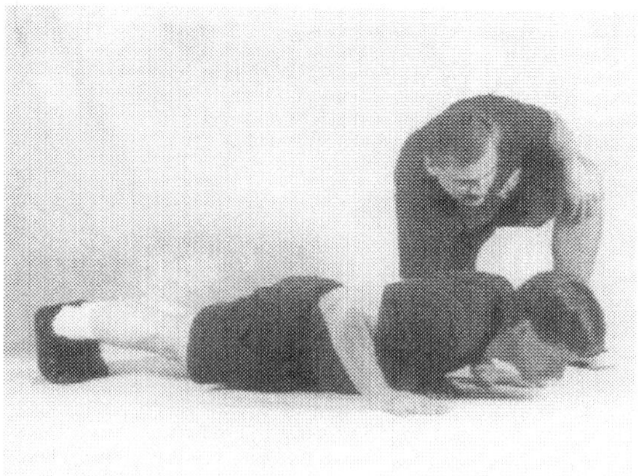

2. Situps

This procedures assesses the strength and endurance of your hip flexor muscles.

As before, you will exercise without pausing for a two-minute time period, or until muscular fatigue occurs. Pace yourself, but do not pause during the procedure.

Begin in the "up" position with your torso vertical, hands crossed over your chest, and knees moderately bent. Have your partner place his/her hands around your ankles to stabilize your lower body. Alternatively, you can place your feet under a sofa, bed, or other piece of furniture.

Lower yourself until your shoulder blades touch the floor, then curl your torso back to a vertical position for one complete repetition. Do not bounce your torso off the floor, or remove your hands from their positions across your chest.

Ask your partner to time the procedure and count the number of situps you perform. Enter the result on the Tally Sheet.

SCORE	**# of Situps**
1	Under 20
2	20 - 30
3	31 - 40
4	41 - 50
5	Over 50

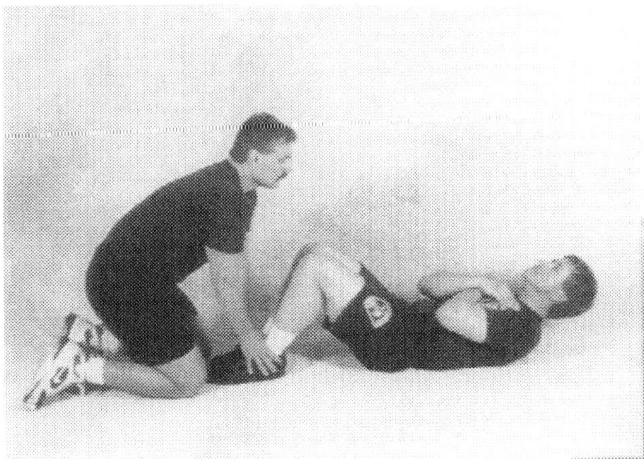

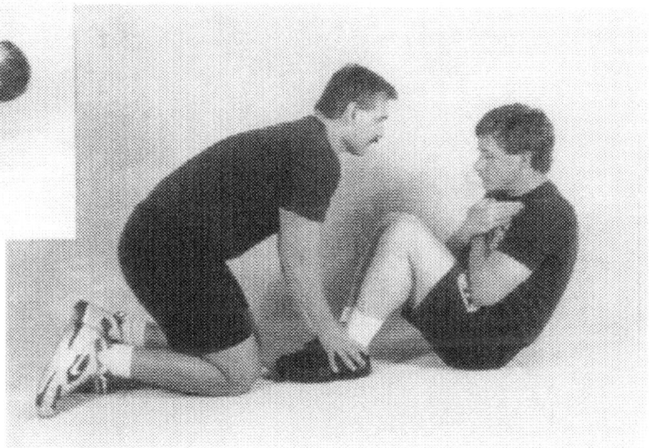

3. Jump and Reach

This procedure assesses the power or explosive force of your lower body muscles—gluteals, thighs, and calves.

Stand beside a smooth wall that's about 12 feet high. Hold a piece of chalk in the hand nearest the wall, or put some chalk dust on your fingertips. Keeping both feet flat on the ground, reach up as high as possible and mark the wall with the chalk or chalk dust. Then sink downward and attempt to jump as high as possible, reaching upward and marking the wall at the peak of the jump.

Using a yardstick or ruler, measure the distance between the two marks to the nearest half inch. Record the best of three trials on the Tally Sheet.

SCORE

1	Less than 9 inches
2	9 - 12.0 inches
4	12.5 - 15 inches
6	15.5 - 18 inches
8	Over 18 inches

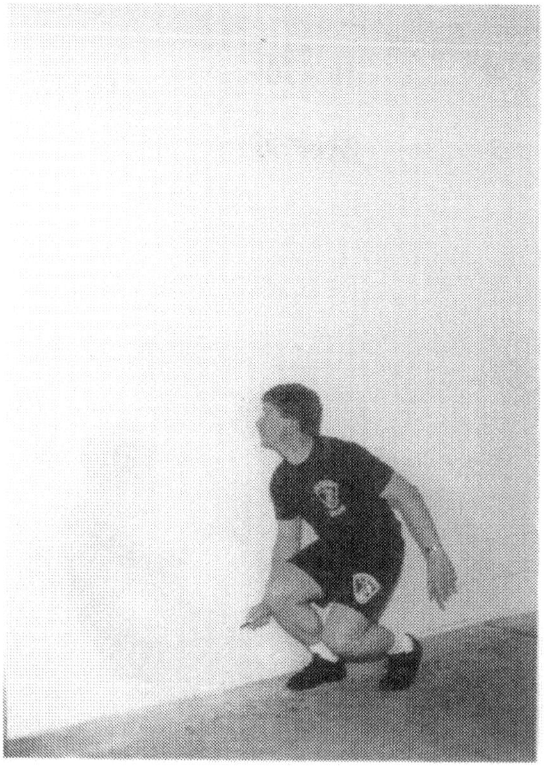

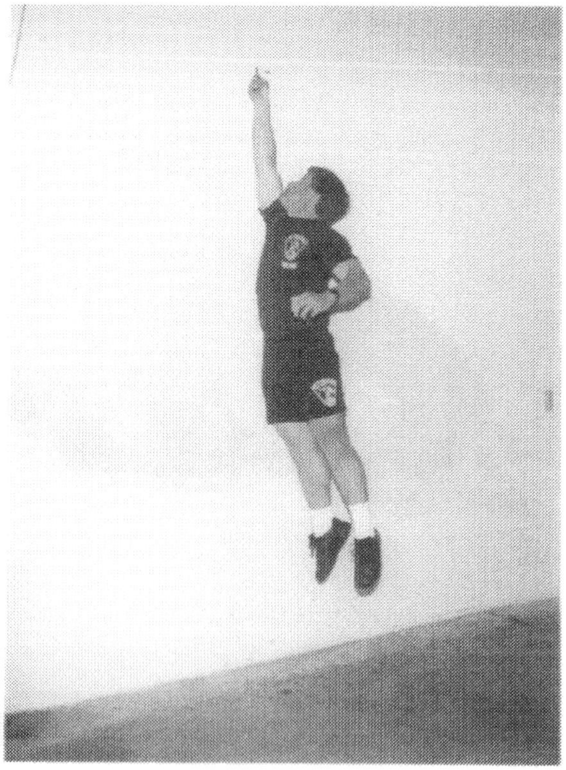

4. Wall Sit

This protocol assesses the strength and endurance of your lower body muscles, especially your quadriceps.

Stand facing away from a wall with your heels approximately 18 inches from it. Then lean backwards until your back rests flat against the wall. Sink slowly into a sitting position, still leaning against the wall, with your thighs parallel to the floor and your lower legs perpendicular (knees forming a 90 degree angle). Cross your arms over your chest.

Once this position is achieved, begin keeping time, using a stop watch or watch with a second hand. Hold this position until muscle fatigue occurs (when the position can no longer be maintained). Record the time you are able to hold the position on the Tally Sheet.

SCORE

1	Less than 30 seconds
2	30 to 60 seconds (1 min.)
4	61 to 90 seconds
6	91 to 120 seconds
8	Over 120 seconds (2 min.)

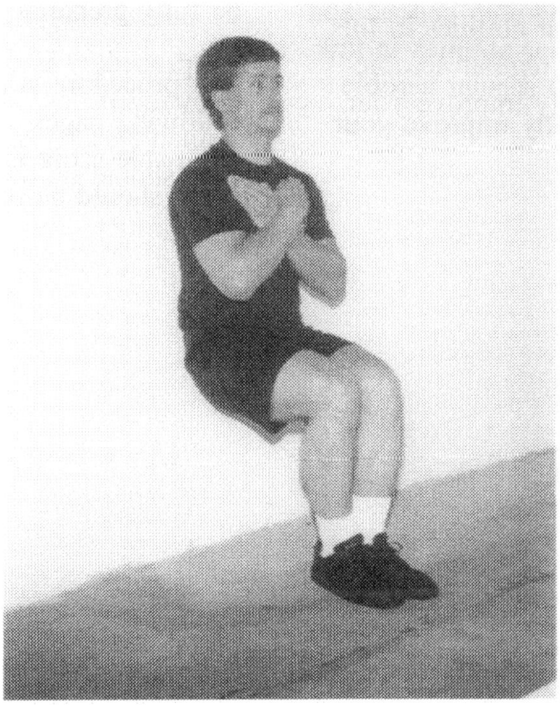

CARDIOVASCULAR FITNESS ASSESSMENT

Continuous vigorous movement requires that your body be able to consume and use oxygen for fuel. The faster you move, the more oxygen your muscles need to sustain the activity over time. As a result, people with higher levels of cardiovascular fitness can walk and jog at a faster pace for extended periods than people with lower fitness levels.

This assessment measures the ability of your heart and lungs to supply your working muscles with oxygen, and your muscles' efficiency in using the oxygen to produce energy. Higher scores indicate a greater level of cardiovascular fitness, which largely determines your capacity to perform vigorous physical activities for long periods of time. Although genetic and age factors affect your abilities in this area, participation in regular aerobic exercise will gradually improve your score.

This assessment requires you to move by walking, jogging, and/or running as far as you can in a 15-minute period. If your level of cardiovascular fitness is high, you will be able to maintain a faster pace, so you can cover more ground during the procedure. The assessment serves to estimate your maximal oxygen consumption ("VO2 Max"), which is the true measure of cardiovascular fitness. (More on this subject is presented in Chapter 4.)

This protocol should be the final component of the assessment. Before beginning, make sure you warm up with gentle stretching and light activity (e.g., brisk walking or marching in place). This reduces the chance of injury and ensures that your body will be fully prepared for exercise.

The procedure is described on the following pages. The maximum attainable score is **31 points**. The score should be recorded on your Tally Sheet.

15-MINUTE WALK/RUN TEST

On a measured, level track, jog, walk, and/or run for exactly 15 minutes, attempting to cover as much distance as possible. Count the number of laps you cover during the time period, being sure to include any fractions of a lap, estimated to the best of your ability.

To determine the total distance covered, multiply the number of laps by the distance per lap, and record the total on your Tally Sheet. Round the results to the nearest tenth (0.1) mile. For example, for a quarter mile track:

7.25 laps x .25 mi. per lap = 1.8 mi.

Then use the chart below to estimate Maximal Oxygen Consumption ("VO2 Max"), which is used to calculate your score on the assessment.

Distance (miles)	VO2 Max
1.0	28.7
1.25	33.5
1.5	38.2
1.6	40.1
1.7	42.0
1.8	43.9
1.9	45.8
2.0	47.8
2.1	49.6
2.2	51.6
2.3	53.5
2.4	55.4
2.5	57.3
2.6	59.2
2.7	61.1

Distance Covered	**VO2 Max**	**SCORE**
Less than 1.33 miles	Less than 35.0	**0**
1.33 to 1.6 miles	35.0 - 39.9	**8**
1.6 to 1.9 miles	40.0 - 45.0	**15**
1.9 to 2.2 miles	45.1 - 51.6	**23**
Over 2.2 miles	Over 51.6	**31**

EVALUATING THE RESULTS

The assessment is now complete. All that remains is to add up your scores for each component of fitness and then for the total assessment. The highest possible score is **100 points**. Enter your calculations on the Tally Sheet.

To determine your fitness level (1, 2, or 3) in each category, use the table at the bottom of the page. Circle the appropriate number on your Tally Sheet.

As you review your assessment scores, keep the following points in mind:

- Summing the separate scores provides a general indicator of overall fitness. However, you can be "fit" in one area and "unfit" in another. **Since all components of fitness are important, a deficiency in <u>any</u> area should be addressed, even if your total score is relatively high.**
- **Since everyone is different, comparing results with others is meaningless or even misleading.** For example, two persons with the same total score could have very different strengths and weaknesses. Consider your score only as a personal baseline—as you get more fit, your score will increase.
- **A fitness assessment is not a substitute or a replacement for a periodic medical examination by your physician.**

After several months, you may wish to repeat the assessment and compare your new and original scores. This can be done using the same Tally Sheet you just used, so keep it in a safe place. The assessment can also be repeated on a periodic basis thereafter. To facilitate long-term comparison of scores, a **Firefighter Physical Fitness Assessment Progress Sheet** (Exhibit 2-2) is provided on the next page.

FITNESS COMPONENT	FITNESS LEVELS Level 1	 Level 2	 Level 3
Body Composition	0, 8 points	15 points	25 points
Flexibility	4-6 points	7-10 points	11-15 points
Muscular Fitness	Under 12 points	12-22 points	23-29 points
Cardiovascular Fitness	0, 8 points	15, 23 points	31 points

Exhibit 2-2

FIREFIGHTER PHYSICAL FITNESS ASSESSMENT
PROGRESS SHEET

NAME____

Key to Scores:

Fat = Body Mass Index
Musc = Muscular Fitness

Flex = Flexibility
C-V = Cardiovascular

	S C O R E S				(Possible 100)
Date	**Fat**	**Flex**	**Musc**	**C-V**	**TOTAL**

CHAPTER SUMMARY

In this chapter, you learned how a physical fitness assessment can be used to refine and enhance your exercise program. You performed a series of simple procedures, or protocols, to measure your capabilities in each of the four components of fitness: flexibility, cardiovascular fitness, muscular fitness, and body composition.

Based on the results of the assessment, your were assigned to one of three fitness level categories, which will be used later for exercise planning. You also totaled the separate scores to get a general indicator of your overall fitness. Finally, guidelines for evaluating and using the results of your assessment were reviewed.

Having completed this chapter, you should now be able to:

- Define the purpose and nature of a physical fitness assessment.
- Describe the benefits and limitations of the CW-F fitness assessment process.
- Identify various techniques and methodologies for evaluating fitness.
- Assess your current level of flexibility, cardiovascular fitness, muscular fitness, and body composition.

BIBLIOGRAPHY

Astrand, Per-Olaf, and Kaare Rodahi, *Textbook of Work Physiology—Physiological Bases of Exercise*, New York: McGraw-Hill Book Company, 1977.

Lohman, Timothy G., Alex F. Roche, and Reynaldo Martorell (Editors), *Anthropometric Standardization Reference Manual*, Champaign, IL: Human Kinetics Books, 1988.

Margaria, R., et. al., "A Simple Relation Between Performance in Running and Maximal Aerobic Power," *Journal of Applied Physiology*, Vol. 8, No. 2, February 1975.

Pollock, Michael L., Jack H. Wilmore, and Samuel M. Fox III, *Health and Fitness Through Physical Activity*, New York: John Wiley & Sons, 1978.

Sharkey, Brian J., *Physiology of Fitness*, Champaign, IL: Human Kinetics Publishers, Inc., 1984.

White, Timothy P., Ph.D., and the Editors of the University of California at Berkeley Wellness Letter, *The Wellness Guide to Lifelong Fitness*, New York: Random House, 1993.

Wilmore, Jack H., *Training for Sport and Physical Activity—The Physiological Basis of the Conditioning Process*, Boston: Allyn and Bacon, Inc., 1984.

United States Fire Administration, *Physical Fitness Coordinator's Manual for Fire Departments*, FA-95, September 1990.

Chapter 3

Physiology and Flexibility: The Science of Stretching

CHAPTER INTRODUCTION

Flexibility is the ability to move a body part through its full and normal range of motion. The stresses placed on the body during physical activity or exercise require adequate flexibility. If muscles are unable to lengthen to their maximum extent, you are more susceptible to sprains, strains, and other injuries.

Flexibility is important to everyone, but particularly fire service personnel whose work involves strenuous physical activity, restrictive areas, slippery or otherwise unsafe conditions, awkward and/or heavy loads, requirements for rapid movement, etc. Studies have shown that greater flexibility reduces the likelihood of back injury in firefighters, the second major cause of premature retirement. (USFA 1990)

This chapter covers principles and techniques for improving your flexibility. You will review the body's major muscle groups and connective tissues, and the elements of an effective workout. A series of safe and effective stretches is introduced. Then you will apply the results of the flexibility assessment in Chapter 2 to develop your own short-term exercise plan. Finally, you will look at factors that promote exercise adherence, which is the ability to stick with your plan and make exercise a regular part of your life.

LEARNING OBJECTIVES

After learning the information in this chapter, you will be able to:

- Identify the major muscle groups and connective tissues in the human body.
- Describe the purpose and benefits of conducting an exercise warm-up and cool-down.
- Conduct a safe and effective flexibility workout.
- Prepare a personal action plan for flexibility exercise that meets your own fitness goals and needs.
- Identify ways to stay motivated and to stick with your exercise program.

THE MUSCULOSKELETAL SYSTEM

The musculoskeletal system's main function is to provide a means of support and locomotion. The word "musculo-skeletal" clearly implies muscles and skeleton (or bones). Muscles that attach to bones provide a series of levers for the movement of body parts.

BONES AND JOINTS

Bones form the framework or "scaffolding" of the body. Despite its rigidity, bone is actually living material that is constantly in a state of turnover as it breaks down old tissue and builds new bone.

If your skeleton was composed of one continuous piece of bone, you wouldn't be able to move. Thus, the skeleton is divided into many individual bones, which meet each other at junctions known as joints or articulations. Common examples of joints are the ankles, knees, hips, vertebrae, shoulders, elbows, wrists, and jaw.

Some joints, called "hinge" joints (e.g., the knee or elbow), permit only limited motion forwards and backwards. Others are "pivot" joints that are capable of rotation, while still others are "ball and socket" joints (such as the hip and shoulder) which allow complex motion in many planes.

In general, joints that are capable of the most complex movements are also the most vulnerable to injury.

MUSCLES AND MUSCLE FIBERS

When you want to perform a certain movement, a message travels from your brain along a nerve to the muscle(s) that will accomplish the motion. Muscle fibers are thin strands of protein that contract and shorten in response to these signals from your nerves. After the contraction, the fibers relax and lengthen again.

Many thousands of these fibers are bound together within a sheath to form individual muscles. When a nerve signal is received, the thousands of muscle fibers shorten, resulting in the contraction and shortening of the entire muscle.

The ends of the muscle attach to different bones on either side of a joint. Another "opposing" muscle attaches across the opposite side of the same joint. In general, contracting one muscle "flexes" the joint (moves body parts closer together), while contracting the opposing muscle "extends" the joint (moves body parts further apart).

Every joint in your body (knee, hip, spine, shoulder, elbow, neck, etc.) is surrounded by a system of opposing muscles which exert their pull on the joint from opposite sides. Common examples include the biceps and triceps of your upper arm or the hamstrings and quadriceps of your thigh (see the following section for a description of the major muscle groups). Good joint alignment is achieved by maintaining a balance in these opposing forces.

LIGAMENTS

Within any joint, the ends of the bones are held together by short, tough fibrous bands known as ligaments. These ligaments function to keep bones in good alignment and in close proximity to each other, while preventing them from moving too far apart. If ligaments become torn or stretched due to injury, the result is a "looser," less stable, and more vulnerable joint.

TENDONS

All muscles gather at each end into tough bands of tissue, known as tendons. These tendons attach the muscle firmly to a bone. Tendons pull on bones at their attachment, effectively transmitting the force of the contracting muscle.

CARTILAGE

A thin coating of material known as cartilage surrounds the ends of most bones. In certain joints that support heavy loads (such as the knees and vertebrae), there are additional thick pads of cartilage **between** bones, acting as an extra protective cushion. The main function of this cartilage is to cover the ends of bones and prevent them from scraping against one another. Thus, cartilage permits smooth and pain-free motion in a joint.

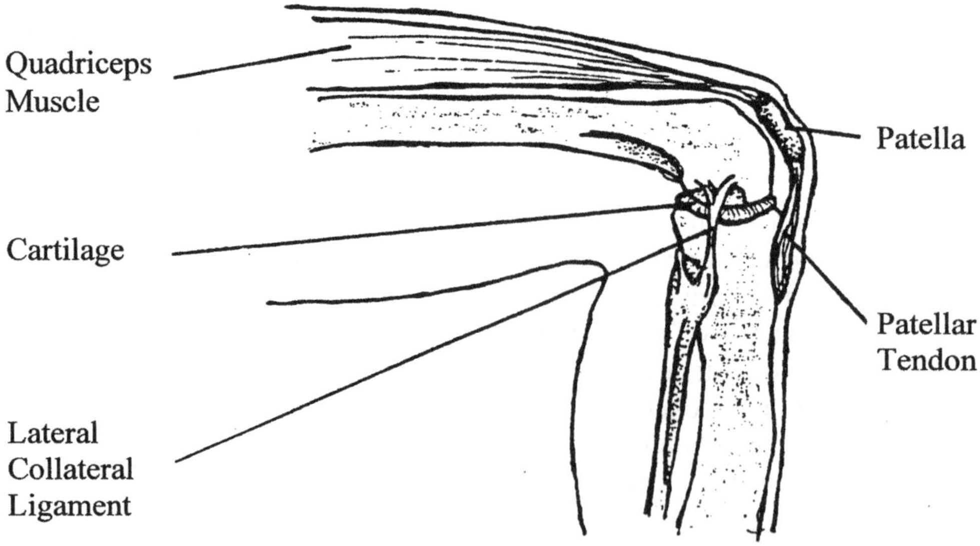

THE MAJOR MUSCLE GROUPS

Trapezius (upper shoulder and neck)

The trapezius (or "traps") attaches along the upper spine and rear of the skull, and runs to the shoulder blade and collar bone. Contracting the trapezius causes a "shrugging" motion of the shoulder.

Deltoid (shoulders)

The deltoid (or "delts") attaches from the top of the shoulder blade and collar bone, runs over the shoulder, and attaches outside the upper arm bone just below the shoulder. Contracting the deltoid raises your arm away from your torso.

Pectoralis (chest)

The pectoralis (or "pecs") attaches from the breast bone, runs across the chest and the front of the shoulder, and attaches outside the upper arm bone just below the shoulder. Contracting it pulls your upper arm forwards and across your chest.

Biceps (front of upper arm)

The biceps attach on the front of the shoulder, run across the front of the upper arm and elbow, and attach on the forearm bones just below the elbow. Contracting the biceps causes your arm to bend (flex) at the elbow.

Triceps (rear of upper arm)

The triceps are three muscles that attach at the back of the shoulder, run along the back of the upper arm and elbow, and attach on the forearm bones below the elbow. Contracting the triceps causes your arm to straighten (extend) at the elbow.

Latissimus Dorsi (upper back)

The latissimus dorsi (or "lats") attaches to the spine, runs across the upper back and under the arm pit, and connects to the outside of the upper arm bone just below the shoulder. Contracting it pulls your upper arm backwards and downwards (the same motion used in pull-ups or rowing).

Abdominals

The abdominals (or "abs") start below the rib cage, run across the front of the stomach, and attach to the bottom of the pelvis. Contracting the abs curls your torso forward, bringing your ribs and pelvis closer together.

Buttocks

The buttocks muscle is also known as the **gluteus maximus** (or "gluteals"). It attaches to the lower spine and back of the pelvis, and runs to the back of the thigh bone. Contracting the buttocks causes "extension" at the hip, like when you stand up from a sitting or crouched (flexed hip) position.

Quadriceps (front of thigh)

The quadriceps (or "quads") consist of four muscles that run from the front of the thigh bone downward across the thigh and over the knee cap. They attach to the front of the lower leg bone just beneath the knee cap. Contracting the quads causes your leg to straighten (extend) at the knee.

Hamstrings (rear of thigh)

The hamstrings (or "hams") are the "biceps in your thigh." They consist of two muscles that run from the back of the pelvic bone across the back of the thigh and behind the knee, attaching to the back of the lower leg bone. Contracting the hams causes your leg to bend (flex) at the knee.

Calves (rear of lower leg)

The calves are more formally known as the **gastrocnemius** (or "gastrocs"). This muscle attaches on the rear of the thigh bone just above the knee, runs down over the back of the lower leg, and attaches underneath the heel. Contracting the gastrocnemius causes you to raise up on your toes ("plantar flexion").

These major muscle groups are shown in the exhibit below. Many other smaller muscles also exist. However, an exercise program that satisfactorily addresses all the major muscle groups listed here generally will be adequate to improve overall muscular fitness.

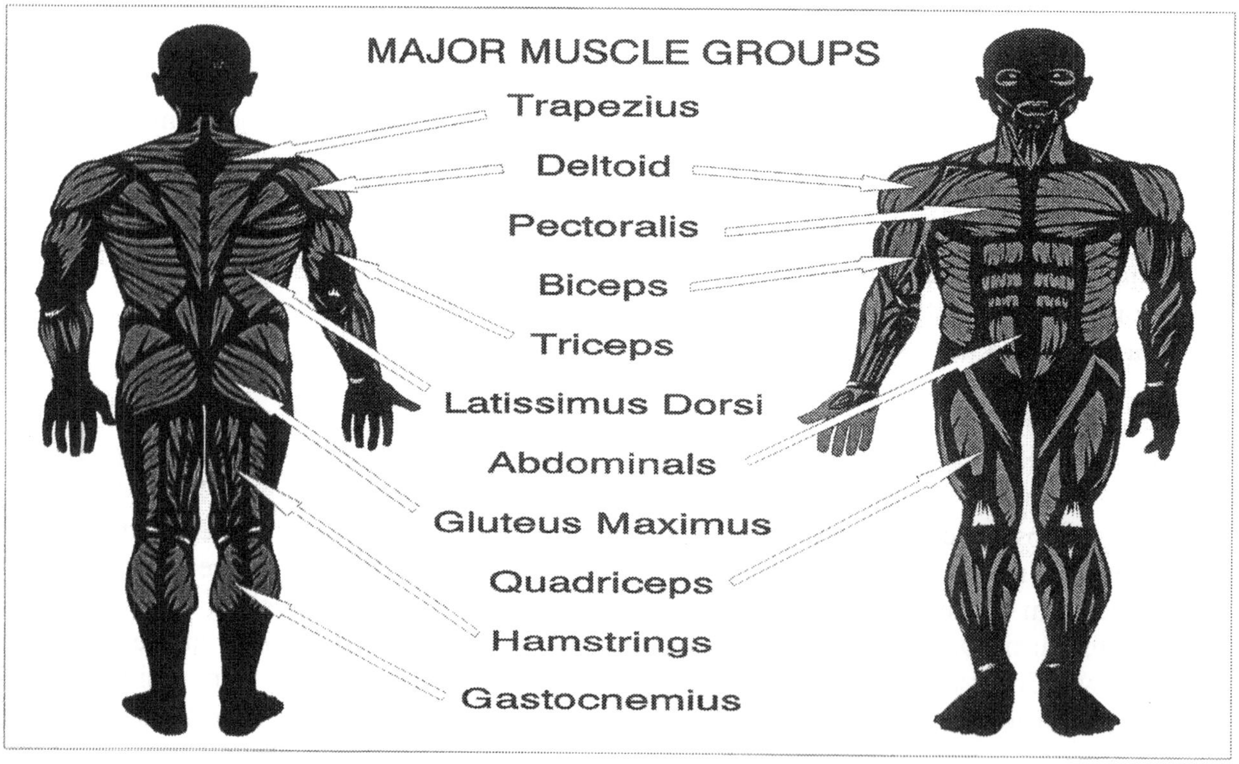

PRINCIPLES OF FLEXIBILITY TRAINING

Flexibility measures the range of motion in a joint, which depends on the pliability of surrounding muscles and connective tissues. If these fibers are too tight, your ability to move will be limited. Activities that cause movement beyond this narrow range of motion can risk straining or tearing your tissues and damaging the joint.

A flexibility training program includes specifically planned exercises to permanently and progressively increase the usable range of motion in a joint or group of joints. This type of program should not be confused with simple stretches that many people use to loosen up before working out. **The frequency, duration, and intensity of warm-up stretching is generally not sufficient to increase the physical fitness component of flexibility.**

The benefits of flexibility training can include the following:

- Relaxation of stress and tension
- Improved body posture and symmetry
- Relief of low back pain
- Relief of muscular soreness
- Better physical and athletic skills
- Heightened job performance
- Injury reduction
- Muscular relaxation
- Union of body and mind
- Personal enjoyment

FACTORS THAT AFFECT FLEXIBILITY

When it comes to flexibility, everyone is anatomically a little different. Some of the factors that affect an individual's flexibility include the following:

Specificity—The amount or range of motion in each joint is somewhat specific. Flexibility of one joint does not ensure flexibility in another.

Heredity—Some persons are naturally more flexible than others, perhaps due to differences in the cellular make-up of their ligaments and other connective tissues.

Gender—On average, women are more flexible than men.

Body Composition—Excess body fat can decrease flexibility.

Occupation and Lifestyle—Persons with sedentary jobs and lifestyles tend to be less flexible.

Age—Joint surfaces degenerate with age, as does the amount and thickness of lubricant (synovial fluid) in the joints. This leads to increased joint stiffness and decreased flexibility.

STRETCHING EXERCISES

In general, everyone is born fairly flexible, but people have a tendency to lose this capacity over time. Flexibility is lost most quickly in those ranges of motion that are not used regularly, either in daily activities or exercise. Gently stretching muscles and tissues causes them to gradually lengthen and improves the movement of the joint.

The most common types of stretches are static and ballistic:

Static Stretches—This type of stretching is the most highly recommended for fitness. Stretches are held to the point of mild tension with no movement for approximately 30 seconds. Stretching beyond mild tension or the use of external force (hands, gravity, a partner, etc.) increases the risk of injury.

Ballistic or Dynamic Stretches—This type of stretching incorporates bouncing movements, which increase the chance of injury to muscles and joints. It also initiates a "stretch reflex," causing the muscle to tighten rather than relax.

GENERAL RULES FOR FLEXIBILITY TRAINING

Stretching exercises should be performed daily in order to improve flexibility. The majority of fitness experts agree that stretching for flexibility is most effective after a warm-up. This is because a warm muscle can be more easily stretched, and gains in flexibility increase with effective stretching. A flexibility exercise session also provides an excellent cool-down activity after a cardiovascular or muscular fitness workout.

Ideally, your flexibility workout should include stretches for all major muscle groups and joints. However, to maximize the training effect or to save time, you may wish to focus on areas that you know to be particularly "tight," either from personal experience or through participation in a flexibility assessment.

To target areas of greater need, first identify the muscles and joints associated with each procedure on which you had a low score in the flexibility assessment from Chapter 2. Then select exercises which address these areas (specific stretching exercises are described later). Spend a greater portion of your workout on these stretches, but don't neglect other requirements for total flexibility training.

General rules for stretching can be summarized as follows:

1. Move into the stretched position SLOWLY.

2. Stretch the muscle only until the point of MILD tension. Trying to over-stretch beyond this point may cause damage.

3. Stay absolutely STILL while holding the stretched position. Do not bounce or jerk.

4. HOLD the stretched position for at least 30 seconds.

5. Ideally, REPEAT each stretch 3-5 times.

6. **NEVER stretch into any position that causes pain.**

Caution: NO GAIN WITH PAIN! Excessive or improper stretching can produce joint instability and increase the risk of dislocation injuries and sprains.

CLOTHES AND EQUIPMENT

Requirements for beginning a flexibility program are minimal. Special attire or footwear is not necessary, although loose-fitting, comfortable clothing that allows free movement is best. You will also need a space large enough to avoid bumping into furniture or other exercisers. A radio or television can be a pleasant addition.

A carpeted area may be preferable since some exercises are performed on the floor. However, exercise mats or carpet squares easily make any physical space suitable. Some programs incorporate towels, bands, or other equipment, but these aids are not necessary for a thorough flexibility workout.

GETTING STARTED/GETTING FINISHED: WARM-UP AND COOL-DOWN

SEQUENCE OF WORKOUT ACTIVITIES

Any type of exercise workout should include the following components:

- **Warm-up**—Moderate movements that allow your body to "get loose" and ready for more vigorous exercise. Many different activities, such as walking and stretching, are appropriate.
- **Workout**—Exercise of sufficient intensity and duration that permits you to attain your health and fitness goals. A balanced exercise program includes both cardiovascular and muscular fitness training, although workouts for each component may be conducted concurrently, sequentially, or separately.
- **Cool-down**—Activities that allow your body to slow down and relax gradually. Again, many moderate exercises are appropriate, although the cool-down period is particularly suited for activities to improve flexibility.

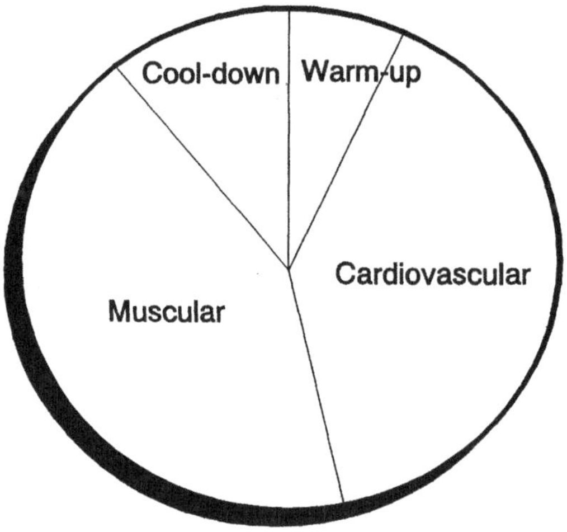

WARM-UP

Compare your muscles to the rubber band around the morning newspaper. When cold, the rubber band is more likely to snap; when warm, it is elastic and easily manipulated. In the same way, cold muscles are susceptible to "tearing" or "ripping." Warm muscles are pliable and flexible, and so can be worked with less chance of injury.

Five good reasons to include a warm-up as part of every workout are:

1. **Muscle Preparation**—Warm-up increases the blood flow to muscles and helps to evenly distribute lubricating fluid around joints. Muscles lengthen and flexibility and elasticity improve.

2. **Increased Heart Rate and Circulation**—As the heart beats faster, blood vessels widen to bring in oxygen and nutrients and to remove waste products. Improved circulation allows more efficient use of oxygen.

3. **Increased Metabolic Rate**—Your metabolic rate increases as your body steps up its production of energy and heat to meet the increased requirements of exercise.

4. **Physical Preparation**—Your body needs time to adjust to the demands of exercise. During warm-up, nerve impulses travel faster and coordination improves. Muscles contract faster, more forcefully, and more efficiently.

5. **Attitude Adjustment**—The warm-up acts as the bridge between work and play. It allows you time to mentally "gear up" for the workout ahead, while leaving the rest of the day and its stressors behind (or ahead of) you.

Principles of Warm-up

Thoughts on the best way to warm up have changed in recent years, leaving some exercisers confused. Several controversies have arisen, such as whether to include stretching as part of warm-up routines. The following summarizes the current recommendations of fitness experts.

WHO needs to warm up? Whether you exercise for fitness or for performance, warming up is a good idea for everyone. Many top athletes believe that a thorough warm-up is critical to high performance. It's especially important for early morning exercisers who have not had the benefit of daily activity to prepare their muscles. Conversely, individuals who have just completed other physical activities may not require as much warm-up. But whatever your exercise goals or routines, a warm-up usually makes your workout more effective and more enjoyable.

WHAT is the best way to warm up? At one time, stretching was considered to be an effective exercise warm-up. Current research suggests that stretching cold muscles alone is not an effective warm-up because it does not stimulate circulation and raise muscle temperatures the way active movement does. However, stretching can help prepare muscles and joints for the special demands of certain types of exercise, particularly competitive sports.

The ideal warm-up depends on your fitness level and the type of workout you are preparing for. Although many different warm-up activities can be useful, the most effective approach is often doing the same movements that you will make during your workout. These "rehearsal" movements may also aid your mental preparation for exercise. Begin at a slow, gentle pace and gradually increase the intensity as the warm-up continues.

HOW LONG should the warm-up last? As the name suggests, you should warm up until you are warm, or just beginning to break a sweat. This usually occurs within five to ten minutes, depending on your individual fitness level and the type of warm-up. If you are preparing for aerobic or cardiovascular exercise, your heart rate should increase to at least 90-120 beats per minute, depending on your age. An aerobic warm-up should gradually increase your heart rate into this "target zone."

Remember: if your warm-up leaves you feeling tired, you're working too hard!

COOL-DOWN

Following a vigorous cardiovascular or strength training workout, it is important to give your body a chance to slow down gradually. The cool-down period allows time for bodily processes to adjust back to normal, and aids in recovery from sustained physical activity.

During exercise, blood flows to the extremities (legs and arms). The rhythmic contractions of the large muscles of the body assist in returning this blood to the heart. This mechanism reduces the heart's workload and helps to eliminate dizziness. A cool-down also acts to prevent the buildup of residual metabolic products.

The length of the cool-down depends on the type and intensity of the activity, the fitness level of the exerciser, and environmental conditions. Generally, three to ten minutes is adequate. A variety of activities may be used, including walking or slow jogging, stretching, and light calisthenics. It's also possible just to slow the pace and intensity of the activity used in your workout. Flexibility routines are especially appropriate because the muscles are already warm, and stretching at this time helps to preserve any flexibility benefit you received during the workout.

FLEXIBILITY EXERCISES FOR FIREFIGHTERS

Flexibility training can easily be tailored to provide important benefits for almost everyone. You can conduct flexibility training separately, or as part of the cool-down after a cardiovascular or strength training workout. Flexibility workouts are most successful following some activity that has prepared the muscles by warming them up.

Like any well-designed exercise plan, you should start off slowly, then add more comprehensive and vigorous exercise options as you become more fit. The diagrams and narratives on the following pages will help you to conduct a thorough flexibility training workout for all the body's major muscle groups and joints.

The stretches in this workout are divided into two sections—lower body and upper body. Each stretch should be held for 15-30 seconds. Every time you perform a stretch, your goal should be to increase your range of motion a small amount. Remember, **no bouncing**—safe stretching uses steady pressure to the point of mild tension! Bouncing or ballistic stretches are less effective, and can actually cause injury to your muscles.

It is recommended that you complete all the exercises in this flexibility training workout at least three times per week. You can perform each stretch 2-3 times before proceeding to the next stretch, or complete the entire workout 2-3 times in a row.

> Remember: Improvement in flexibility comes slowly. Just keep trying, and your flexibility will improve. However, it's important to gauge your success from where you are when you first begin this type of flexibility workout. You may not ever be as flexible as someone else you see doing the same workout. Follow the three P's to ensure success:

PRACTICE

PERSISTENCE

PATIENCE

LOWER BODY STRETCHES

1. Hamstring Stretch

The first stretch is for the hamstrings or the back of the thigh. Many people have tight hamstrings because they sit so much during the day.

Sit on the floor with one leg straight; pull the heel of the other leg in toward your groin. Keeping your upper body as straight as possible, lean out, moving your chest toward the knee of your straight leg. It's important to keep both hips on the floor, and stretch only to the point of mild tension; back off if it's painful.

Throughout the exercise, keep your knee as straight as possible, and point your toes straight up to prevent the hip from rotating. Pointing the toes also allows you to feel a stretch through the back of your calf and through the achilles tendon over your heel.

It doesn't matter where the other foot is placed or whether the knee of the bent leg touches the floor. Keeping your head up helps eliminate the tendency to bend forward. You may want to place your hands on the ankle of your leg to help you keep your back straight. Tilting the pelvis forward puts more of a stretch on the hamstring rather than the back.

It is not safe to try this stretch with one leg bent back (see the second photograph). This position is dangerous to the knee, and should only be done in certain types of athletic training, not for general fitness.

Repeat the stretch with the other leg. It's not unusual to find that one side is more flexible that the other.

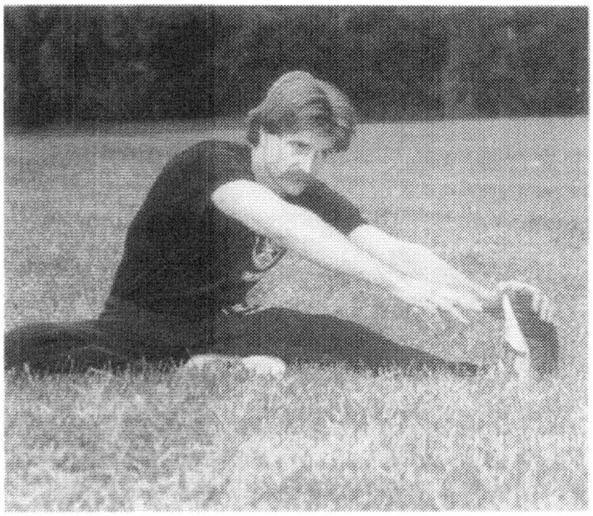

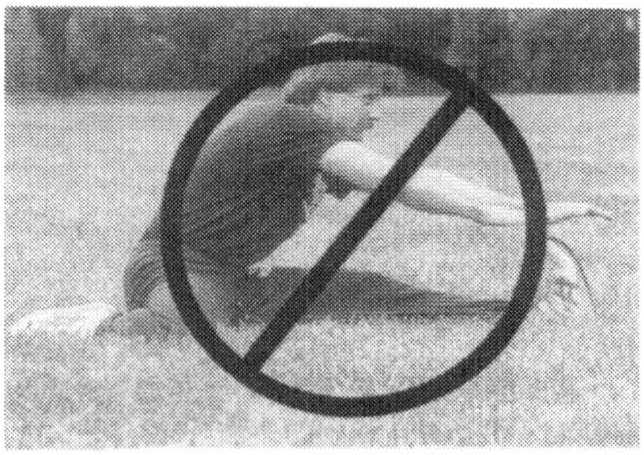

2. Quadriceps Stretch

This stretch is for the front of your thigh, or quadriceps, muscle. Lay on your side, leaning on your elbow and upper arm. Keeping the bottom leg fairly straight, bend the top leg at the knee, and press it backwards. Your goal is to get the knee behind the hip to stretch the front of your thigh.

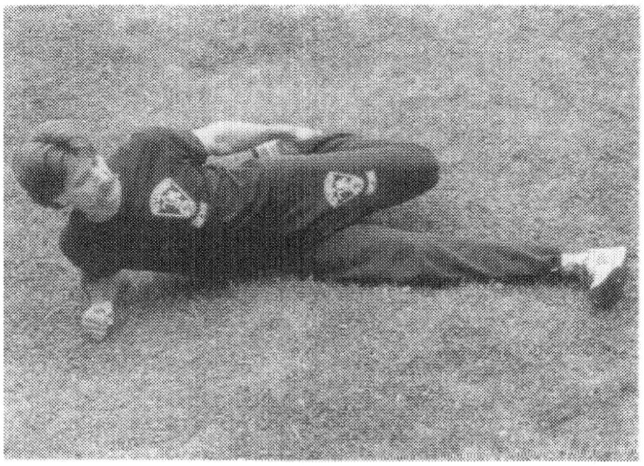

If you aren't flexible enough to grab your shoe over the laces, try grabbing your heel or just pressing the knee back by placing your hand in front of your body for balance. During the stretch, press back with the knee to the point of mild tension. Avoid pulling too hard on your foot. Roll over to the other side to stretch the other leg.

3. Toe Tower

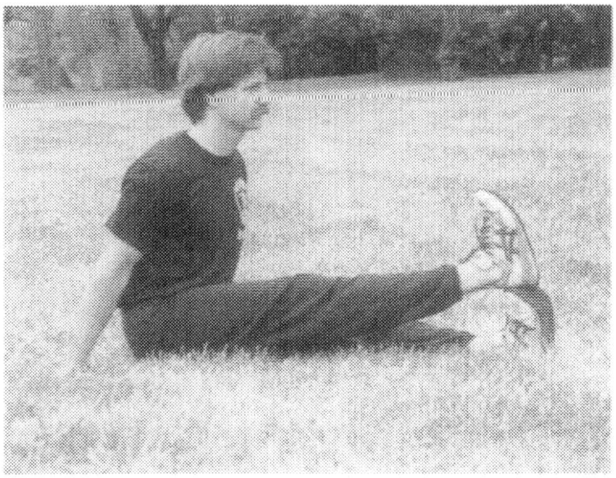

The next exercise is a stretch for the hamstrings or back of the thigh. Sitting on the floor and keeping your hands next to your sides for balance, place the heel of one foot on top of the toes of the other. Try to keep your top leg as straight as possible.

Point the toes of the top leg toward you and gently lean forward from the hips. Keep your chin up, and your back as straight as possible. You may also choose to bring your hands forward if you wish to hold the calf or foot of your top leg. Switch feet positions to stretch the other leg.

4. Lower Back Stretch

These excellent exercises can help you avoid lower back problems. Although best performed on a hard surface, they can even be done before you get out of bed in the morning or before you go to sleep at night.

Lay on your back with both legs extended. Pull one knee in toward your chest, keeping the other leg straight. Grab the back of your thigh below the knee and pull the knee towards your chest. You should feel a stretch in your lower back and a stretch in the buttocks and groin area of the extended leg. Remember to hold under the leg, not the knee. Switch legs and do the same stretch with the other leg.

For the final part of the stretch, pull both knees in toward your chest. It's important to pull on the thighs, not over the knee. You may lift your head to increase the stretch through the entire spine. Since this requires some abdominal strength, you may want to wait a while before adding this option.

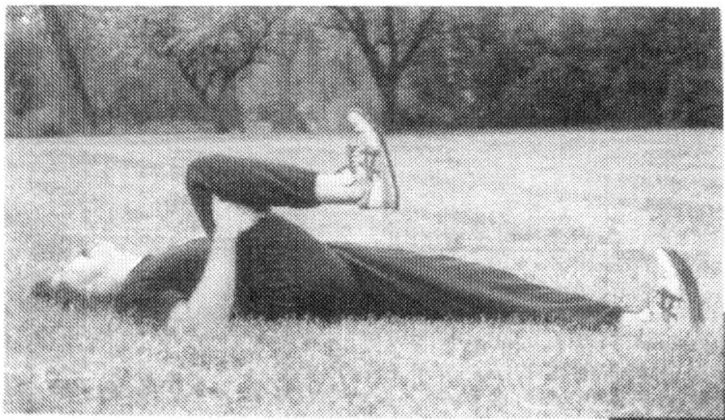

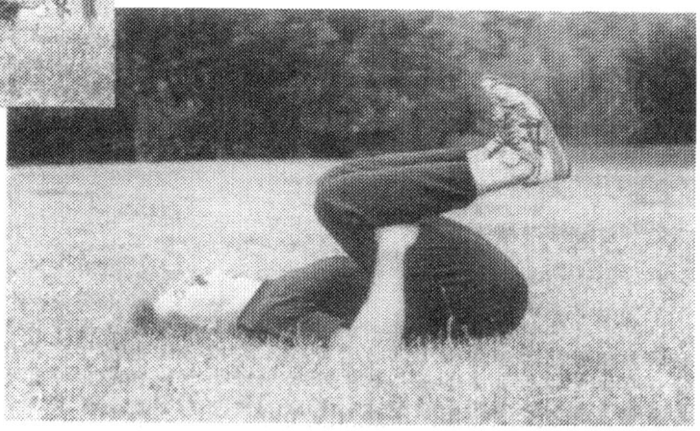

5. Abdominal Stretch

The abdominals are the opposing muscle group to your back muscles, and many back problems are due to weak abdominals. Although this exercise is not a back stretch, it extends your spine and increases the mobility of your lower back.

Lay on your stomach with both legs extended all the way out. Place your palms close to your shoulders and gently raise your upper body off the floor, coming up onto your elbows. In order to stretch the entire abdominal area, lift your head gently backwards, tilting your chin toward the ceiling. If you are flexible enough, you can increase this stretch by straightening your arms further. Remember to breathe normally throughout the exercise.

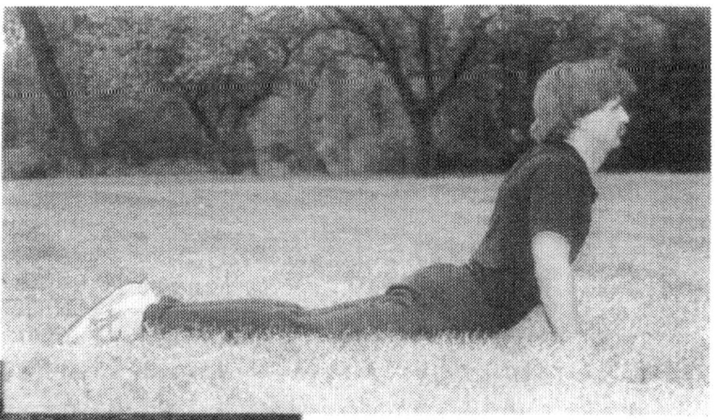

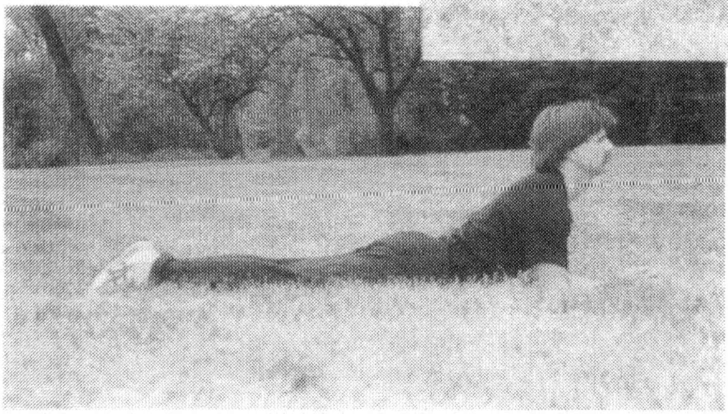

6. Calf Stretch

Good flexibility in the calves helps you absorb shock when running and minimize shin splints. In a seated position, extend your legs to the front. Place your hands at your sides for balance. Straighten your legs and bend your ankles so that your toes come back toward your nose. This will stretch the backs of your calves.

You can increase the stretch by lifting your heels off the floor. You can also lean forward slightly to feel more stretch through your hamstrings.

The second step is to stretch the front of the calves by pointing and pressing the toes forward. Remember to keep your knees straight, and lean forward if it's comfortable. Keep pressing down with your toes to the point of mild tension.

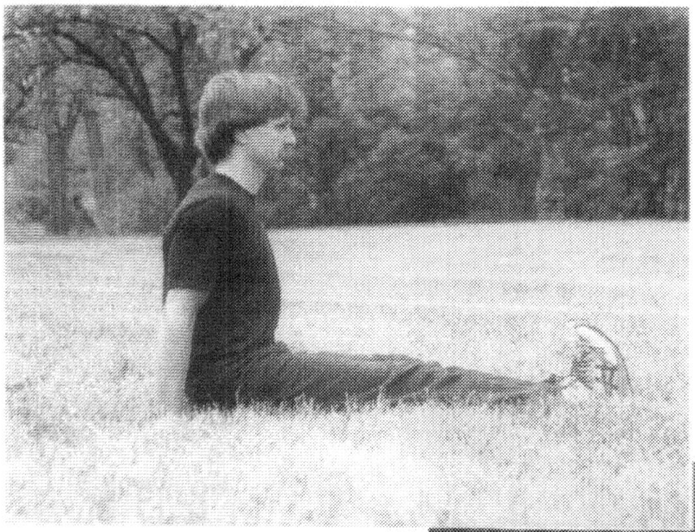

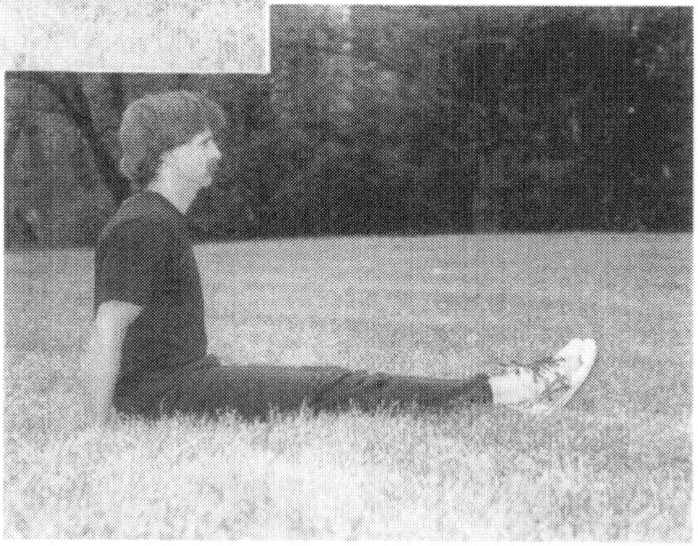

7. Inner Thigh Stretch

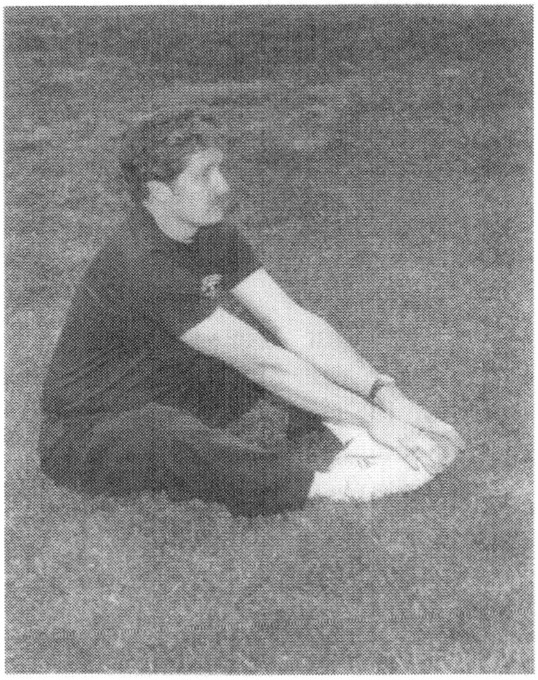

This exercise stretches the inner thigh, another area that is often inflexible. While sitting, start with a modified stretch by bending your legs slightly and rotating them outward. Bring the heels of your shoes together.

Keeping your back as straight as possible (leading with your chin), bend from the hips and reach toward your toes. Alternatively, lay your elbows on your knees and place your forearms along the lines of your calves. Lean gently forward. If you are more flexible, you may be able to grab your ankles and pull yourself into the stretch.

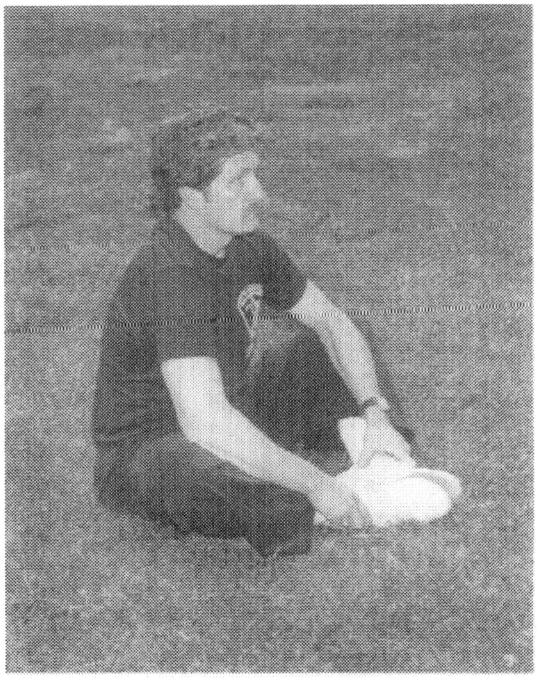

For the second part of this stretch, gradually slide your heels in along the floor toward your groin, as far as you can to the point of mild tension. Gently press your knees outward, toward the floor. Your knees do not have to touch the floor. It also doesn't matter how far you pull in your feet.

If your knees are off the floor and you want to gently press down on your legs with your elbows or hands for a better stretch, just remember to exert gentle, even pressure, and not to press directly on the knee. Lowering your head will also stretch the cervical vertebrae in the back of your neck.

8. Crossover Hip Stretch

The next stretch is a great total body stretch, especially for the hip, waist, and back areas. It also incorporates some of the muscles of the upper body.

Sit on the floor and cross your left leg over your right. Your left hand should be close to your hip; keeping the hand close to the hip helps you remember to sit up straight. Turn your right shoulder toward your bent leg, placing your right forearm outside the upper thigh.

As you rotate your torso towards the left, try to keep your left foot and both hip bones on the floor. You should look down toward your left hand, and gently exert pressure on the crossed leg with your forearm until you feel a stretch through the outside hip.

Don't pull on your knee—make sure the pressure is on the thigh, closer to the hip. Press to the point of mild tension and hold. Return to the front and repeat on the opposite side.

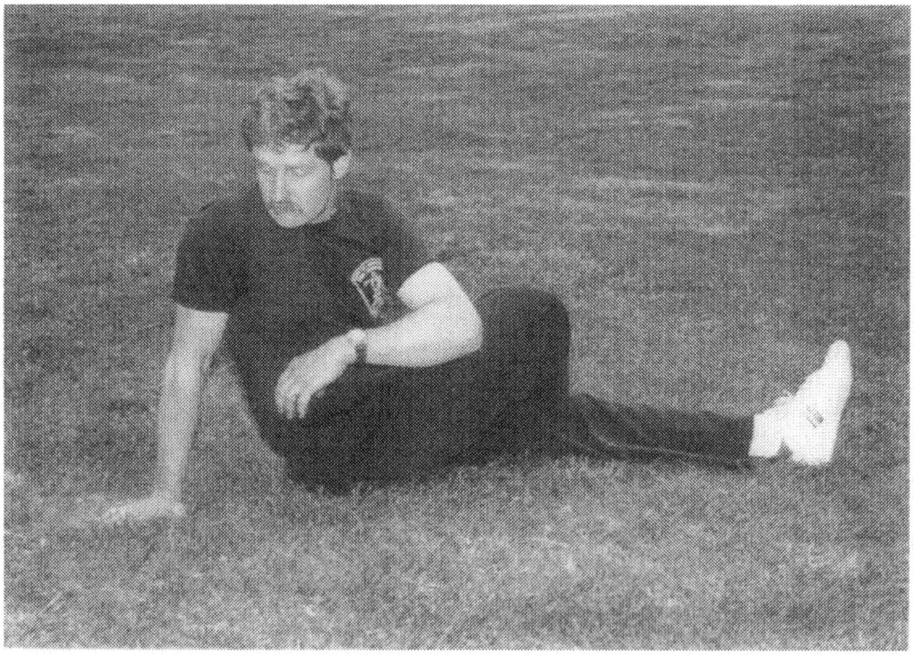

UPPER BODY STRETCHES

9. <u>Overhead Shoulder and Chest Stretch</u>

Laying the palm of one hand over the fingertips of the other hand, and placing your chin on your chest, gently press your arms back as in the photograph. Your arms should be slightly bent, with your chin pressing gently downward to stretch the back of your neck. You should feel this stretch through your chest and the front of your shoulders.

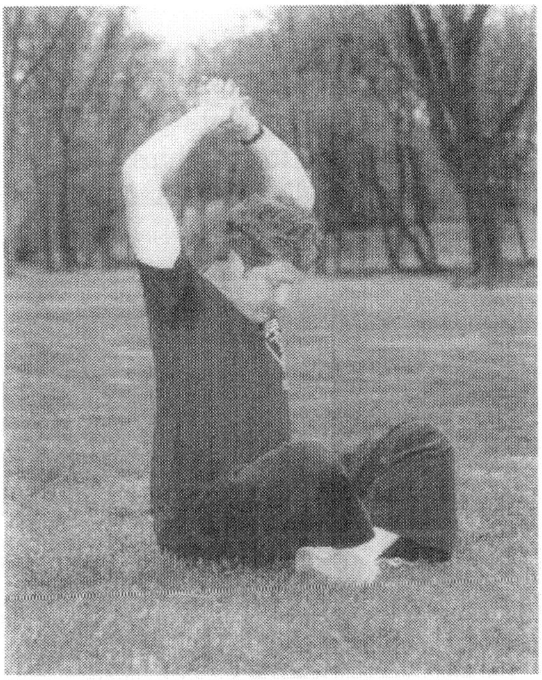

10. <u>Chest, Back, and Shoulder Stretch</u>

Place your hands on your shoulders, and gently press your elbows back, stretching through the chest. Keep your neck relaxed, head forward, and chin up.

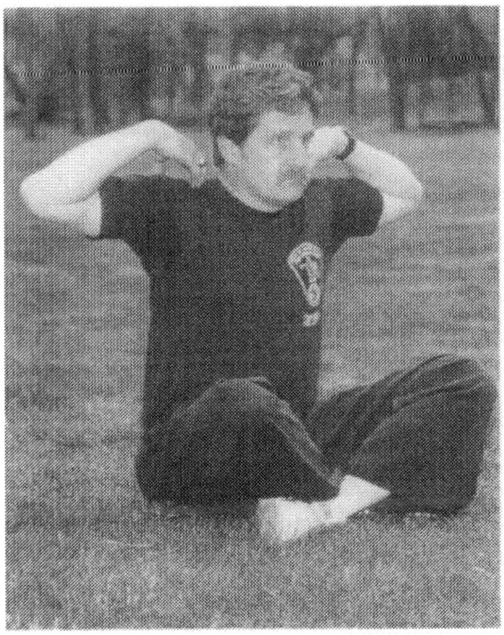

To stretch the opposing back muscles, bring your elbows to the front, gently pressing them toward each other, while lowering your chin to your chest. If you lean gently forward from the hips, you can include your lower back in this stretch.

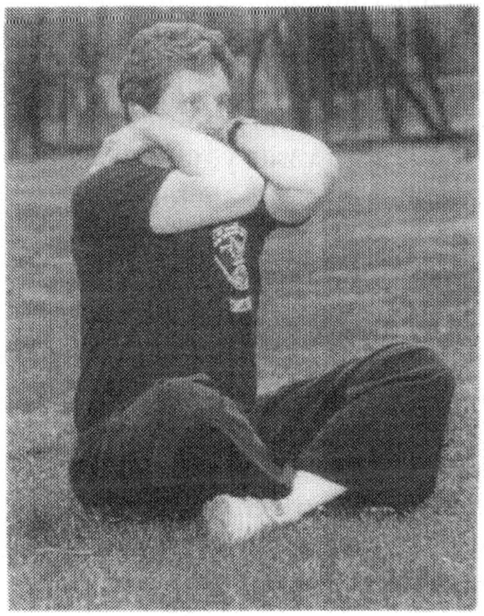

11. Back, Waist, and Shoulder Stretch

This stretch is for the back, waist, and shoulders. Begin by putting one hand on the floor close to your hips. Place the fingertips of the other hand lightly on the back of your head. Lean gently to the side, keeping your back straight to help stay in the proper position.

Keep both hip bones on the floor and try not to lean into the stretch. If you want to stretch the upper back further, you may extend the entire arm over your head. Bring the arm back down and switch to the other side. Remember not to lean forward.

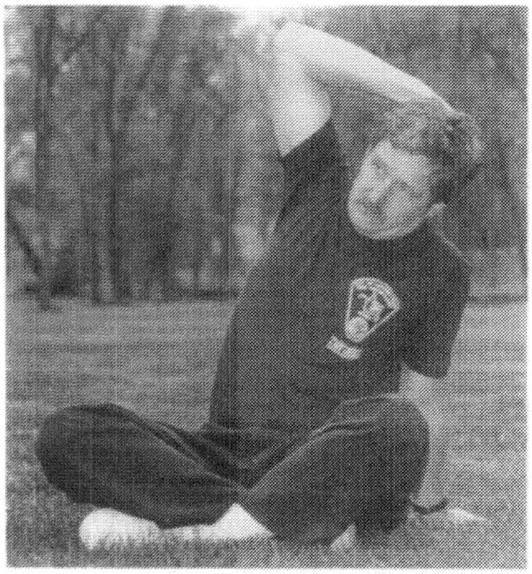

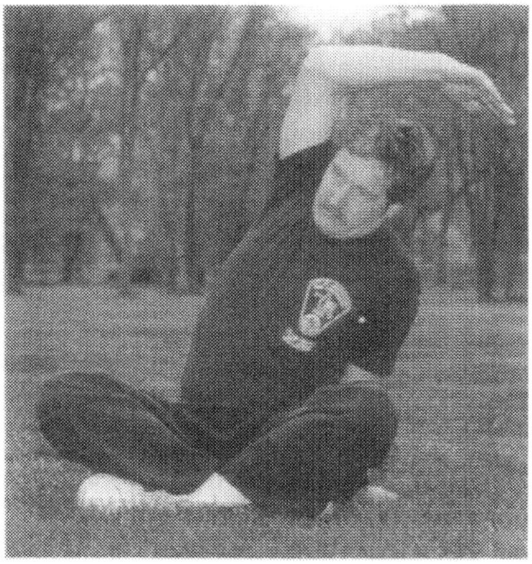

12. Crossover Shoulder Stretch

To stretch your shoulder muscles, bring one arm across the front of your body, placing the fingertips of the other hand on the upper arm. Gently pull the arm towards you until you feel the stretch across the shoulder.

Keep your shoulders level, and don't let the shoulder come up toward your ear. You can either keep the free hand extended or rest it on the other shoulder. Make sure to face forward and don't turn at the waist. You will also feel some stretch in the triceps muscles (back of your upper arm). Repeat the stretch on the other side.

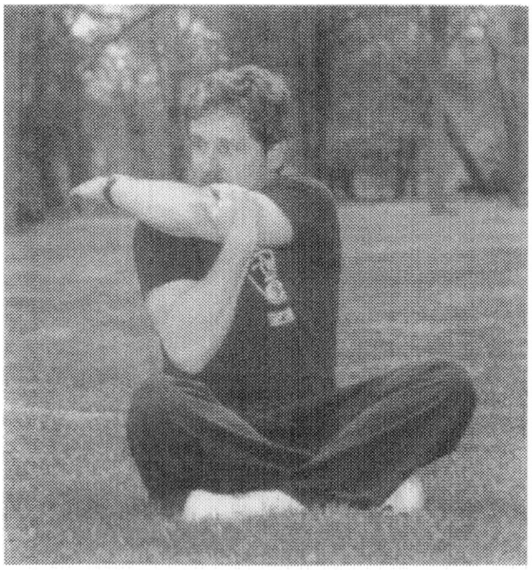

13. Triceps Stretch

This stretch is for the back of the upper arm. Take one arm up over head, bend at the elbow, and aim your fingertips toward the back of your opposite shoulder.

The idea is to sit up straight and keep your head back, using your head to exert the pressure needed to stretch the back of your upper arm. You may use your other hand to help you hold the proper position or to increase the stretch. Repeat the stretch with the other arm.

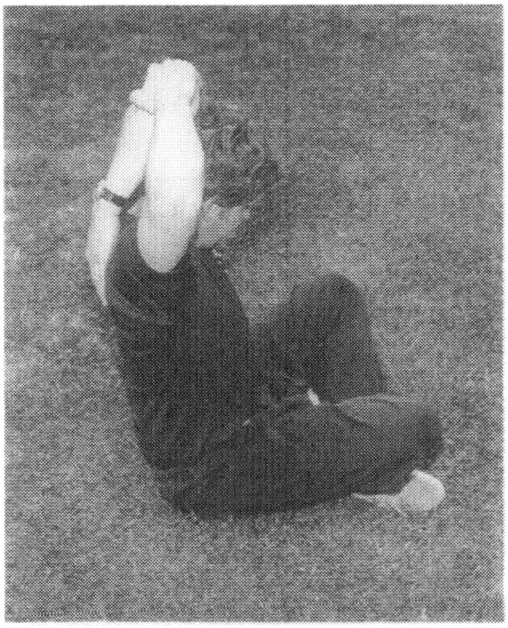

14. Biceps Stretch

Begin this stretch by placing your hands on the floor behind your hips, leaning back as far as you can, while keeping the elbows straight. Your fingertips should be pointing away from your body.

Increase the stretch by rotating your torso gently **away** from one arm, looking over your shoulder. Repeat the stretch for the other arm by looking over the opposite shoulder.

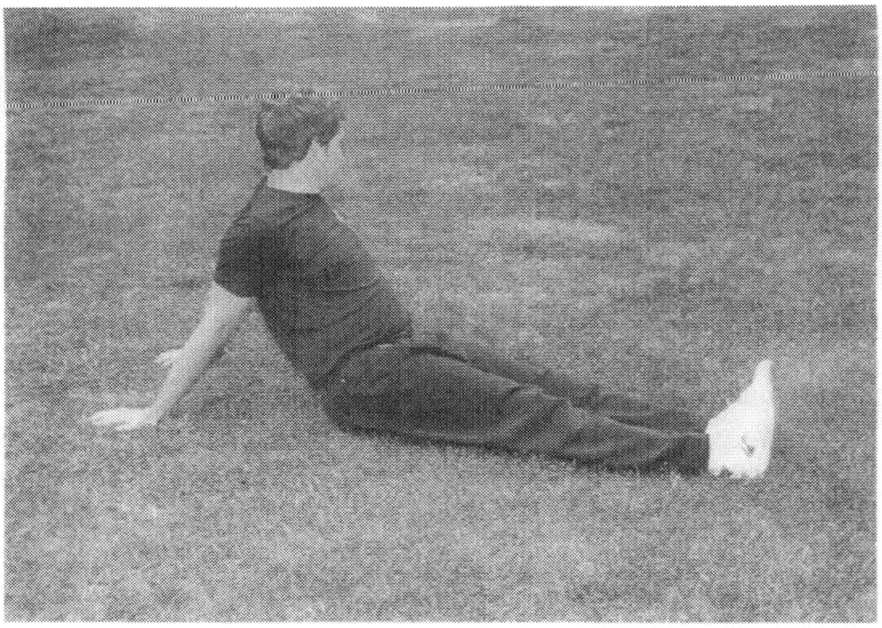

15. Neck Stretches

End your flexibility workout with a few stretches for your neck. Stress, tension, and everyday activities can cause these muscles to become tight. Sit up straight and tilt your chin forward to your chest, feeling the stretch through the cervical vertebrae in the back of your neck. Don't let your torso sag forward, and keep both hips on the floor. You may use your fingertips to gently press on the back of your head to increase the stretch, or just use the weight of your head to feel the stretch through your neck.

Stretch the sides of the neck by tilting your ear toward your shoulder, keeping your head up. It's important to sit up straight and keep your chin lifted. Don't let your head rotate forward. Gently relax and bring your head back to center and over to the other side. Remember not to lean into the stretch. Keep breathing. If you wish to exert more pressure, take the fingertips of your hand and gently press your head downward toward the shoulder.

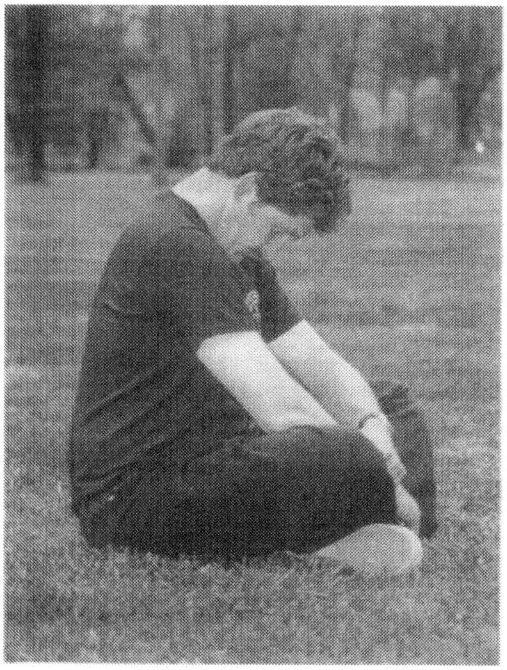

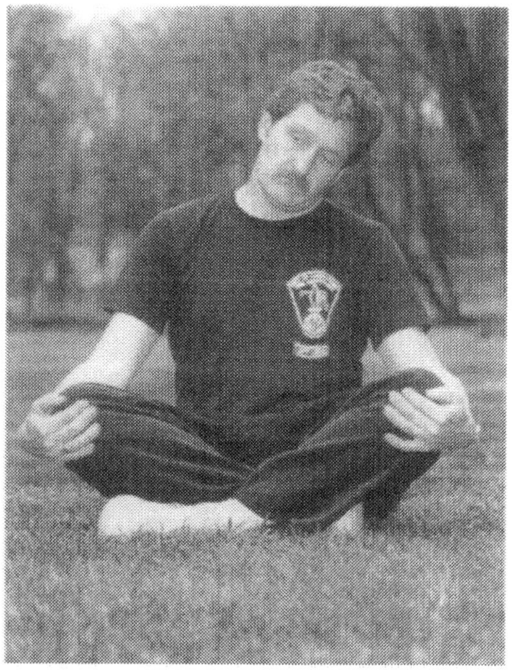

Complete the flexibility workout with a few deep breaths. Just lift and circle your shoulders as you inhale and exhale, letting your arms fall loosely at your sides. Congratulations, you're finished! You should be feeling relaxed. Remember, these exercises can be repeated 3-5 times each as you go through the sequence, or you may choose to just repeat the entire sequence straight through.

Activity 3-1

FLEXIBILITY EXERCISE PLANNING

This planning activity provides a simple approach for estimating how long you need to work out, based on your current fitness level and personal exercise goals.

FITNESS LEVELS AND GOALS

Any personal exercise plan must take into account your current level of fitness. Fortunately, you estimated your flexibility fitness level as part of the assessment process described in Chapter 2. As you recall, you fell into one of three categories: Level 1—Basic Conditioning; Level 2—General Fitness; or Level 3—Performance Fitness.

You also need to decide your personal fitness goals for flexibility training. In using this approach, the options are defined as follows:

- **Bronze Medal**—Maintain at least minimum levels of fitness to promote good health.
- **Silver Medal**—Achieve gradual, progressive improvement beyond minimum or current levels of fitness.
- **Gold Medal**—Significantly exceed basic fitness and health requirements: "be all that you can be."

The goal you choose is important, so think it through carefully. **It must be realistic—a goal you are willing and able to achieve**. Considerations might include the time you have available, other personal or work commitments, personal motivation and interest, past history of exercise, obstacles you expect to encounter, support (or lack of it) from family and friends, etc. Remember: the goal you select governs how long you will need to work out.

PLANNING INSTRUCTIONS

1. Follow the directions in Part A of the worksheet on the next page to estimate the amount of time (in minutes) you need to spend during each flexibility workout.

2. Transfer the results from Part A to Part B to develop a weekly action plan for your flexibility program. Use the following guidelines:

- Plan at least three combined flexibility workouts each week.
- List additional workouts, as desired. (Stretching is best conducted every day.)
- After several weeks, consider adding five or ten minutes to your workout as you become more fit.

Activity 3-1 (Continued)
WORKSHEET

A. FLEXIBILITY WORKOUT TIME

Based on your flexibility fitness level (1, 2, or 3) and personal fitness goal (gold, silver, or bronze), estimate the time (in minutes) for your flexibility workout by circling the appropriate number in the table below. **Warm-up time is not included.**

YOUR FITNESS GOAL	YOUR FITNESS LEVEL		
	Level 1	Level 2	Level 3
Gold	20	25	30
Silver	15	20	25
Bronze	10	15	20

B. WEEKLY ACTION PLAN AND PROGRESS CHART

Develop an exercise action plan using the first half of each column (P = Planned) below. Transfer the time estimate from Part A for each day you will work out. Use the second half of the column (A = Actual) to record the time you actually spend exercising.

DAY OF WEEK	WEEK 1		WEEK 2		WEEK 3		WEEK 4		WEEK 5		WEEK 6	
	P	A	P	A	P	A	P	A	P	A	P	A
DAY 1												
DAY 2												
DAY 3												
DAY 4												
DAY 5												
DAY 6												
DAY 7												

EXERCISE ADHERENCE

Developing an exercise plan is only the first step on the road to fitness. Staying with the program, commonly called **exercise adherence**, continues to be a major problem for many people. Studies show that the likelihood of maintaining an exercise program for more than a year is less than 50 percent. Some experts feel that even this figure is optimistic.

Many of the reasons people commonly give for exercising—fear of illness or disease, increased health benefits, desire for control, and personal vanity—have proven to be poor motivators for long-term exercise adherence. The answer seems to lie in whether the exercise is enjoyable, rather than unpleasant. That's why exercise equipment designers often add electronic panels to their machines—the computer graphics and digital readouts provide feedback and entertainment during the workout.

The key to long-term exercise adherence is matching your personality and interests with your exercise program. Thus, the success (or failure) of your fitness plan will probably depend on the nature of the program you implement. When planning your fitness program, think through your own personal needs and preferences, and make decisions accordingly. In this way, you will ensure that the program will be both enjoyable and maintainable.

Some important factors for exercise adherence can be categorized under the three basic phases of your fitness program:

- Planning your workouts
- Beginning your exercise routine
- Maintaining your exercise program

PLANNING YOUR WORKOUTS

When planning your fitness program, it's important to think through your reasons and strategies for exercising. Some considerations are described below.

Motivation

What are your reasons for getting in shape? Is it your health, your job, your appearance, your stress level? You will be more successful if you clearly define why you want to start exercising. Your job as an emergency responder should provide you with one good reason: you need to be physically fit in order to safely and effectively perform the activities and tasks required by your profession. Others' lives, and your own, may depend on your level of physical conditioning.

Type of Exercise

What type of exercise appeals to you? Do you like general recreational activities, or does exercise need to be competitive for you to enjoy it? Both types of exercise can be included in a fitness program. Look for exercise activities that meet your needs. Some questions you might ask yourself include:

- Is the activity fun? Do I like other activities better?
- Is it convenient for me to workout?
- Is cost (equipment, clothes, travel, etc.) a factor?
- Does the program offer enough variety?
- Am I in good enough condition to participate?
- Am I satisfied with my level of performance, or can I improve?

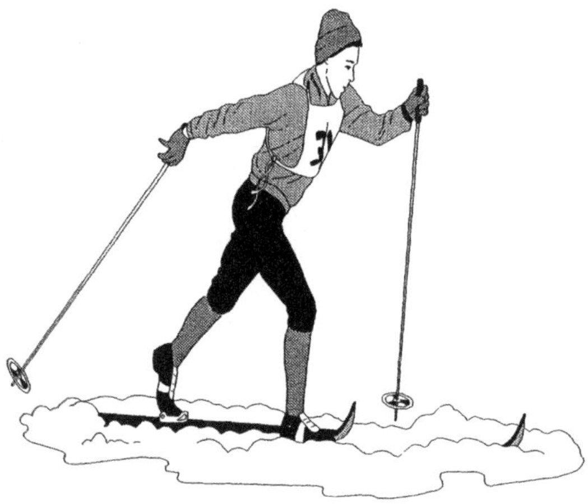

Workout Conditions

Your exercise routine should fit your personality: social preferences, how you feel at different times of the day, choice of surroundings, and so forth. For example, some people like to exercise with friends, and others prefer to be by themselves. In order to have a successful program, you may need to recruit a partner, or nicely tell someone you'd rather work out alone.

Are you an early morning, afternoon, or evening exerciser? Even though your personal or professional schedule may force you to exercise at certain times, it's best to try to exercise when the workout feels best. Forcing your body to go against its natural "time table" might be enough to keep you from sticking with the program.

Do you prefer to exercise at home, in a fitness facility, at work? Would you rather exercise indoors or outdoors? Many well-intentioned exercisers find that home settings can be distracting or uninspiring—an estimated 70 percent of home exercise equipment is not used after the first 30 days. You will need to decide where you exercise best.

BEGINNING YOUR EXERCISE ROUTINE

For many people, the early stages of an exercise program are the hardest. After some initial excitement, personal doubts or fears creep in. Exercise might feel unpleasant at first, or progress may seem too slow.

Some suggestions for getting through this difficult initial period follow.

- **Start gradually.** It takes a long time to get out of shape, and it will take a while to get fit again. Set realistic goals. If you push too hard, you could injure yourself, a sure program "killer."

- **Listen to your body.** A philosophy of "no pain, no gain" is not only unnecessary, it can be dangerous. Rest if you need to, or reduce your activities when you become sore or lose energy.

- **Keep a record of your activities.** A workout log helps you analyze your exercise program, and provides an incentive by reminding you of your commitment. This process is especially important when you experience "plateaus" in your progress.

- **Build a support network.** Peer pressure can be a strong incentive (or disincentive) at this stage. Associate with people who support your effort, and avoid "naysayers." Don't make the process harder than it has to be.

- **Reward yourself for small accomplishments.** The benefits of exercise may take a while to realize, so plan some rewards to reinforce your efforts along the way. Pick something specific and appealing.

- **Employ prompts and cues.** Behavior is often influenced by the situation or the environment. Identify and use signals that help you with your fitness program, e.g., posters in the exercise room, a calendar with workout days marked, readily available exercise equipment, etc.

- **Avoid negative self-talk.** How you "think about things" strongly influences your behavior. Try to emphasize positive statements about fitness and exercise. In particular, analyze your excuses and set up plans to deal with them.

MAINTAINING YOUR PROGRAM

After you have been working out for a while, you will begin to experience some of the benefits of exercise. You will feel better and have more energy. You may lose weight, or notice an improvement in your performance at work. You will also begin to enjoy your workouts more. At this time, you need to work on making exercise a normal part of your daily routine.

Many of the earlier suggestions for promoting exercise adherence apply at this stage, too. If you have been monitoring your progress since the program began, you will know which methods work for you. But everyone encounters obstacles from time to time. Most problems can be easily handled if you actively address them. Some long-term strategies follow.

Goal Setting

After initial successes, improvements in fitness may come slowly or in stages. Establishing goals helps by providing personal incentives and "benchmarks" for evaluating your progress over time. Monitoring gains (e.g., changes in the length of your workout, resting heart rate, increases in strength) can give you a psychological "boost." Goal setting also helps you recognize when you have reached a fitness level that's satisfactory to you. Then the goal changes from small incremental gains to long-term exercise maintenance.

Overtraining

Exercising too hard can reduce the pleasure of your workout and cause unnecessary discomfort. Research also shows that overtrained people have lower levels of glutamine, an amino acid that fuels the immune system. The resulting physical and psychological symptoms (see box on next page) can interfere with your exercise routine and cause you to quit the program.

If you think you may be experiencing the "burnout" caused by overtraining, it's time to step back a little. Take a day off or reduce the intensity of your workouts. Remember, situations in life change; you may need to modify your routine when other priorities (job, family, health, etc.) take precedence. Be especially careful when restarting your program after a break due to illness, injury, vacation, personal situations, and so forth.

BURNOUT SYMPTOMS

According to the American Running and Fitness Association, mood changes and lingering general fatigue are the first signs that you are training too hard. Other symptoms include:

Signs in Your Training

- No desire to train
- Cutting sessions short
- Performance going down
- Unusual muscle soreness
- Recovery taking longer
- Fatigue lingering during workout

Signs in Your Life

- Increased tension, anger, irritability
- No interest in enjoyable activities
- Changes in sleep patterns
- Increased thirst

Signs in Your Health

- Increased infections, colds, illnesses
- Inexplicable weight changes
- Constipation or diarrhea
- Elevated morning pulse
- Cuts and scars taking longer to heal

Enjoying Yourself

Your goal is to establish an exercise program that you can maintain for the rest of your life. That won't happen unless your workouts are enjoyable and effective. To make sure, continue to monitor your reactions to the exercise program, and be open to improvements. Don't get stuck in a rut; try different exercises and new exercise patterns.

Also, be reasonable in your expectations. The purpose of the program is to feel good and be fit, not necessarily to win the New York City Marathon. Accept the fact that you will have occasional "off days" when exercise doesn't feel good and performance declines. Make a commitment to working through minor problems and staying with your program. The results may well be a lifetime of fitness and health!

CHAPTER SUMMARY

In this chapter, you first reviewed some basic information about the anatomy and function of the musculoskeletal system. Principles for conducting a safe and effective flexibility exercise program were examined. You learned about the components of a comprehensive workout, and reviewed some excellent stretches for all the major muscle groups. Finally, you prepared a short-term flexibility training plan, and identified personal considerations that may affect your ability to maintain the program in the months and years ahead.

Having completed this chapter, you should now be able to:

- ♦ Identify the major muscle groups and connective tissues in the human body.
- ♦ Describe the purpose and benefits of each component of a comprehensive workout (warm-up, exercise, cool-down).
- ♦ Conduct a safe and effective flexibility workout.
- ♦ Prepare a personal action plan for flexibility exercise that meets your own fitness goals and needs.
- ♦ Identify ways to stay motivated and to stick with your exercise program.

BIBLIOGRAPHY

Alter, Michael J., *Science of Stretching*, Champaign, IL.: Human Kinetics Books, 1988.

American Running and Fitness Association, "New Thoughts on Overtraining," *Running & Fitness News*, Volume 11, Number 6, June 1993.

Asken, Michael J., PhD., "Fire Psychology: How to Stay with Your Fitness Program," *Firehouse*, July 1993.

Baeta, Al, *Fire Fitness*, Presentation at the Phoenix Fire Department's Health, Fitness, & Safety Training Seminar, June 15-18, 1993.

Eller, Daryn, "Flex Time," *American Health*, April 1993.

Maryland Department of Health and Mental Hygiene and Maryland Army National Guard, *Getting Fit Your Way: A Self-Paced Fitness Guide*, 1983.

McArdle, W., et al., *Exercise Physiology*, Philadelphia: Lea and Febiger, 1986.

National Fire Protection Association, *Standard on Medical Requirements for Firefighters* (NFPA 1582), 1992 Edition.

O'Conner, Jack II, PhD., "Fire Fitness—Improving Flexibility," *VFIS News*, June 1993.

Pollock, Michael L., Jack H. Wilmore, and Samuel M. Fox III, *Health and Fitness Through Physical Activity*, New York: John Wiley & Sons, 1978.

United States Fire Administration, *Physical Fitness Coordinator's Manual for Fire Departments*, FA-95, September 1990.

Weineck, Jurgen, *Functional Anatomy in Sports*, Chicago: Year Book Medical Publishers, Inc., 1986.

White, Timothy P., Ph.D., and the Editors of the University of California at Berkeley Wellness Letter, *The Wellness Guide to Lifelong Fitness*, New York: Random House, 1993.

COMPREHENSIVE WELLNESS FOR FIREFIGHTERS

Chapter 4

Cardiovascular Fitness: Run (or Walk) For Your Life

CHAPTER INTRODUCTION

CARDIOVASCULAR FITNESS

Firefighters and emergency rescue personnel routinely undertake physically demanding tasks, such as dragging hose, carrying victims, hauling heavy equipment, and ventilating roofs. These tasks are performed for sustained periods of time while wearing up to 50 pounds of personal protective equipment. Extremes of heat and cold are routine.

Studies show that this type of work requires high levels of cardiovascular fitness. This critical component of health and performance measures the ability of your heart and lungs to supply working muscles with oxygen, and your muscles' ability to use that oxygen to produce energy. Thus, your cardiovascular fitness largely determines your ability to participate in vigorous physical activities for extended periods of time.

In this chapter, you will learn the basic terminology of the body's energy system, and discover why a high level of cardiovascular fitness is necessary for public safety occupations. You will also learn how to conduct an effective exercise program to increase your aerobic capacity. Finally, you will apply the results of your fitness assessment to develop a personal program for effective cardiovascular conditioning.

LEARNING OBJECTIVES

After learning the information in this chapter, you will be able to:

- Define cardiovascular fitness and its importance in firefighting and rescue work.
- Identify basic differences between anaerobic and aerobic activities.
- List minimum criteria for exercise to improve cardiovascular fitness.
- Implement a safe and effective walking/running aerobic conditioning program.
- Identify planning considerations for cardiovascular exercise (hot and cold environments, activity options, etc.).
- Develop a personal exercise plan for cardiovascular exercise.

PRINCIPLES OF CARDIOVASCULAR FITNESS

FIREFIGHTING AND CARDIOVASCULAR FITNESS

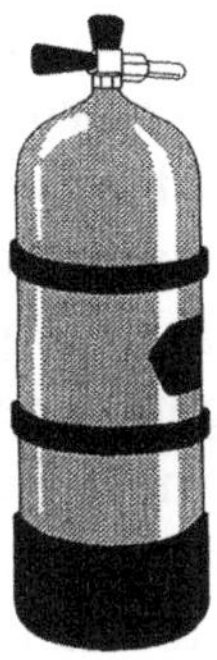

Numerous studies have shown that high levels of cardiovascular fitness are particularly important for firefighters' health, performance, and safety. An article in the Journal of Occupational Medicine summarized these studies as follows (Sothmann 1992):

- During fire suppression, heart rate levels increase, often to near-maximal levels, for periods that average from 12 to 14 minutes. Oxygen consumption requirements and respiratory demands greatly increase.
- Even the best available respiratory protection equipment presents both a resistance to airflow and a limited rate of air delivery. These factors increase the work of breathing and may result in workers with marginal lung capacity being unable to ventilate adequately.
- Firefighters often are exposed to excessive heat. Protective gear impedes efficient heat dissipation, resulting in increased body temperatures. Effective cardiovascular functioning is necessary to dissipate this heat.
- Protective gear worn by firefighters has been shown to increase oxygen consumption and heart rates by approximately one-third and to reduce maximal physical work capacity from 17.5 to 27 percent.
- Speed is often critical in fire suppression activities, for example, to ventilate a building before flashover occurs. Firefighters with lower levels of aerobic fitness have longer performance times on simulated fire suppression tasks, a factor with important implications for personal safety and property conservation.
- Studies show that older, more experienced firefighters do not perform the physical tasks "differently," but demonstrate similar cardiorespiratory needs when compared with younger, less experienced firefighters.

The study concluded that aerobic capacity is so important to firefighter performance that it provides "an independent and necessary indicator" of the physical fitness of firefighters to perform the more critical elements of their job. **In other words, without cardiovascular fitness, you can't do your job either safely or well.** Unfortunately, "a large percentage of municipal firefighters beyond the age 40 years do not meet (cardiorespiratory requirements) unless there is a concerted effort to maintain fitness levels." (Sothmann 1992)

THE BODY'S FUEL SUPPLY

All movements and activities require the contraction of muscles. In order for a muscle to contract, fuel must be available for energy. Otherwise, the contraction cannot occur.

There are two basic types of fuel that your muscles use for energy. One is called **anaerobic** (which means "without oxygen"). The second type is called **aerobic** (which means "with oxygen"). Muscles are always using a combination of both anaerobic and aerobic fuels for energy, but the proportion of each depends upon the intensity and duration of the activity being performed.

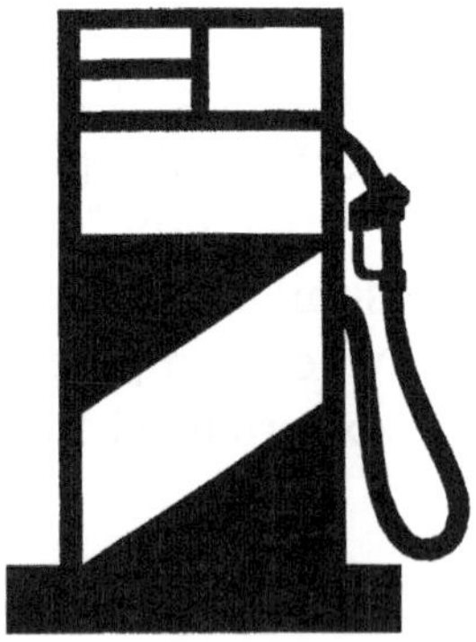

Anaerobic Fuel

This fuel comes from carbohydrates in the diet and is stored within the muscle as glycogen. When glycogen is burned as fuel, it releases a great deal of energy, so it is used primarily for high-intensity activities. In other words, the more vigorous the activity, the greater the proportion of glycogen being used for energy.

Muscles can store only a limited amount of glycogen. Since the supply of anaerobic fuel is limited, large proportions of anaerobic fuels can only be used for relatively brief activities (under 10 minutes). For activities that last longer than 10 minutes, a greater proportion of fuel must come from the aerobic system.

Although glycogen is an anaerobic fuel, it is burned incompletely without oxygen, resulting in a waste product called "lactic acid." When enough lactic acid builds up in the muscle, fatigue sets in rapidly and you must temporarily decrease activity.

Aerobic Fuel

This fuel comes from fat stores in the body that break down and enter the bloodstream, traveling to the muscle where they are burned and converted to energy in the presence of oxygen.

The aerobic system is always working, supplying energy to the body. In fact, the aerobic system is responsible for resupplying the muscle's glycogen stores when they get low.

Anaerobic Fuel	Aerobic Fuel
♦ Main energy source: glycogen (stored in muscle and available immediately)	♦ Main energy source: fat (stored in fat cells and transported through bloodstream)
♦ Vigorous activities	♦ Low- to moderate-intensity activities
♦ Short duration	♦ Long duration

Muscles cannot store aerobic fuel, and when burned, fat releases less energy than glycogen. Thus, the aerobic system is used primarily for low- to moderate-intensity activities. However, the amount of fat available in the body is very large, so the source of energy for the aerobic system is practically limitless. Therefore, larger proportions of aerobic fuels are used in relatively long duration activities (over 10 minutes).

Working muscles create a demand for fuel. At low intensities, the aerobic system can easily supply enough fuel to meet the demand. As the intensity of the activity increases, the demand continues to rise. At some point, the intensity of the activity raises the demand so high that the aerobic system can no longer supply enough fuel, i.e., the aerobic system has reached its "ceiling." Then anaerobic fuel sources must make up the difference. But since anaerobic fuel sources are rather limited, the demand for fuel may eventually outstrip the supply, leading to exhaustion.

Oxygen Consumption

In the lungs, oxygen combines with red blood cells to be transported through the bloodstream. As needed, the oxygen exits from the bloodstream for use by tissues such as working muscles. When fat is burned to produce energy, oxygen must be present. Since the amount of available fat stored for fuel in the body is very large, **the limiting factor in the processing of aerobic energy is the ability to transport and utilize oxygen.**

Because the aerobic system depends on the bloodstream to deliver oxygen, the ability to uptake, transport, and utilize oxygen is referred to as "cardio-vascular fitness." A higher level of cardiovascular fitness means a higher "ceiling" to the aerobic system's ability to supply fuel and energy. As cardiovascular fitness increases, this ceiling increases as well.

RELATIONSHIP BETWEEN FUEL SOURCE AND ACTIVITY TYPE

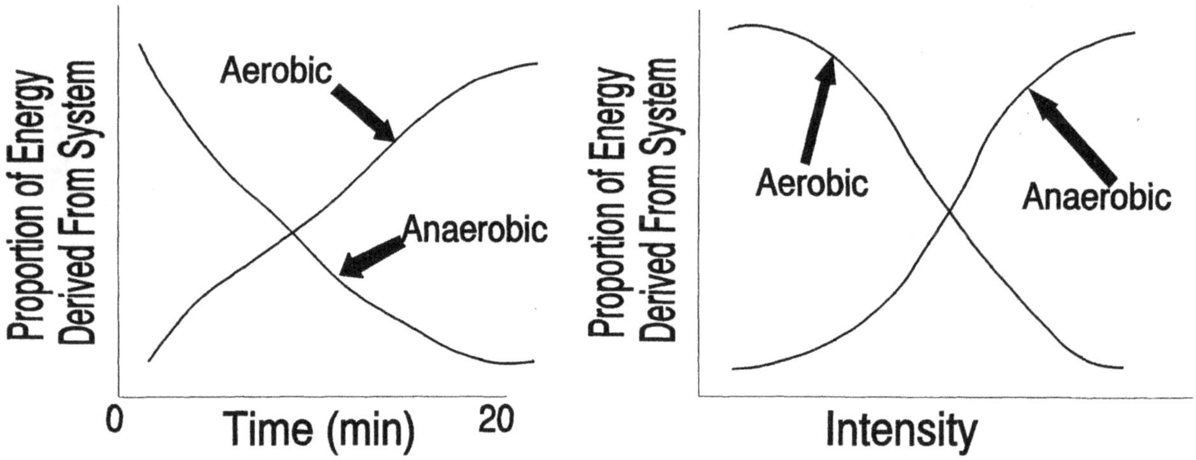

This concept is also called "oxygen consumption," which is represented scientifically as "VO_2" (the **V**olume of **O**xygen consumed every minute). VO_2 is expressed in milliliters of oxygen per kilogram of lean body weight per minute (ml/kg/min.) To simplify things, it is easier to refer to oxygen consumption in terms of "units" of oxygen consumed.

Any activity involving muscular work requires that your cardiorespiratory system be able to transport oxygen through your bloodstream to feed working muscles. Generally, the more vigorous the activity, the more "units" of oxygen your bloodstream must deliver every minute.

For example:

- A relatively easy job (such as sweeping a stairwell) might require 20 units of oxygen per minute.
- A harder job (such as digging ditches) might require 35 units of oxygen every minute.
- Firefighting and rescue work require that you be able to deliver <u>at least 45 units of oxygen</u> through your bloodstream every minute.

The 45 units of oxygen required every minute during fire and rescue work is a level of fitness somewhat above average for most Americans. If you are "out of shape" (i.e., your cardiovascular fitness level is too low to deliver this amount of oxygen), then your muscles will literally "starve" for oxygen, and they will tire out. The higher your level of cardiovascular fitness, the more units of oxygen your body will be able to transport and use.

Maintaining Cardiovascular Fitness

Once you've developed a sufficient level of cardiovascular fitness, you must continue to follow a regular exercise program to maintain this level. No exercise, or insufficient exercise, causes a progressive loss of the cardiovascular fitness you've gained. As someone once said, *if you don't use it, you'll lose it.*

Furthermore, numerous studies show that cardiorespiratory capacity in both firefighters and the general population decreases with age. Cardiac output is reduced approximately one percent per year after maturity, or 25-45 percent by age 65, due to declines in maximal attainable heart rate, stroke volume, and oxygen extraction by working muscles. A substantial portion of this decline is due to lifestyle. The decline may be reduced to 20 percent with moderate physical activity and to 10-15 percent with long-term, high-intensity exercise programs.

Your goal is to keep your level of cardiovascular fitness at or above the minimum needed for your occupation. **Studies show that merely performing the duties of a firefighter or rescue worker will not develop or maintain the fitness required for these occupations. Only a regular program of physical conditioning can accomplish this goal.**

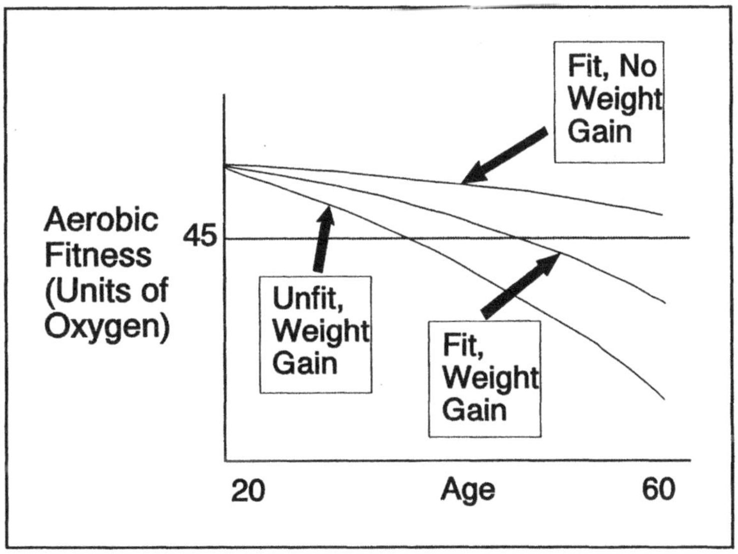

GUIDELINES FOR AEROBIC EXERCISE

PHYSICAL CONDITIONING FOR CARDIOVASCULAR FITNESS

Some firefighters train very sporadically. They might exercise in preparation for an upcoming fitness test, but stop training once the test is over. However, physical fitness must be maintained year round, since the need to perform demanding firefighting and rescue tasks may arise at any time.

To increase your level of cardiovascular fitness, you must undertake a regular program of sustained aerobic exercise. To be effective, this program must meet certain criteria. These criteria are collectively referred to as the "**FITT principle,**" standing for the important characteristics of the exercise program:

- Frequency
- Intensity
- Time
- Type of exercise

Frequency

Studies on aerobic exercise show that a positive training effect is received only if exercise is performed on a regular basis. Specifically, the aerobic exercise must occur a minimum of three days per week, every week. Exercise that is performed less frequently will not improve your level of cardiovascular fitness.

Intensity

The most critical factor for improving the cardiovascular system is the intensity of the activity. Exercise carried out at a low intensity is ineffective for causing an improvement in cardiovascular fitness (no effort, no gain). Conversely, exercise carried out at too high an intensity does not let you sustain the exercise session long enough to be effective (see "Time" below). Thus, **moderate exercise intensity is optimal—not too easy, not too hard—for the entire exercise session.**

Time

The activity must be sustained at this moderate intensity for a minimum of 20 minutes to effectively challenge the cardiovascular system. Aerobic exercise sessions of shorter duration will not produce a training effect.

Type

The most effective exercises for producing an improvement in cardiovascular fitness are those that are performed continuously while using large muscle groups. These exercises cause an increased volume of blood to be pumped throughout the body. Activities that meet this criteria include jogging, brisk walking, cycling, stair climbing, rowing, rope skipping, aerobics, cross country skiing, swimming, etc. As long as you keep moving at an adequate intensity for a sufficient period of time, the type of exercise you choose is really not that important.

PROGRESSION

A vital element of an effective cardiovascular exercise program is **progression**. After several weeks of regular sustained aerobic exercise, your cardiovascular system will adapt by improving itself somewhat, bringing you to a slightly higher level of cardiovascular fitness.

To improve further requires that you do one or more of three things: exercise more frequently, exercise a little longer during each workout, or exercise at a slightly higher intensity. By making incremental changes in your workout every few weeks, your level of cardiovascular fitness will steadily increase. Once you stop making these increments, your level of fitness cannot improve any more—no further stimulation means no further adaptation.

With respect to increments in intensity, you'll notice as the weeks go by that you have to exercise at a slightly higher intensity just to maintain the same "feel" to your workout. In other words, the level of intensity you once maintained no longer feels very difficult; thus, you naturally exercise a little more intensely to get the same effect. This is a sure sign that you're getting in better shape!

Increments in exercise intensity must occur gradually. The body cannot adjust instantly to sudden leaps in workload, which often result in injury. Improving your level of fitness should be approached as a long-term project that requires dedication, discipline, and patience.

The greatest amount of improvement in cardiovascular fitness is usually experienced in the first six to eight weeks of the exercise program. After this initial time period, improvements continue to occur, but at a slower rate.

Remember: most machines wear out with repeated use. The human body is the only machine that gets better with use. Regular exercise keeps the body youthful and functioning well.

Exhibit 4-1

SAMPLE AEROBIC EXERCISE PROGRAM

Week 1-2	**Week 3-4**	**Week 5-6**	**Week 7-8**
15 min.	20 min.	25 min.	30 min.
Exercise at **moderate intensity**.			
Week 9-10	**Week 11-12**	**Week 13-14**	**Week 15-16**
30 min.	30 min.	30 min.	30 min.
Gradually increase the intensity of each workout.			
Beyond Week 16			
Maintain the program you've established at the end of Week 16. By then, you will have been exercising for nearly four months, and your fitness level will have improved significantly! Small increases in duration or intensity can be made occasionally, especially on days when you feel extra good and want to do a bit more than your usual workout.			

WARM-UP AND COOL-DOWN

Any cardiovascular exercise workout should include an effective warm-up and cool-down period. A wide variety of activities, including walking and flexibility exercises, are appropriate for this purpose.

Warming Up

Warming up prior to aerobic exercise is critical for two reasons. First, warming the muscles helps reduce the chance of injury. Second, it is important to realize that the aerobic system cannot instantly meet a sudden increase in the demand for fuel. Your body must gradually "gear up" to a higher capacity, and this process takes several minutes. Warming up allows the aerobic system to keep pace with the gradually increasing demand for fuel and oxygen. Otherwise, the anaerobic system must make up the difference. This situation, referred to as "oxygen deficit," usually leads to early exhaustion.

Cooling Down

Just as it is important to warm up prior to exercise, allowing your body to make a gentle transition into an active state, it is vital to end the exercise session gradually.

During aerobic exercise, the repeated contractions of large muscle groups act as a secondary pump to circulate blood throughout your body. If you stop exercising suddenly, the secondary pumping action of the muscles ceases abruptly, leading to "pooling" of blood in the extremities and lower body. This means less blood returning to the heart and head, which can result in dizziness or fainting. Thus, after exercising, it is important to **keep moving**, gradually slowing down your movements over a period of several minutes.

Workout Components

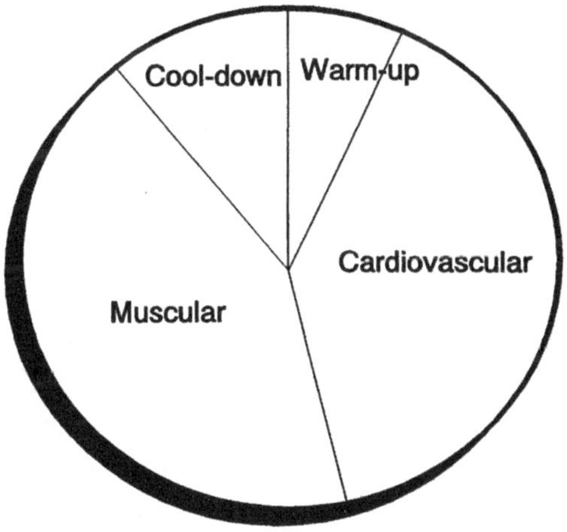

MONITORING EXERCISE INTENSITY

What level of intensity is right for you? The ability to monitor and adjust exercise intensity is essential to the safety, effectiveness, and enjoyment of aerobic exercise. "High" levels of intensity may contribute to injury, fatigue, and exercise burnout. "Low" levels will produce little or no cardiovascular effect. Monitoring intensity also helps exercisers document their increasing levels of fitness, which serves as an incentive to keep working out.

For safe and effective cardiovascular workouts, many fitness experts recommend exercising at an intensity equal to 60-80 percent of your maximum heart rate. Although heart rate can provide a helpful guide, people are different, so general rules don't always apply. Several other limitations to this method exist:

- ♦ Fitness gains depend to some extent on your current level of fitness. If you are unfit, you will begin to achieve cardiovascular benefits at intensity levels below 60 percent. If you are in great shape, you may need to work at higher-intensity levels to show improvement.
- ♦ Some people—including cardiac patients, those with high blood pressure, diabetics, and pregnant women—do not have a "normal" heart rate response to exercise.
- ♦ Antihistamines, cold medications, antidepressants, and tranquilizers have an effect on the heart rate that might make monitoring inaccurate.
- ♦ Caffeine and nicotine affect heart rates in ways that can influence this type of monitoring technique.

For these reasons, it is recommended that you use a simple "talk test" or "exertion awareness check" to ensure that you maintain a **moderate** level of intensity during your workout.

Talk Test

You should be able to breathe comfortably, deeply, and rhythmically during aerobic exercise—even be able to carry on a conversation. If you are gasping or short of breath, or if you can't talk or answer a question, you probably should reduce your exercise intensity.

Exertion Awareness Check

During exercise, use any simple method to evaluate on a "gut level" how hard you are working. A numerical scale might be as follows:

0 Nothing
1 Very light
3 Light
5 Moderate
7 Heavy
9 Very heavy
10 Near maximum

RECREATIONAL SPORTS INSTEAD OF AEROBIC EXERCISE?

Many firefighters and rescue workers choose to spend most, if not all, of their "physical conditioning" time playing recreational sports, such as basketball, tennis, or volleyball. These people often experience high injury rates associated with playing sports. Conversely, some emergency personnel perform only aerobic exercise (like jogging) while neglecting to do stretching or strength training. Again, injuries are common.

This is no coincidence. Recreational athletes are often injured simply because they are out of shape. When someone is not in condition and tries to play a strenuous game, they get injured. Playing sports with weak muscles, tight muscles, or an unfit cardiovascular system leads to injury. If someone is also carrying extra weight (the more you weigh, the more impact there is with each step), injuries are practically guaranteed.

Another prime reason for injury is games that are played too aggressively. For whatever reason, many people use recreational sports as an opportunity to demonstrate their athletic prowess, trying to impress their friends...and end up hurting themselves or others needlessly. Too often, in sports at any level, excessive aggression is used to make up for lack of skill.

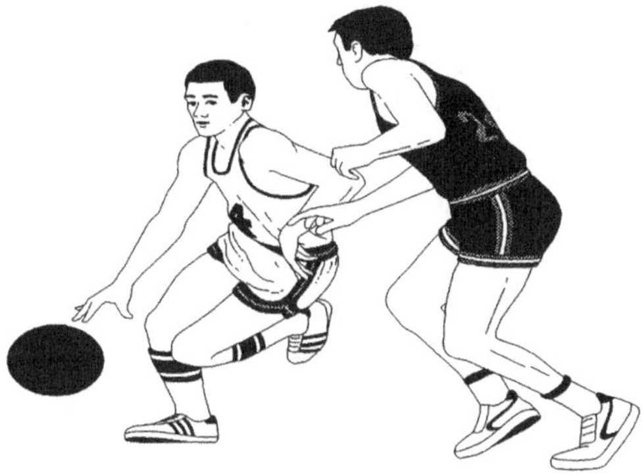

Physical training is very specific—it only works if you do it correctly:

- To increase or maintain muscular flexibility, you must perform static stretching exercises...without them, muscles gradually become tighter.
- To increase or maintain muscular fitness, you need to perform strength training exercises... otherwise, strength is progressively lost as time goes by.
- To increase or maintain cardiovascular fitness, regular aerobic exercise is necessary...otherwise, your cardiovascular system gets more and more "out of shape."

Basketball, tennis, and volleyball are games designed more for fun and competition than for fitness. During these games, no static stretching is going on, and there certainly isn't any strength training involved, either. Sports also fall short of aerobic exercise for improving the cardiovascular system because intensity levels are not steadily maintained throughout the game. Your heart rate falls as soon as the ball goes out of bounds, or is passed to another player, or whenever time-outs occur, etc.

In short, playing sports is not effective training—it typically has little positive effect on your physical conditioning, and your chances of getting injured are higher. Therefore, sports should not be used to get in shape—you should be in shape <u>before</u> you play sports. Playing sports is not a very efficient method for <u>staying</u> in shape either. That's why stretching, strength conditioning, and aerobic exercise are all known as "training." The only thing that playing a sport can do is make you better at that particular game, plus burn up a few calories in the process.

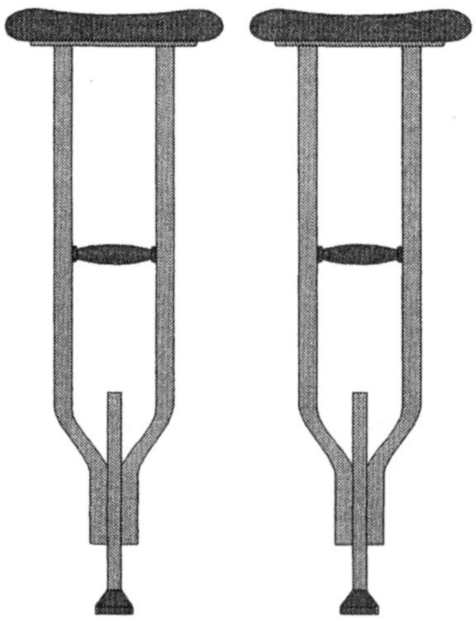

THE R.I.C.E. PRINCIPLE

Proper physical conditioning can help prevent injuries, but sooner or later, most people experience strains or sprains. If an injury occurs, the acronym R.I.C.E. (Rest, Ice, Compression, Elevation) is often used to describe general guidelines for immediate (first 48 hours) treatment.

- ***Rest***—The activity should be discontinued as soon as pain or injury is noticed. Continued exercise may further aggravate the injury. Listen to your body—it's trying to tell you something. Use the concept, "Train, don't strain; if stressed, get rest," instead of "no pain, no gain." Rest should continue until symptoms of pain and injury subside.

- ***Ice***—An ice pack should be applied immediately to a new injury. Ice constricts blood vessels, decreasing swelling and blood flow, and reducing pain and inflammation. Ice should be used for the first 48 hours, 20 minutes on followed by 20 minutes off. Ice should not be applied directly to the skin; wrap the ice in a towel and move its location frequently to avoid frostbite. Remember: during the first 48 hours or until swelling has subsided, the application of heat can actually make an injury worse.

- ***Compression***—Compressing the injured area reduces swelling and the pooling of blood. At first, a wet wrap may be used to provide compression. Start away from the injury and wrap toward the heart. Later, an elastic bandage can be used. The area should be wrapped firmly, but not so tight as to cut off circulation. During the early stages of severe swelling, the wrap should be loosened every 30 minutes, then reapplied. Compression is not necessary at bedtime unless pain interferes with sleeping.

- ***Elevation***—Initially, elevate the injury so it is higher than the heart whenever possible (even during sleep). Continue elevation until swelling has subsided. Gravity prevents pooling of the blood and other fluids.

See a physician immediately if:

1. **Pain is severe.**
2. **Pain persists for more than two days.**
3. **The injured area cannot be moved.**
4. **An injury does not seem to be healing after reasonable home treatment.**

WALKING/RUNNING EXERCISE PROGRAMS

Whether you are a beginner or an advanced exerciser, a good walking program can be beneficial. For beginners, it's an easy way to start a cardiovascular exercise program. For de-conditioned exercisers, it's a safe way to begin the journey back to fitness. For others, walking can serve as an effective warm-up or add variety to a cross-training program. It's free, easy, safe, and appropriate for almost everyone!

Jogging or running provides a more intense (and effective) cardiovascular workout than walking. Although appropriate for many people, running puts greater strain on muscles and joints, and demands higher levels of cardiovascular conditioning. Thus, many walkers need to gradually get in better shape before embarking on a vigorous running program.

WHERE, WHEN, AND HOW

Where

Indoors. If weather or personal preference finds you indoors, use a pedometer to calculate the desired distance at a local shopping mall. Indoor tracks and gymnasiums also provide potential locations. Local fitness centers often have treadmills for indoor exercise; less expensive versions can be purchased for in-home use.

Outdoors. Outdoor distances can also be calculated using a pedometer or car odometer. Look for routes that are scenic and safe, with a minimum exposure to car exhaust fumes and other sources of air pollutants. If a group is exercising together, consider routes with long, straight stretches to keep each other in view. For safety's sake, walk or run facing traffic with an appointed leader on the outside of the group. Advanced groups may wish to include steps or hills in their route.

When

Safety should be your primary consideration in deciding what time of day to exercise. During warm weather, you may prefer to work out in the early morning or late afternoon.

How

Walk or run with your shoulders back and relaxed, chest lifted, eyes straight ahead, and chin up. Swing your arms naturally and rhythmically. Rotate the hips naturally to avoid stress on the knees and ankles. Strike down on the front foot with the heel as you push off with the big toe of the back foot. Then roll the weight along the outer sole of the foot to the big toe to prepare for the next push-off.

EQUIPMENT

Shoes

Although many people exercise in street shoes, aerobic shoes, or tennis shoes, special walking and running shoes have been designed to provide maximum support, shock absorbency, and durability. A good pair of athletic shoes is an investment in your exercise program, and may decrease your chance of injury. It is also recommended that you wear thick socks, or more than one pair.

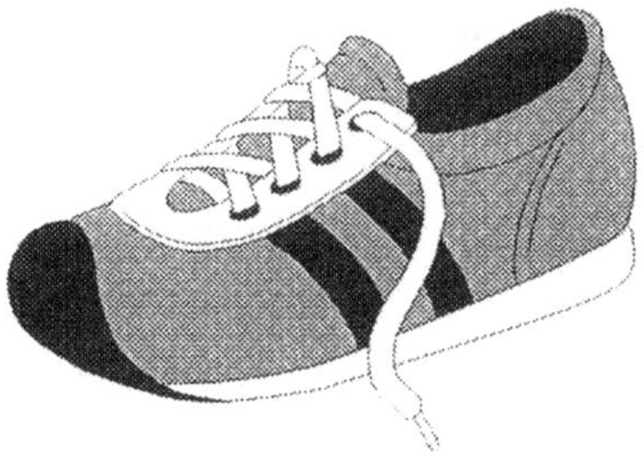

If your hips, knees, and ankles are not within normal alignment, or if walking or running is biomechanically stressful, it may be necessary for you to use orthotics (shoe inserts). If you have any discomfort in your joints, consult a podiatrist, physical therapist, or sports medicine specialist for advice.

Clothing

Clothing is a matter of personal preference. Some exercisers like Spandex, others wear sweats. Let comfort and weather guide your clothing selection. When possible, stay cool during your workout—the hotter you are, the less likely you will feel like working hard. When your intensity is lower, you receive fewer cardiovascular and calorie-burning benefits. Comfortable, non-chafing clothing is best. Layered clothing, such as shorts under sweats and T-shirts under sweatshirts will allow you to remove layers as the body warms up (see the following sections). A reflector vest or tape is advised if you are walking along roads when visibility is poor (daybreak, dusk, fog, etc.). In cold weather, cover your head and hands, and dress in layers. Everyone should wear sunscreen on bright days.

BUILDING INTENSITY

When starting a walking/running program, choose a routine based on your current fitness level. Adopt a basic walking program if you are currently a non-exerciser or if you exercise infrequently. Begin by walking slowly to warm up, then more briskly at a comfortable pace. Twenty minutes at medium to high intensity at least three times a week is the minimum duration needed to receive a cardiovascular benefit. You should always be able to "talk while you walk."

As you become more fit, increase the duration of your workout or add another workout to your weekly schedule. Alternatively, you can increase the intensity of your workout.

Some options include:

1. **RUSH Walking**—Walk quickly. Imagine being late for an important appointment.

2. **RUSH Walking with Arms**—Rush walk with exaggerated arm movements to incorporate upper body work.

3. **Hills, Stairs, or Curbs**—Add a long hill, flight of stairs, or stepping up and down on a curb as part of your workout.

4. **Power Walking or Race Walking**—Walk as quickly as possible without jogging—one foot is always in contact with the ground. Keep hips low, walk with a heel-to-toe striking movement on every step. Maintain good posture with the head, shoulders, hips, and heels in a vertical line.

As your conditioning improves, intersperse walking and running as appropriate. For example, run one minute for each three to five minutes of walking. Increase the time running as you become more fit. Eventually, you should progress until you can jog or run for the entire workout.

Hand Weights

Another method to add intensity is to use hand weights. However, for beginners, hand weights may push the heart rate above a safe target level. For this reason, weights should only be used by those with adequate endurance to complete at least a 20-minute brisk walk using exaggerated arm movements. In addition, persons with hypertension or back, knee, or other musculoskeletal problems should not use hand weights.

If you use hand weights:

- Make sure your upper body muscles are warmed up before you use them.

- Hold weights with a light grip. Forceful gripping causes muscle fatigue and produces a "pressor response," increasing blood pressure.

- Arm movements should be controlled, without momentum. Don’t swing your arms above your head or allow your elbows to lock. Keep your arms moving, but not swinging.

- To avoid joint trauma, never put weights on your ankles, waist, or legs while walking.

- Never run with weights. Running is a high-impact activity. Weights increase the load on bones and joints.

EXERCISE IN HOT WEATHER

To understand how your body deals with hot weather, it is important to keep the following points in mind:

1. Your body is always trying to maintain a constant internal temperature. To accomplish this, the body must rid itself of any excess heat that it generates.

2. Heat flows from warmer areas to cooler areas.

3. Body fluids serve as the medium by which your body transports heat and dissipates it.

Heat Gain

Your body gains heat in one of two ways. First, it produces its own heat all the time from your metabolism, the basic chemical processes required to maintain life and to produce energy. Any time you work or exercise, your metabolism accelerates, producing more heat.

The other way your body gains heat is from the environment. If the temperature of the air around you is higher than your skin temperature, heat radiates into your body. Your body also receives direct heat by absorbing sun light—the brighter the sun, and the more direct its rays, the more radiant heat your body will gain.

Heat Dissipation

When your body builds up heat, blood flow increases to the skin. Warm blood loses its heat at the skin and cooler blood is returned. The main way in which your body dissipates this heat is through the evaporation of sweat. As sweat evaporates, the body is cooled.

Sweat is produced all the time, but you usually don't see it because it evaporates instantly, keeping you cool. For sweat to evaporate properly, the surrounding air must be low in moisture content (low humidity) so that it can accept more moisture in the form of evaporation.

When the surrounding air already has a high moisture content (high humidity), sweat can't evaporate readily, and sweat beads up on the skin until it drips off. Sweat that drips off does not cool the skin because sweat must evaporate to have a cooling effect. If it can't evaporate due to high humidity, it doesn't cool you.

As a result, high temperature and high humidity make it difficult for your body to dissipate heat. Of the two, high humidity is the most important. It is very common for people to become overheated on days with high humidity, even when the air temperature is not particularly warm.

The clothing you wear is also an obstacle to heat loss. Your skin must be exposed to the air in order for sweat to evaporate effectively. The more skin you cover, the less surface area is available for evaporation. Tight-fitting clothes in particular don't allow air to circulate over the skin.

Preventing Overheating

During warm and/or humid weather, it is very common for people to become overheated. Sometimes, this can become a very serious and life-threatening situation.

The most critical factor causing someone to overheat is the volume of body fluid. Once your body loses too much fluid, you can't cool yourself properly until that fluid is replaced.

Whenever you sweat, whether that sweat evaporates or drips off your skin, you are losing fluid. This fluid comes from the blood that circulates throughout your body. Circulating blood acts like the coolant in your car. If you lose too much fluid from your blood-stream, you become "dehydrated" and can overheat, just like your car will overheat if the water level in the radiator is too low.

The good news is that overheating is almost always preventable—just make sure your body has plenty of fluid at all times. To do this, you should drink plenty of plain cold water. Plain water is the most essential factor to maintaining body fluid volume at its proper level.

Any time you are working or exercising in a hot or humid environment, be sure that you allow yourself access to plenty of cold water **before, during, and after the activity**. The water should be cold because this factor speeds the emptying of your stomach, permitting water to be absorbed rapidly into your system.

Substances dissolved in the water only slow down the absorption rate, so you may wish to avoid the use of so-called "sports drinks" or sugared drinks such as sodas to replace lost body fluid. Alcoholic beverages (such as beer) are particularly to be avoided, since alcohol promotes (rather than prevents) fluid loss.

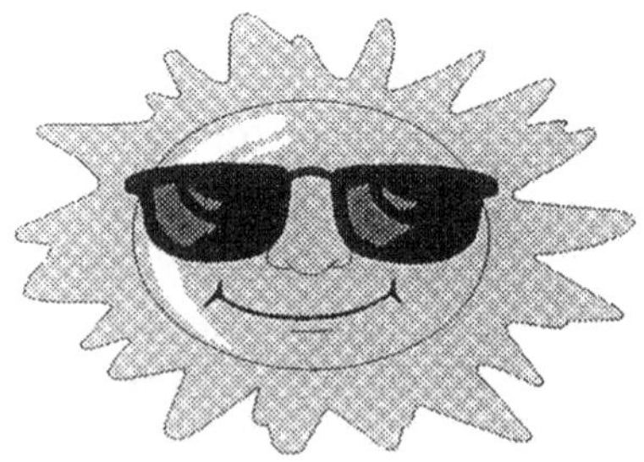

Never rely on your sensation of thirst to tell you when you need to drink water. Quenching your thirst will only supply about half the fluid that your body actually needs. So drink cold water frequently on hot or humid days, even if you don't feel thirsty. It's almost impossible to drink too much water.

Other important points to remember:

- Try to exercise during the time of day when the sun's rays are least intense (i.e., in the morning and late afternoon).
- Wear light-colored clothing on sunny days. Light colors reflect sun light, while dark colors tend to absorb heat.
- Be sure that your clothing is loose-fitting and doesn't cover more than necessary (thus maximizing the skin's ability to evaporate sweat).
- Either postpone exercise on days when the heat or humidity is very high, or exercise at a reduced intensity.

EXERCISE IN COLD WEATHER

Unlike hot and humid conditions, you have little to be concerned about when exercising in cold weather. When your skin is exposed to a cold environment, its blood vessels narrow, reducing blood flow to the skin and extremities. But as you exercise, your muscles produce heat, which warms the blood. As this warm blood reaches the extremities, the blood vessels respond by dilating, thus restoring normal blood flow to these outer regions.

Typically, your muscles generate plenty of heat during exercise to keep warm blood flowing throughout your body. This mechanism prevents any area from getting too cold. However, in severe conditions, you can run the risk of exposure, which means that your body loses heat faster than you can generate it. With this in mind, it is wise to take certain precautionary measures.

Clothing

When exercising in cold weather, moisture and wind are your main enemies. If your clothing becomes wet, it loses up to 90 percent of its ability to insulate. That's why it's important to dress in layers, so you can peel off a layer as you begin to heat up and before you sweat a lot.

Sweaty clothing will refrigerate your body very quickly, especially if the wind is blowing. Later, when you are finished exercising and beginning to cool down, you can replace the layer of clothing. **The rule to follow is STAY DRY, or if you become wet, dry off as soon as possible.**

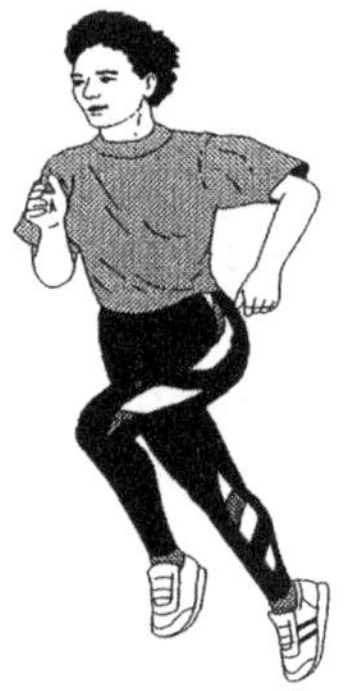

Wind is the other main problem. Any breeze on a cold day robs your body of heat just that much faster. This effect is much more severe if you're moving forward into the wind. Therefore, it is a good idea to try to move with the wind (i.e., have the wind at your back) during exercise. If this is not possible, then start your exercise moving into the wind, and finish by moving with the wind. This will greatly reduce the wind's chilling effect, especially if you should begin to perspire heavily during your workout.

Always be aware of this "wind chill" factor. As a general rule, if the wind chill is -20 degrees (F) or less, don't exercise outside that day. Otherwise, you run a risk of exposure and frostbite. (See Exhibit 4-2.)

Proper clothing is your best protection. For the hands, mittens are better than gloves because mittens trap the warmth of your hand in one single, oven-like compartment. A wool hat is also important because an uncovered head can lose up to 40% of the body's heat.

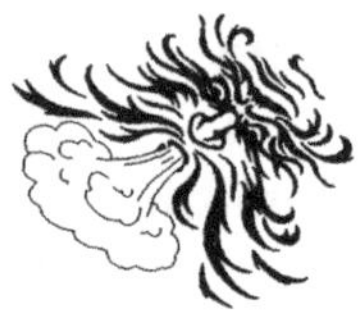

Since leg muscles tend to be working constantly during most exercise sessions, they generate their own heat and require only one layer of clothing, such as a good pair of nylon pants.

In cold weather, the torso should be dressed in layers. A layer of clothing acts as a mesh of fibers that traps warm air and provides a barrier to heat loss. Thus, several light layers work better than a single bulky one. Also, dressing in layers means you can peel off one thickness as you begin to heat up or open a layer for ventilation.

Three layers of clothing is optimal. Ideally, the innermost barrier should be made of polypropylene or silk, since these materials draw moisture away from your skin so that it can evaporate. Cotton should not be used for this innermost layer, since cotton quickly becomes soaked with sweat and collapses against your skin, stealing heat. The middle layer should consist of a wool shirt or sweater. All you usually need for the outer layer is a light windbreaker.

Other Considerations

Many people wonder about the risk of injury to their throat and lungs from breathing cold air. While there is very little chance of any actual harm to your breathing passageways, it is still common to experience a drying sensation or irritation in the mouth and throat. To prevent this, wear a bandanna, scarf, or surgical-type mask over your mouth and nose. This will trap the warm vapor in your expired air, thus serving to warm and humidify your next incoming breath. This is especially important for people who experience exercise-induced asthma.

Finally, when preparing to exercise in the cold, be aware that your pre-exercise warm-up is especially critical. Warming up prior to exercise will not only increase your body temperature, but will also increase the extensibility of your muscles. Muscles are much more likely to be torn when they're cold, just as a rubber band is more likely to break if it has been stored in the freezer. Warm muscles are more pliable and less prone to injury during a workout on a cold day.

Exhibit 4-2

WIND CHILL GUIDE

Ambient Temperature (Degrees Fahrenheit)

Wind Speed	40	35	30	25	20	15	10	5	0	-5	-10	-15	-20	-25	-30	-35
5	35	30	25	20	15	10	5	0	-5	-10	-15	-20	-25	-30	-35	-40
10	30	20	15	10	5	0	-10	-15	-20	-25	-35	-40	-45	-50	-60	-65
15	25	15	10	5	0	-10	-20	-25	-30	-40	-45	-50	-60	-65	-70	-80
20	20	10	5	0	-10	-15	-25	-30	-35	-45	-50	-60	-65	-75	-80	-85
25	15	10	0	-5	-15	-20	-30	-35	-45	-50	-60	-65	-75	-80	-90	-95
30	10	5	0	-10	-20	-25	-30	-40	-50	-55	-65	-70	-80	-85	-95	-100
35	10	5	-5	-10	-20	-30	-35	-40	-50	-60	-65	-75	-80	-90	-100	-105
40	10	0	-5	-15	-20	-30	-35	-45	-55	-60	-70	-75	-85	-95	-100	-110

ZONE 1
Little danger of cold injury.

ZONE 2
Increasing danger—flesh may freeze within 1 minute.

ZONE 3
Great danger! Flesh may freeze within 30 seconds.

Note: Winds above 40 mph have little additional effect.

Source: USFA 1990

AEROBIC EXERCISE OPTIONS

Walking or running can provide a good foundation for a cardiovascular fitness program because, for most people who take basic precautions, these activities are safe, easy, and effective. However, some people find walking too time consuming and running too high impact. Others want more variety in their workout program. Still others simply prefer different types of aerobic exercise.

Fortunately, many other options exist for building and maintaining cardiovascular fitness. Which activity you choose doesn't really matter as long as the activity is aerobic. By definition, aerobic exercise means SUSTAINED, UNINTERRUPTED MOVEMENT, preferably using the larger muscle groups of the lower and middle body.

Common exercise activities (other than walking and running) which are considered aerobic include:

- Cross-country skiing
- Cycling (bicycles or stationary machines)
- Dance exercise or aerobics
- Rope skipping
- Rowing (water craft or stationary machines)
- Jogging or running
- Stair climbing
- Step aerobics
- Swimming

EXERCISE CRITERIA

Unlike almost all recreational sports, aerobic activities like those listed provide an efficient and effective cardiovascular workout without significant risk of injury. However, these activities differ from each other in other respects. Some considerations include:

- **Aerobic Intensity**—Exercises which involve larger muscle groups and which require more vigorous exertion use more oxygen, thereby improving aerobic fitness faster.

- **Force of Impact**—Some aerobic activities place more physical demands on the musculoskeletal system than others; higher impact means greater risk of injury.

- **Calories Burned**—Some activities burn more calories in a given amount of time than others, thus contributing more to weight loss and control.

- **Body Region Used**—Most aerobic activities use the large muscles of the lower body; however, some provide the added benefit of a middle or upper body workout.

CHOOSING AEROBIC ACTIVITIES

These characteristics are summarized for the major aerobic activity options in Exhibit 4-3. **But even more important are factors that relate to your own personal interests and satisfaction.** In the long run, the chances are greater that you will stick with an exercise program if you find the activities enjoyable, rather than inconvenient or unpleasant. Therefore, you need to identify activities that most match your interests and personality.

Some guidelines for selecting aerobic exercise activities include the following:

1. Consider your reasons for exercising. Do you want to improve your health, job performance, weight, physical appearance, stress level, etc.? Choose activities that promote these personal goals.

2. If possible, choose several different activities to add variation and interest to your program. Cross-training also provides for more complete body conditioning.

3. Make it easy on yourself. Choose activities that are convenient and affordable.

4. Select activities with an intensity level that's right for you. As a guideline, choose lower-intensity activities if you are starting an exercise program or haven't worked out in a while; choose higher-intensity activities if you are in good condition and want to further improve your cardiovascular conditioning.

5. Determine whether you like to work out with a partner, in a group, or by yourself. Then choose activities accordingly.

6. Consider the exercise efficiency of different activities. If you work out at a higher intensity, you need less time for the same aerobic benefit.

7. Most importantly, select activities that are fun for you, or at least ones that you don't mind doing.

Exhibit 4-3

CHARACTERISTICS OF AEROBIC ACTIVITIES

ACTIVITY	AEROBIC INTENSITY	FORCE OF IMPACT	CALORIES BURNED	BODY REGION USED/ OTHER COMMENTS
Walking				Primarily lower body; add arm movements or hand weights for upper body benefit
3.5 mph	Low	Low	Low	
5.0 mph	Moderate	Low	Moderate	
Uphill hiking	Moderate	Low	Moderate	
X-Country Skiing				Good upper body; very efficient aerobic workout
Slow	Moderate	Low	Moderate	
Fast	High	Low	High	
Cycling				Works limited muscle groups; some machines incorporate upper body workout
5.5 mph	Low	None	Low	
9.4 mph	Moderate	None	Moderate	
Racing	High	None	High	
Dance Exercise				Many variations, levels of intensity; upper body workout possible
Traditional	Mod. to High	High	High	
Low-impact	Mod. to High	Moderate	Moderate	
Rope Skipping				Limited upper body; very efficient aerobic workout
Slow	Moderate	Moderate	High	
Fast	High	High	High	
Rowing				Excellent total body workout, using upper and lower body
Slow	Moderate	None	Moderate	
Fast	High	None	High	
Running				Limited upper body; very efficient aerobic workout
11:30 mile	Moderate	High	Moderate	
8:00 mile	High	High	High	
Stair Climbing				Limited upper body; very efficient aerobic workout
Slow	Moderate	Moderate	Moderate	
Fast	High	Moderate	High	
Step Aerobics				Limited upper body; very efficient aerobic workout
4-6 inch bench	Moderate	Moderate	Moderate	
8-10 inch bench	High	Moderate	Moderate	
Swimming				Total body workout with emphasis on upper body
Slow	Moderate	None	Moderate	
Fast	High	None	High	

Activity 4-1

CARDIOVASCULAR AND FLEXIBILITY EXERCISE PLAN

Hopefully, you have been following the flexibility workout plan you developed in Chapter 3. This activity expands on that plan to include aerobic exercises like those just discussed. The stretching exercises are used as an effective cool-down after your cardiovascular workout.

This planning approach again provides guidelines on the amount of time you need to exercise. The time for flexibility training is simply transferred from Chapter 3. The time required for the cardiovascular component of your workout is based on three factors:

- Your cardiovascular fitness level (1, 2, or 3), which you determined as part of the assessment in Chapter 2;
- Your fitness goal (gold, silver, or bronze) for cardiovascular conditioning (which may or may not be different than your flexibility fitness goal); and
- The type and intensity of the aerobic activities you choose.

Like before, the goals you select are important, so think them through carefully. Remember: the higher your goals, the longer you have to work out to reach them.

Other general cardiovascular planning requirements, based on the **FITT Principle** learned earlier, include:

Frequency—A minimum of three workouts per week; others can be added as desired.

Intensity—Determined by the activities you choose (see Exhibit 4-3).

Time—A minimum of 15-20 minutes, depending on your aerobic fitness level, fitness goal, and the intensity of the activities chosen (higher-intensity activities require less time for the same benefit).

Type—Selection among the various aerobic activity options should be based on your personal preferences and interests (see Exhibit 4-3).

Planning Instructions

1. Follow the directions on **Worksheet 1** to select aerobic activities for your exercise program and to estimate how long you need to work out.

2. Follow the directions on **Worksheet 2** to develop a weekly action plan for your cardiovascular and flexibility workout program.

Activity 4-1 (Continued)
WORKSHEET 1

A. CARDIOVASCULAR WORKOUT TIME

In the spaces below, fill in your cardiovascular fitness level from the assessment process. Next, decide on your personal cardiovascular fitness goal. Then fill in the type and aerobic intensity of the activities you select from Exhibit 4-3. Finally, use the table below to estimate the time (in minutes) you need to exercise for each type of activity chosen.

1. Cardiovascular Fitness Level (1, 2, or 3) __________
2. Cardiovascular Fitness Goal (Gold, Silver, or Bronze) __________
3. Aerobic Activities Selected (from Exhibit 4-3)

Type	Aerobic Intensity	Time
______________________	______________________	__________
______________________	______________________	__________
______________________	______________________	__________

YOUR FITNESS GOAL	ACTIVITY'S AEROBIC INTENSITY	YOUR FITNESS LEVEL		
		Level 1	Level 2	Level 3
Gold	High	N/A	30	40
	Moderate	25	35-40	50
	Low	30	45	60
Silver	High	N/A	25	30
	Moderate	20	30	40
	Low	25	35-40	50
Bronze	High	N/A	20	25
	Moderate	15-20	20-25	30-35
	Low	20	30	40

Activity 4-1 (Continued)
WORKSHEET 2

B. WEEKLY ACTION PLAN AND PROGRESS CHART

To develop a four-week exercise plan, 1) fill in the type of exercise you will conduct under "Aerobic Activity(ies) Selected"; 2) using the first half of each weekly column (P = Planned), transfer the time estimates from Worksheet 1, as appropriate; and 3) add a time estimate for the Flexibility/Cool-down portion of the workout from Chapter 3. Use the second half of each weekly column (A = Actual) to record the time you actually spend exercising.

DAY OF WEEK	AEROBIC ACTIVITY(IES) SELECTED	WEEK 1		WEEK 2		WEEK 3		WEEK 4	
		P	A	P	A	P	A	P	A
DAY 1 MONDAY									
	Flex/Cool-down								
DAY 2 TUESDAY									
	Flex/Cool-down								
DAY 3 WEDNESDAY									
	Flex/Cool-down								
DAY 4 THURSDAY									
	Flex/Cool-down								
DAY 5 FRIDAY									
	Flex/Cool-down								
DAY 6 SATURDAY									
	Flex/Cool-down								
DAY 7 SUNDAY									
	Flex/Cool-down								

CHAPTER SUMMARY

This chapter introduced some of the basic principles of cardiovascular fitness, including its importance in fire and rescue work, basic terminology, and related concepts. You learned the FITT principle (frequency, intensity, time, type), which is useful in planning an effective exercise program, and the RICE principle (rest, ice, compression, elevation), which provides basic guidelines for treating common exercise injuries.

Then you reviewed aerobic activity options, with an emphasis on walking and running programs. Finally, you applied this knowledge to prepare your own personal cardiovascular and flexibility exercise program.

Having completed this chapter, you should now be able to:

- Define cardiovascular fitness and its importance in firefighting and rescue work.
- Identify basic differences between anaerobic and aerobic activities.
- List minimum criteria for exercise to improve cardiovascular fitness.
- Implement a safe and effective walking/running aerobic conditioning program.
- Identify planning considerations for cardiovascular exercise (hot and cold environments, activity options, etc.).
- Develop a personal exercise plan for cardiovascular exercise.

BIBLIOGRAPHY

American Running and Fitness Association, "Monitoring Exercise Intensity," *Running & FitNews*, Volume 11, Number 6, June 1993.

Gilman, William D., and Paul O. Davis, "Fire Fighting Demands Aerobic Fitness," *NFPA Journal*, March/April, 1993.

McArdle, W., et al, *Exercise Physiology*, Philadelphia: Lea and Febiger, 1986.

National Fire Academy, "Unit II: Firefighter Health and Physical Fitness," *Firefighter Safety and Survival: The Company Officer's Responsibility*, NFA-SM-FSCO, 1988.

Pollock, Michael L., Jack H. Wilmore, and Samuel M. Fox III, *Health and Fitness Through Physical Activity*, New York: John Wiley & Sons, 1978.

President's Council on Physical Fitness and Sports, *Walking for Exercise and Pleasure*, Government Printing Office, 1992.

Sothmann, M.S., Ph.D., F. Landy, Ph.D., and K. Saupe, M.S., "Age as a Bona Fide Occupational Qualification for Firefighting," *Journal of Occupational Medicine*, Vol. 34, No. 1, January 1992.

United States Fire Administration, *Physical Fitness Coordinator's Manual for Fire Departments*, FA-95, September 1990.

University of Maryland, *Development of a Job-Related Physical Performance Examination for Firefighters*, September 1977.

Van Gelder, Naneene, *Aerobic Dance-Exercise Instructor Manual*, San Diego: International Dance-Exercise (IDEA) Foundation, 1987.

Weineck, Jurgen, *Functional Anatomy in Sports*, Chicago: Year Book Medical Publishers, Inc., 1986.

Wilmore, Jack H., and David L. Costill, *Training for Sport and Activity*, Dubuque, IA: Wm. C. Brown Publishers, 1988.

Chapter 5

Muscular Fitness: Building Strength Safely and Effecively

CHAPTER INTRODUCTION

Muscular fitness is an entirely separate and unique area of physical fitness, different from flexibility and cardiovascular fitness. The physical demands of firefighting and rescue work require a high degree of muscular fitness.

Muscular fitness is your muscles' ability to contract and produce **force**. It encompasses three properties of muscle tissue:

- **Strength**—the maximum amount of force a muscle can generate during a single contraction.
- **Power**—the rapid generation of force, or the ability to move loads quickly.
- **Endurance**—the ability of a muscle to perform repeated contractions for a prolonged period of time.

In this chapter, you will learn the principles of physical conditioning for the muscle groups in your body. You will also learn proper techniques and safety precautions for various types of strength training exercises. Finally, you will prepare a short-term personal exercise plan to improve your muscular fitness.

LEARNING OBJECTIVES

After learning the information in this chapter, you will be able to:

- Describe muscular fitness and its role in health and performance.
- Identify and apply eight principles of strength training in muscular fitness exercises.
- Identify common causes of back injuries and basic precautions for avoiding problems.
- Use proper technique in performing various strength training exercises.
- Develop a personal exercise plan for strength training and comprehensive fitness.

PRINCIPLES OF STRENGTH TRAINING

MUSCULAR FITNESS

Someone who performs only aerobic exercise (for example, jogging) is doing a lot of good for their cardiovascular system...but that's about all. Many firefighters and rescue workers believe that jogging is all you need for overall conditioning. However, to increase strength, muscles must contract repeatedly against a relatively high resistance. This type of workout does not occur during jogging, so muscular strength is not increasing. Unless regular strength training is included in your fitness program, your muscles will gradually weaken over time.

Strength

Strength is the ability to produce force. Whenever a muscle contracts, tension is developed within the muscle, and this tension creates force. When a muscle becomes stronger, it can produce more tension during a contraction, thus generating more force.

Firefighting involves a great deal of muscular strength. Pulling charged hoses, climbing stairs in full gear, dragging or carrying victims, chopping through doors or roofs, pulling ceilings, removing debris, throwing ladders, vehicle extrication...all of these activities require strong muscles.

Strength is also important for proper physical conditioning. For example, during jogging, an impact equal to five to six times your body weight is created each time you land on your front foot. Muscles act as the body's shock absorbers—the stronger the muscles, the more shock they can absorb. When muscles are weak, the shock must be absorbed by the bones and joints, often leading to pain and injury in ankles, knees, hips, back, etc.

Muscles also act like a suit of armor. They surround and support your joints. Thus, strong muscles contribute to a well-protected joint, and fewer and less severe injuries. Weak muscles are associated with high injury rates in physically demanding jobs such as firefighting and rescue work.

Lastly, because muscles attach to bones on either side of a joint, stronger muscles increase the amount of pull on those bones. Your bones respond to this tension by growing thicker and stronger. Strength training also results in thicker and stronger ligaments, which act to hold the various bones in a joint together.

Strength Training

Strength training is the method of using specific exercises to increase the strength of muscles. Most exercises are designed to stimulate and improve the strength in one particular muscle group. Different exercises must be used to strengthen different muscle groups.

It is important to realize that **when you increase a muscle's strength, you also increase its power and endurance:**

- **Power**—A muscle that can produce more force will also be able to move loads more quickly than a weak one.
- **Endurance**—A stronger muscle expends less effort during a contraction. Thus, more repeated contractions can be made before muscular fatigue occurs.

Of all the components of physical fitness, strength training is the area in which the most misinformation exists. Everyone seems to have a different theory about what works best for making your muscles bigger and stronger. This section is designed to eliminate some of the confusion by reviewing important concepts of strength training. These concepts can be remembered by using the acronym "***PROGRESS***":

Progression
Resistance
Opposing muscle groups
Good form
Range of motion
Exhaustion
Sets
Speed of movement

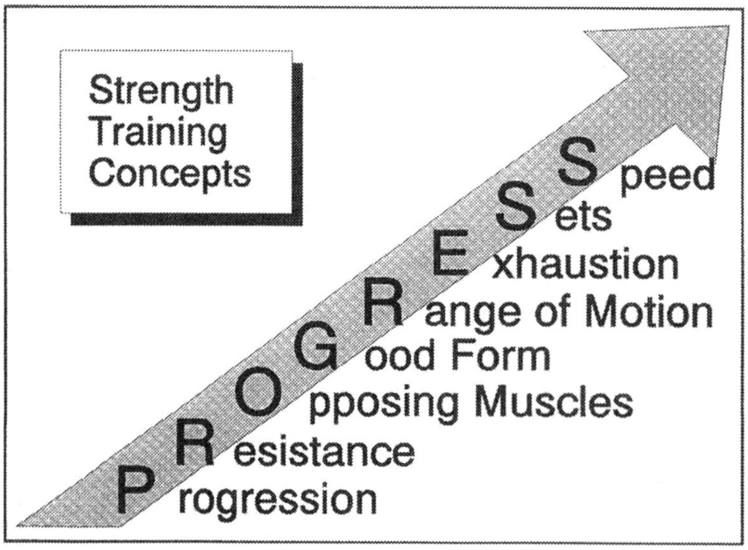

PROGRESSION

If you follow a program of regular strength training, your muscles will gradually grow stronger. This means that in time you'll be able to lift or move larger amounts of weight. A weight that once seemed heavy and required maximum effort to lift can now be lifted many times.

Muscular strength is gained gradually in an almost stepwise fashion. When you train at a high level of intensity—one that is challenging for your level of muscular fitness—your muscles adapt and grow stronger. You are then able to work out at this higher level of intensity with ease. At this point, you must again increase the intensity of your workout to stimulate further gains in strength.

In other words, if you keep your workout the same during future strength training sessions, you won't get any stronger. **A muscle only adapts itself to develop just enough strength for whatever load it regularly encounters. If that load doesn't increase, the muscle won't be stimulated to grow stronger.**

Therefore, throughout your strength training program, you need to periodically increase the amount of weight used during your workouts. This concept is called **progression**.

RESISTANCE

The only way to increase the strength of a muscle is to subject it to a higher amount of tension than it is normally accustomed to. In other words, some additional external **resistance** must be applied. Strength training is basically asking your muscle to contract against an increased resistance, which creates a high level of tension in the contracting muscle. High tension acts as a stimulus; your muscle responds by building new muscle tissue and growing stronger.

Load

There are many factors that cause a muscle to increase in strength, but the most important is the amount of resistance, or "load," that is used. This resistance can take many forms: weights, springs, elastic bands, manual force, etc. Although weights are referred to in this discussion, the principles apply equally to other forms of resistance.

An absolute requirement for successful strength training is to use fairly heavy weights. "Fairly heavy" means a weight that can be lifted repeatedly about 10 times. A lighter load that can be lifted repeatedly more than ten times will develop less tension within the muscle, and thus will provide less of a stimulus for improving strength. A load that is too heavy can potentially cause injury to your muscles.

Repetitions

When a weight is lifted and then lowered, this is referred to as one **repetition**. Contracting your muscles repeatedly against a fairly heavy load will cause your muscles to work very hard for a short period of time before they eventually fatigue. This muscular fatigue should occur after about ten repetitions.

In other words, the first few repetitions should feel fairly easy, the next few should feel increasingly difficult, and the last few should require maximum effort to complete. At this time, total muscular fatigue should occur, forcing you to stop. After the tenth repetition, you shouldn't be able to lift the load again, even if you wanted to.

Remember: Strength training should not be "easy." It should feel like hard work, requiring powerful contractions and a significant amount of effort. Otherwise, it won't be very effective for producing an increase in strength.

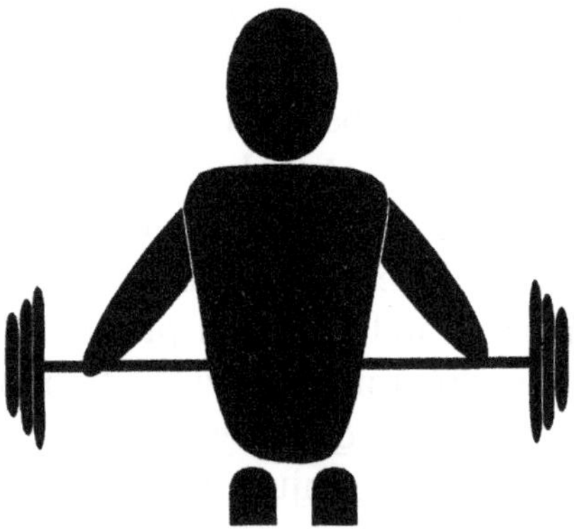

OPPOSING MUSCLE GROUPS (TOTAL BODY STRENGTHENING)

Muscle groups exert a pull across joints. Every muscle group attaches across one side of a joint, while another ("opposing") muscle group attaches across the opposite side of the same joint. In general, contracting one muscle group "flexes" the joint (moves body parts closer together), while contracting the opposing group "extends" the joint (moves body parts further apart).

A common example of opposing muscle groups are the biceps and triceps of the upper arm. The biceps attach across the front of the elbow. When the biceps contract, the elbow bends (flexes), drawing the upper arm and lower arm closer together. The triceps, conversely, attach across the back of the elbow. When the triceps are contracted, the elbow straightens (extends), moving the upper arm and lower arm away from each other.

Every joint in your body (knee, hip, spine, shoulder, elbow, neck, etc.) is surrounded by opposing muscle groups. Opposing muscle groups exert their pull on the joint from opposite sides. **Good joint alignment is achieved by maintaining a <u>balance</u> in these opposing forces.**

Firefighting and rescue work involve complex tasks that use many of the body's different muscle groups. Strength is needed in **all** of these muscle groups so that you can handle the various heavy loads and external forces encountered on the job. **Hence, strength training must be performed for every major muscle group to ensure optimal fitness and performance.**

A typical strength training exercise is designed primarily to strengthen only **one** muscle group. In order to strengthen **all** of your body's major muscle groups, you must perform many different exercises, each one focusing on a different muscle group.

This concept is referred to as **total body strengthening**. If you only work a few muscle groups and neglect the opposing muscle groups, the stronger group will create an unbalanced and excessive pull on one side of the joint. This "muscle imbalance" is a leading cause of joint pain and musculoskeletal injury. Therefore, you should strive for a good balance of strength in all your muscle groups by following a program of total body strengthening.

GOOD FORM

Employing proper form in strength training exercises is critical for several reasons. As noted before, each exercise is designed to strengthen primarily one muscle group. Using improper form, or "cheating," allows other muscle groups to take over some of the load. Thus, the original muscle group doesn't have to work as hard, leading to slower gains in strength.

Using improper form can also result in injury by placing part of the body in a vulnerable position to be strained or damaged. Back injuries are common when improper form is used. The spine can only support loads when the vertebrae are kept in proper alignment. Poor lifting form causes improper alignment of the vertebrae and leads to back injuries. Other types of injuries are also possible.

RANGE OF MOTION

When performing a particular strength training exercise, it is important to allow the muscles and joints to move through their **full range of motion**. A muscle group will get stronger at every position in its range of motion only if resistance is applied at every position.

For example, during a biceps curl, the weight should be lifted from a position in which the arm is totally straight until the elbow is completely bent. If this is done, the biceps muscle generates tension through the full range of motion and is strengthened at every angle. However, if you neglect part of the exercise (partial range of motion), the muscle will remain weaker in the ranges you leave out.

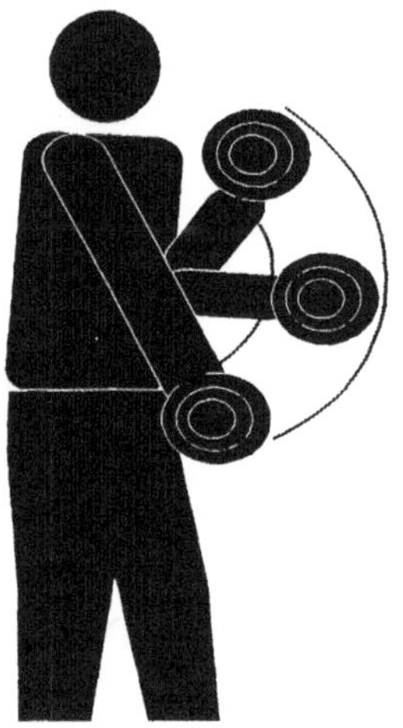

Firefighting and rescue work frequently involve moving your body into different positions; therefore, all your muscles need to be strong at every position within their normal range of motion.

EXHAUSTION (REST)

Productive strength training occurs when a muscle is repeatedly contracted against fairly heavy resistance until total muscular **exhaustion** and fatigue occur. After about ten repetitions, your muscle should be so exhausted that another contraction against that resistance cannot be made. At this point, you must **rest** the muscle before attempting to perform the exercise again.

Two types of rest are important to strength training: rest between sets, and rest between workouts.

Between Sets

When you perform ten repetitions of an exercise and then rest, this is referred to as one "set" of ten repetitions. Some people perform only one set of an exercise, while others perform multiple sets (see discussion in the next section).

If you are performing more than one set of a given strength training exercise, it is important to allow your muscles sufficient time to rest between sets. If you begin the next set too soon, your muscles will still be fatigued from the set you've just completed. This means that you'll have to use lighter loads, and thus you won't be able to work very hard. If each set doesn't feel like hard work, it won't be very productive towards stimulating an increase in strength.

About 90 seconds of rest between sets is usually sufficient. However, you shouldn't start that next set until you feel ready to work hard again and give maximal effort. Productive strength training only results from your ability to work hard!

Between Workouts

It is important to realize that your muscles don't get stronger during the strength training session. Muscles adapt by building new tissue **between workouts**, while you are resting and recovering.

Building new muscle tissue is a chemical process in your body that takes at least 48 hours to complete. Therefore, once you have stimulated a certain muscle group with high-intensity strength training exercise, that muscle group should not be stimulated again for at least 48 hours.

Ideally, you should conduct strength training exercises for each muscle group at least three times per week. However, for any single muscle group, you should never perform a strength training exercise more frequently than every other day.

SETS

Some people perform only one set of a strength training exercise, others do multiple sets, and still others complete dozens of sets! Which is best?

For any strength training exercise, perform a "warm-up set" if you will be using heavier weights than you are used to. In other words, do one set using a light weight in order to prime the muscle group for the high-intensity work to follow.

How many sets of high-intensity work should you then perform with your "fairly heavy" weight? Performing only one set of ten repetitions will certainly produce an improvement in strength for any muscle group. But if you have the time, a few more sets will add a little extra strength in the long run.

Research seems to show that for optimum strength development, **three sets** of exercise using a fairly heavy load will produce the most rapid gains in strength. More than three sets confers little if any extra gains in strength, so why spend the additional time and effort?

SPEED OF MOVEMENT

During any repetition, there are two phases: the initial "raising phase" when the weight is lifted against the force of gravity, and the "lowering phase" when the weight is returned to the starting position.

Raising Phase

During the **raising** portion of the repetition, it is important that you attempt to contract the muscle quickly by lifting the weight as rapidly as possible. Since you are using a fairly heavy load, you probably won't be able to physically move the load very quickly no matter how hard you try, but you should attempt to.

That's because each muscle in your body is composed of essentially two types of fibers. One type contracts slowly and relatively weakly (low tension). The other kind contracts quickly and powerfully (high tension).

This second type, the fibers that produce powerful and fast contractions, is the type that responds to high tension by becoming thicker and stronger. In order to stimulate these fibers, you must attempt to contract your muscles quickly when raising the load. When these fibers are stimulated, muscular strength gradually improves.

Raising the weight slowly means that the other type of muscle fiber is used more. You'll have to use less resistance, since these fibers cannot generate enough tension to handle a heavier load. Less tension within the muscle means a reduced stimulus for improving muscular strength.

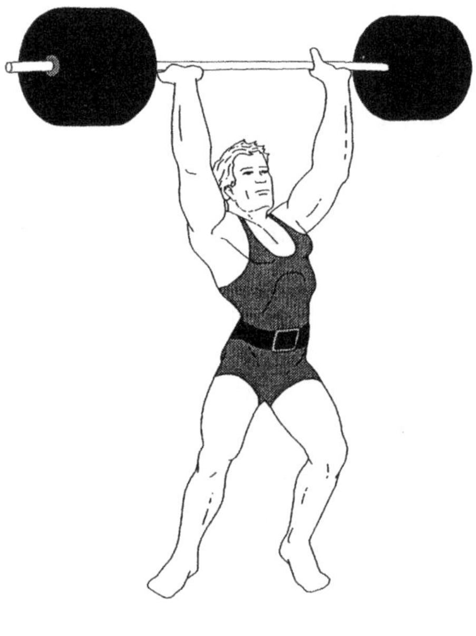

Lowering Phase

After the weight has been raised, it should be lowered slowly and in control. You should expend some effort to return the weight to the starting position much less quickly than it was raised. For most exercises, lowering the weight should take about three to four seconds to complete.

Lowering the weight slowly is strongly recommended in order to prevent injury. Allowing the weight to come crashing down, rather than controlling its rate of descent, may lead to pulled muscles, torn ligaments, and crushed body parts.

Remember the acronym "**PROGRESS**." The eight critical elements—progression, resistance, opposing muscle groups, good form, range of motion, exhaustion (or rest), sets, and speed of movement—all play a vital role in building muscle strength. In the following sections, other aspects of strength training are discussed.

INCREASING MUSCLE SIZE

Muscle Fibers

Strength training produces new muscle tissue, which is then available to contract and generate force. More muscle tissue means that each individual fiber becomes thicker (larger diameter). Since muscles are made up of thousands of fibers, increased strength results in more muscle tissue and greater muscle size.

This increase in muscle size depends upon many things other than just effective strength training. The number of fibers a muscle contains is very important—the more fibers you have, the bigger your muscles can become. If you are born with fewer fibers, the potential to increase muscle size is not as great. The number of muscle fibers is genetically determined and cannot be increased.

Testosterone

Another critical factor in building muscle size is your level of the hormone testosterone. This hormone plays a large role in the development of new muscle tissue. A higher level of testosterone means that a greater potential exists for increasing muscle size. Again, the level of testosterone circulating in your body is genetically determined.

Some women worry that strength training will produce big, bulky muscles that they find unattractive. However, for most females, a great deal of muscular strength can be developed **without** a proportional increase in muscle size. This is probably due to the fact that, on average, females are born with fewer muscle fibers and have about one tenth the level of circulating testosterone.

How Fast Can I Gain Muscle Mass?

Certainly, as a muscle's size increases, so will its weight. Over time, this results in an increase in body weight proportional to the increase in muscle mass. The rate at which this change occurs varies greatly between individuals for the reasons just stated.

In general, it's a rather slow process. Even for the most highly motivated person with a genetic tendency for building large muscles, regular high-intensity strength training can produce an increase in muscle mass of no more than about one half pound per week. If you are gaining weight faster than this, you are probably eating more calories than you need.

STEROIDS

Some people are always looking for an easier way to get strong. Since it is well known that testosterone levels affect muscle strength and size, they resort to taking synthetic testosterone, known as "steroids." Use of these substances appears to be increasing, not only among athletes, but in other occupations, including the fire service.

Steroids, taken either in pill form or injected with a hypodermic needle, have two basic properties: anabolic, meaning that they build tissue, and androgenic, meaning that they produce male sex characteristics. Producers try to chemically alter these drugs to minimize their androgenic properties, and to maximize their anabolic benefits, but **all steroids exert both effects on the user**.

There is little doubt that steroids do what they are supposed to:

- Extra testosterone increases protein synthesis, leading to a quicker build-up of muscle tissue.
- Steroids induce the body to retain fluid, making muscles appear larger.
- Steroids can increase aggression, which some people channel by exercising more intensely.
- Steroids can shorten the rest and recovery period needed between workouts, so steroid users can lift weights more frequently.

However, there is a flip side to the coin: unwanted "side effects" and dangerous dependency. These problems can be summarized as follows.

"Less Serious" Side Effects

In male steroid users, some of the extra testosterone may be converted by the body into estrogen, the female sex hormone. The result is the appearance of breast tissue, a condition known as gynecomastia. Too much testosterone in the bloodstream triggers the testicles to reduce their own natural production. The end result is that the testicles shrink (testicular atrophy) which can lead to impotence and sterility.

For the female user, suddenly higher testosterone levels seem to confuse the body into thinking it is male: breasts shrink, the clitoris enlarges (often becoming painful), hair begins to grow on the face and body, the voice deepens, and the menstrual cycle is disrupted. Except for the latter effect, these changes are usually irreversible.

In **both sexes**, steroids cause acne, balding, and aggressive behavior. Steroids can disrupt the brain's chemistry, and documented cases of steroid-induced psychosis are growing.

"More Serious" Side Effects

The water retention induced by steroids leads to higher blood pressure and kidney damage. Steroids also affect the liver, resulting in higher blood cholesterol. The process of atherosclerosis is accelerated, so that heart attacks and strokes have occurred in users who are only 20-30 years old. In fact, steroids are so toxic that liver cells begin to die with even small doses. Liver tumors and various forms of cancer are also linked to steroid use.

People tend to be impatient, wanting a quick fix or a magic pill to speed up progress. No such thing exists. Regular strength training and a balanced diet should be considered long-term projects, requiring dedication and discipline.

Dependency, Cumulative Damage

As with any drug, steroid users quickly develop a tolerance—they must take ever larger doses to achieve the same effect. Steroids also tend to be psychologically addicting because users feel weak and depressed without them. They don't like to see their muscles shrinking when they stop taking the drug.

The end result is that steroid users tend to take larger doses for longer periods of time, and damage to the body mounts. Experts now conclude that long-term, high-dose steroid usage comes with a steep price tag: an average fifteen-year life expectancy.

DIET SUPPLEMENTS

There is no question that a complete, balanced diet is critical to health, physical fitness, and performance. Americans are fortunate to live in a country where food is plentiful and nutrients are abundant. By eating a balanced diet with a wide variety of foods, nutrient requirements can be easily met. Even top athletes undergoing intense physical training do not need anything beyond a balanced diet to supply the nutrients their bodies need.

Unfortunately, some exercisers seem to adopt the philosophy that "if some is good, more is better." People with this attitude often spend hundreds of dollars on dietary supplements. Popular examples include protein powders, sports drinks, amino acids, various herbs, large doses of vitamins and/or minerals, and many others. They believe these supplements will "fill in the gaps" of their diet, or give them an advantage in gaining strength, muscle mass, stamina, peace of mind, etc. However, the body extracts from the diet just enough to meet its needs and is unable to use any more. The excess either ends up in the toilet or is stored as fat.

Since these diet supplements don't even work theoretically, the following blanket statements are generally true:

1. Virtually all diet supplements are ineffective.

2. Most don't contain anything that can't be found in common foods.

3. Some can actually be toxic (too much of anything is toxic).

4. Most folks who purchase them are fooling themselves, or at least wasting money.

In controlled laboratory studies, the vast majority of these products have never been shown to have any beneficial effect on strength, endurance, health, longevity, etc. As mentioned before, the typical American diet has more than enough nutrients to satisfy the needs of even the most active people. Eating more is like adding extra gas to your car when you're only driving to the corner.

Dietary supplements are not the answer...they just mean less money in your wallet.

EQUIPMENT

Many different types of strength training equipment are available in stores and health clubs, including free weights (barbells, dumbbells), specialized machines, elastic bands, and tubing. Does the type of strength training equipment you use matter? Are free weights superior to machines? Are certain machines better than others?

Remember, your muscles respond to an external load which creates tension when they contract against resistance. As long as the load is heavy enough, the muscle will adapt and become stronger...regardless of what was used to create it.

Muscles only feel tension, not the method used to create the tension. Therefore, all strength training equipment works equally well for producing gains in strength. You should use the type of equipment you prefer or have available.

In fact, you can perform strength training without any equipment. In this system, called "manual resistance," you work with a partner. While you contract a certain muscle group, your partner applies resistance to your movement. This resistance acts as the load necessary to stimulate gains in strength.

Free Weights vs. Machines

Using free weights typically requires a "spotter" or partner to assist the lifter so that he/she doesn't become "stuck" underneath a heavy barbell. Free weights also require that you learn a certain amount of technique and develop strength in accessory muscles to control the movement of the load.

Strength training machines, on the other hand, offer some extra degree of safety. They don't require a spotter, since the load is supported and balanced within the frame of the machine. The apparatus can be entered and exited without fear of having a heavy weight drop accidentally. However, since the load is controlled by the configuration of the machine, accessory muscles are not used or strengthened.

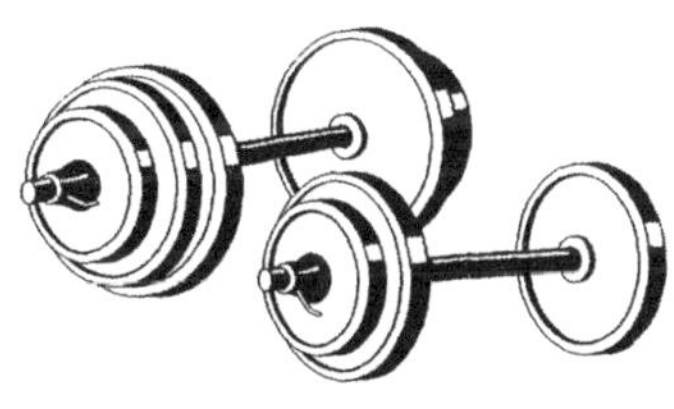

In the real world of firefighting and rescue work, the weight of objects—such as equipment and unconscious victims—is not balanced or controlled as it is in machines. These loads act as free weights. Thus, if your desire is to condition your muscles for specific job tasks, free weights may be better for training. However, if you're just starting a strength program or if safety is more of a concern, machines may be preferable.

Gloves, Belts, and Wraps

Padded leather gloves can be worn when using free weights (barbells and dumbbells) to prevent developing callouses on the hands. The material may also improve your grip on the metal bars. Wearing lifting gloves is strictly a matter of personal preference.

Lifting belts are thick bands of leather or other strong material worn tightly around the waist. They are intended to increase pressure inside the torso, possibly conferring some small amount of protection to the spine. However, their main benefit is making the lifter more aware of this vulnerable area, and thus less likely to make movements or assume positions that could cause a back injury. **It is important to realize that these belts, despite their firm construction, provide very little actual support or protection**. Don't make the mistake of thinking you can use heavier weights or improper form when you wear a belt!

Similarly, many lifters wrap long sections of cloth around their knee joints, mistakenly thinking that this practice will support and protect them. Again, wrapping a joint primarily serves to increase your awareness of that area of the body. Such wraps can not make up for poor body mechanics, nor provide the ability to use excessive weights.

STRENGTH TRAINING EXERCISES

This section describes a variety of exercises you can use in your strength training program. Although other exercises and options exist, those listed here address the major muscle groups of the body. Each exercise should be performed exactly as described to ensure safety and to isolate the appropriate muscles for effective conditioning. Performing the exercises incorrectly will allow other muscles to substitute for the weaker ones...the strong will get stronger, while the weak gets weaker.

General notes on strengthening exercises:

- For greatest improvement, exercises should be performed three days per week.
- Proper form must be maintained.
- Once fatigue develops, rest until it subsides.
- **Discontinue any exercise that causes pain.**
- As strength improves, add slightly more resistance...otherwise, no further gains in strength will occur.

Strengthening exercises for specific muscle groups begin on the next page. Photographs are included with the descriptions. Exercises are divided according to major areas of the body:

Midsection

Legs

Chest

Shoulders

Back

Arms

Within each area (except Midsection), a choice of exercises is provided so you can tailor your program according to the equipment you have available and/or your personal preferences:

- Barbell exercises
- Dumbbell exercises
- Manual resistance exercises (requires partner)

MIDSECTION EXERCISES

1. Curl-ups (strengthens abdominal muscles)

Lie on your back with your arms at your side. Your legs may be either straight or bent slightly. Starting with your head and then your shoulders, slowly curl your torso forward, reaching forward with your arms as you do so. Continue curling forward until your shoulder blades are off the floor. Pause briefly, then uncurl to the starting position. As your strength improves, perform this exercise with arms crossed over your chest, and eventually with your arms behind your head.

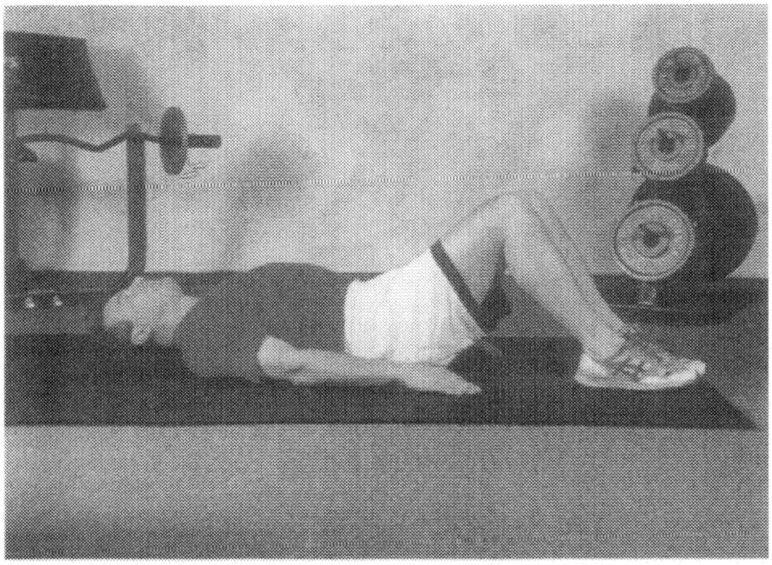

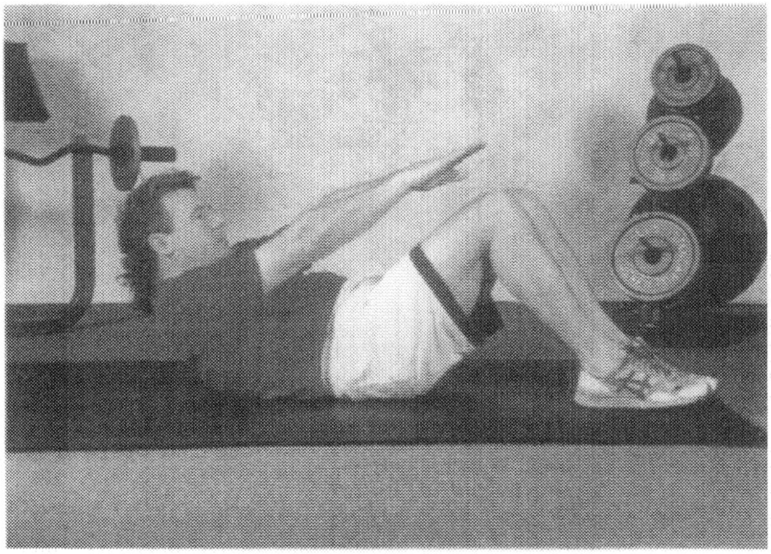

2. Oblique Curl-ups (strengthens abdominal muscles)

Lie on your back with your arms at your side. Your legs may be either straight or bent slightly. Starting with one shoulder (while reaching forward with your arms), slowly curl your torso forward, turning at the waist so that one shoulder clears the floor before the other. Continue curling forward until the second shoulder blade clears the floor. Pause briefly, then uncurl to the starting position, "untwisting" as you go down.

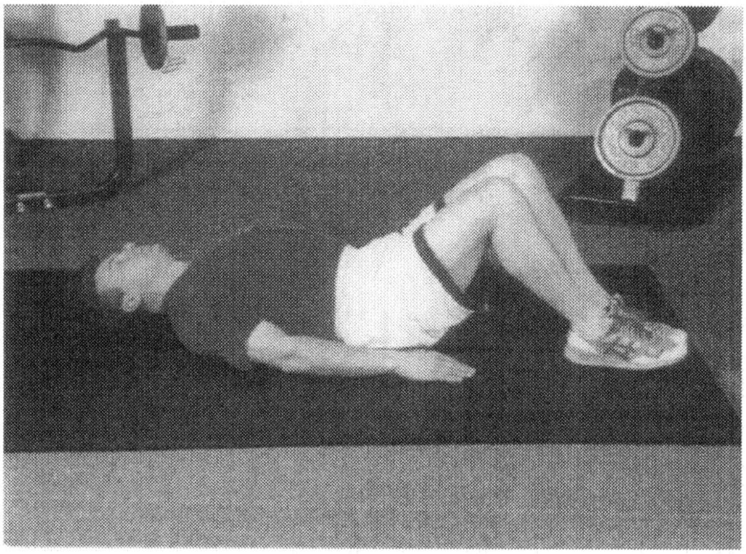

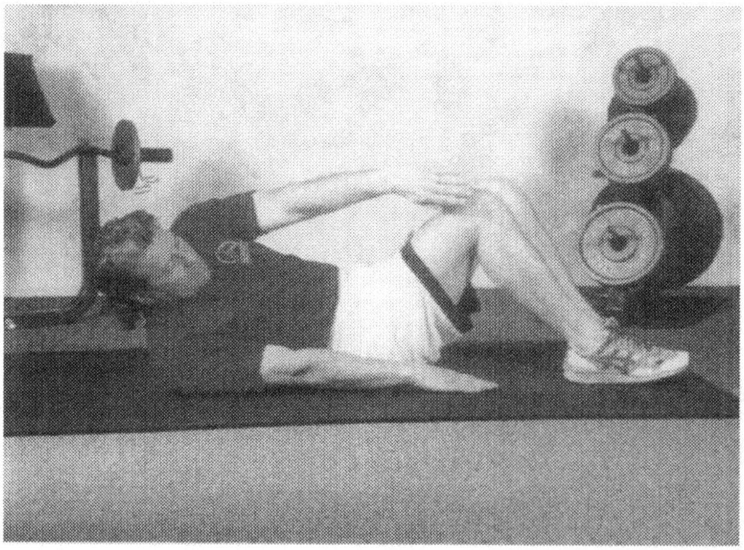

LEG EXERCISES

1. <u>Barbell or Dumbbell Half Squat</u> (strengthens buttocks, front of thigh)

Approach a weighted bar resting on its support racks, positioned slightly lower than shoulder height. Place the bar across the back of your shoulders, resting it just below the base of your neck **(A dumbbell on each shoulder or held at hip level can be substituted, holding one dumbbell in each hand.)** Grasp the bar with your hands six inches wider than your shoulders. Remove the bar from the rack and take a few steps backwards. Spread your feet to shoulder width. You may wish to use a 1/2-inch block of wood beneath your heels.

Keep your head up and do not bend forward or twist at the waist. Bend at the knees and sink slowly downward, pausing when your thighs are parallel to the floor (your knees should be bent no further than a 90 degree angle). Return to the starting position by straightening your legs and pressing from your heels, keeping your head up and back straight.

Spotter: Stands behind lifter, assisting only if required. When needed, the spotter grasps the lifter around the waist with both arms, giving only a minimum amount of assistance so that the lifter can complete a repetition. At the end of the set, the spotter helps guide the lifter and bar back to the support racks, being sure the bar is set firmly in the racks before releasing it.

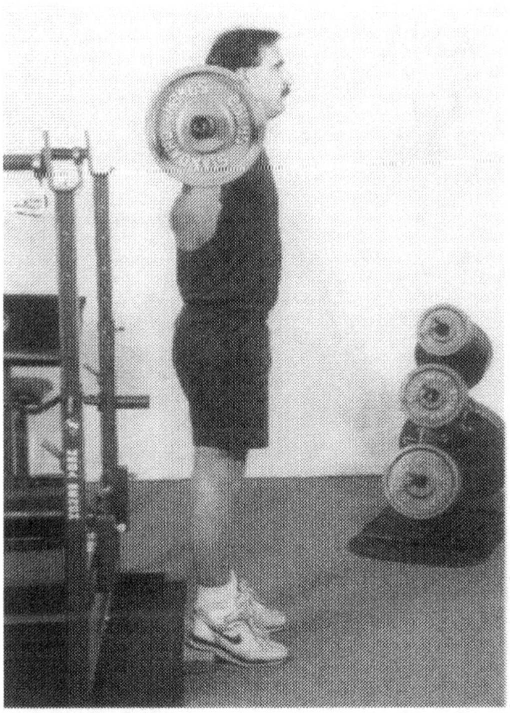

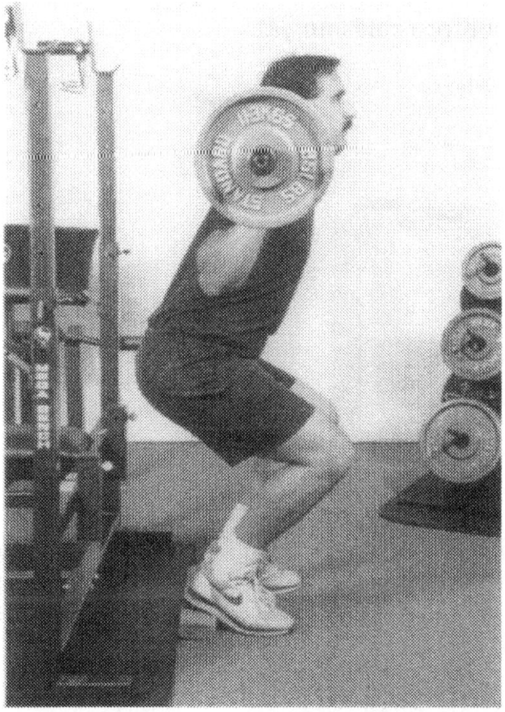

LEG EXERCISES (continued)

2. Barbell or Dumbbell Lunge (strengthens buttocks, front of thigh)

Approach a weighted bar resting on its support racks, positioned slightly lower than shoulder height. Place the bar across the back of your shoulders, resting it just below the base of your neck **(A dumbbell on each shoulder or held at hip level can be substituted, holding one dumbbell in each hand.)** Grasp the bar with your hands six inches wider than your shoulders. Remove the bar from the rack and take a few steps backwards.

Assume a normal stance and step forward with one foot. Bend at the knees and lower yourself until your back knee almost touches the floor behind you. Be sure that your front foot and front knee are pointing directly ahead. Press upwards, pushing off your front foot in a toe/heel manner and straighten your front leg, returning to the standing position. It is best to complete one entire set of repetitions with the same forward leg, then switch and complete another set with the other leg.

Spotter: Stands behind lifter, moving forward and back as he/she performs each lunge. When needed, the spotter grasps the lifter at the waist with both hands, giving only a minimum amount of assistance so that the lifter can complete a repetition. At the end of the set, the spotter helps guide the lifter and bar back to the support racks, being sure the bar is set firmly in the racks before releasing it.

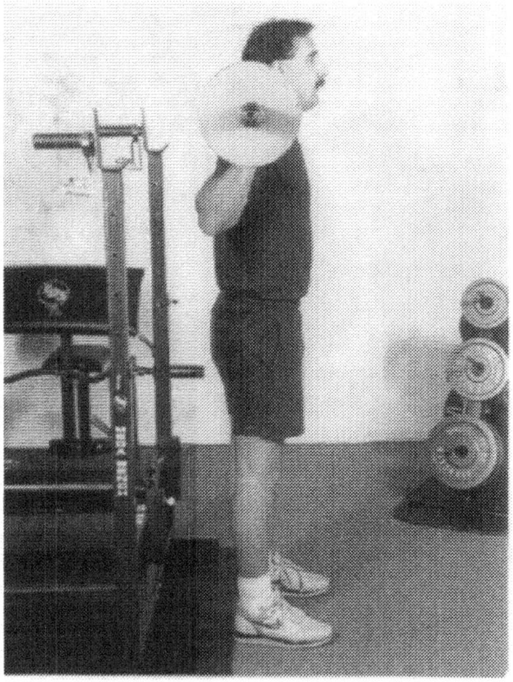

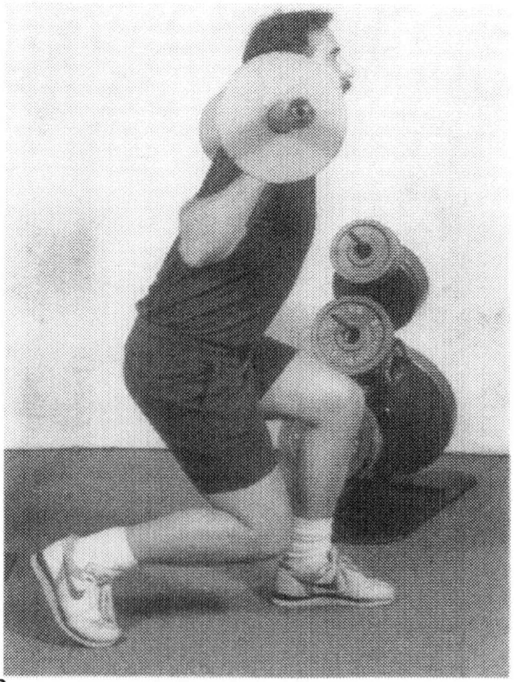

LEG EXERCISES (continued)

3. <u>Barbell or Dumbbell Toe Raise</u> (strengthens calf)

Approach a weighted bar resting on its support racks, positioned slightly lower than shoulder height. Place the bar across the back of your shoulders, resting it just below the base of your neck **(A dumbbell on each shoulder or held at hip level can be substituted, holding one dumbbell in each hand.)** Grasp the bar with your hands six inches wider than your shoulders. Remove the bar from the rack and take a few steps backwards. Spread your feet to shoulder width, toes pointed directly forward.

Keeping your knees completely straight and locked, raise up on your toes. Pause briefly, and then slowly lower to the starting position. To increase the difficulty of this exercise, place the balls of your feet on a block of wood or small step, or work one leg at a time.

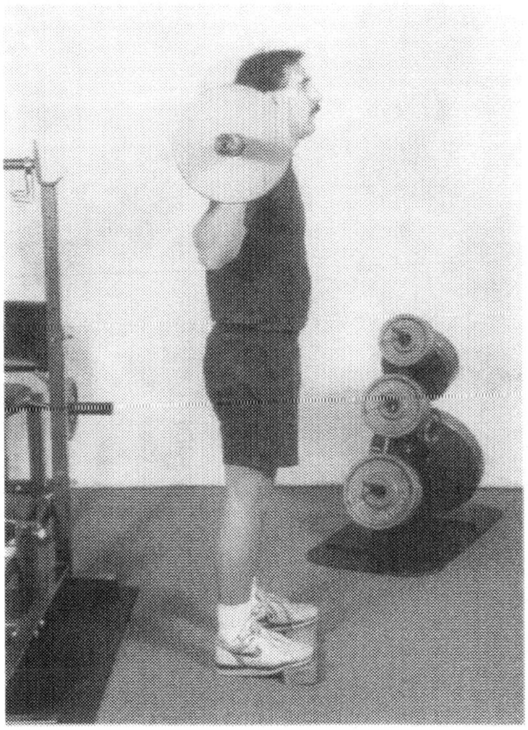

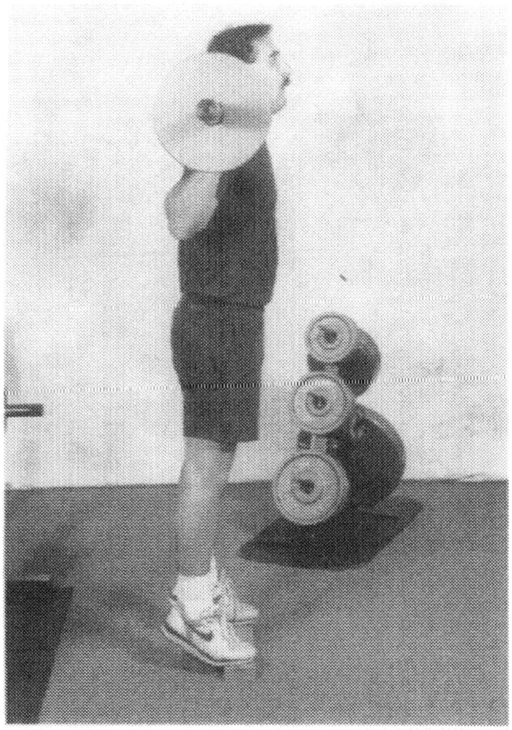

LEG EXERCISES (continued)

4. <u>Manual Resistance Knee Extension</u> (strengthens front of thigh)

Sit on a table so that your lower legs hang over the side. Your partner should stand in front of you and place his/her hand on one of your ankles. Straighten one leg completely while your partner applies resistance at your ankle. Your partner should apply enough force so that muscular exhaustion occurs after about 10 repetitions. As you get stronger, your partner will need to apply more force. Resistance should be applied by your partner as you are straightening your leg and while you are lowering it.

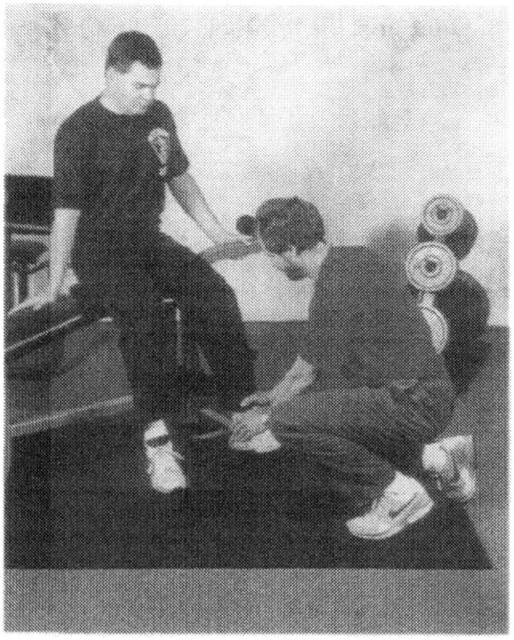

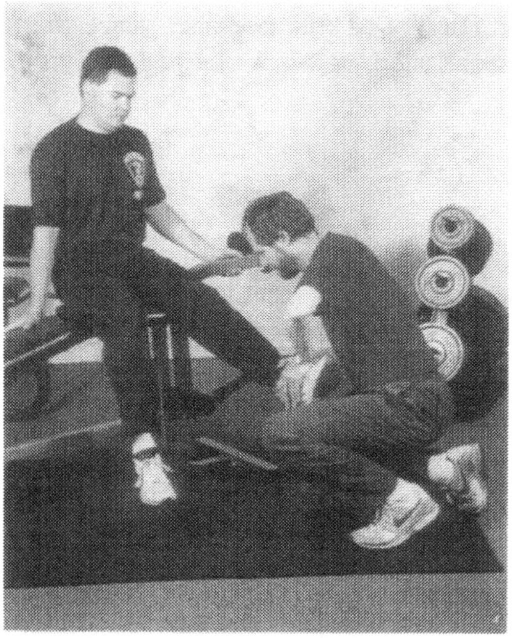

5. <u>Manual Resistance Knee Flexion</u> (strengthens back of thigh)

Lie on your stomach. Your partner should kneel behind you and place his/her hand on one of your ankles. Bend one leg, bringing the heel toward your buttocks, while your partner applies resistance at your ankle. Your partner should apply enough force so that muscular exhaustion occurs after about 10 repetitions. As you get stronger, your partner will need to apply more force. Resistance should be applied by your partner as you are bending your leg and while you are lowering it.

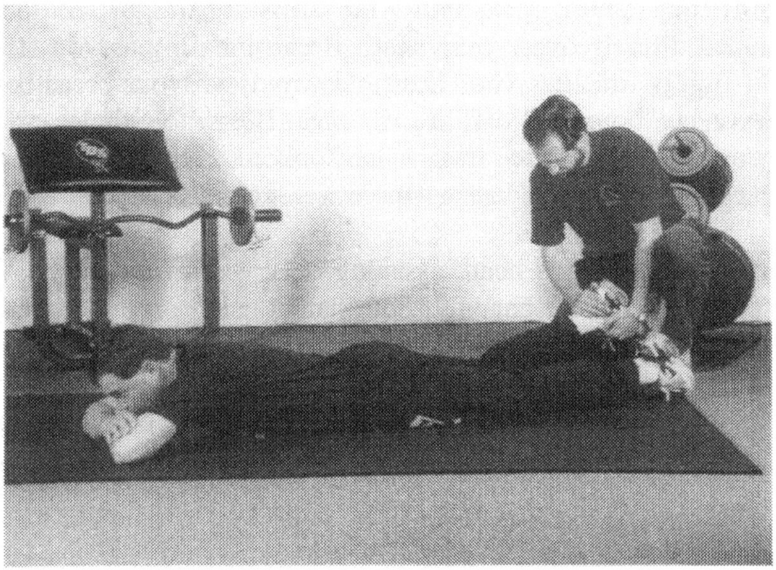

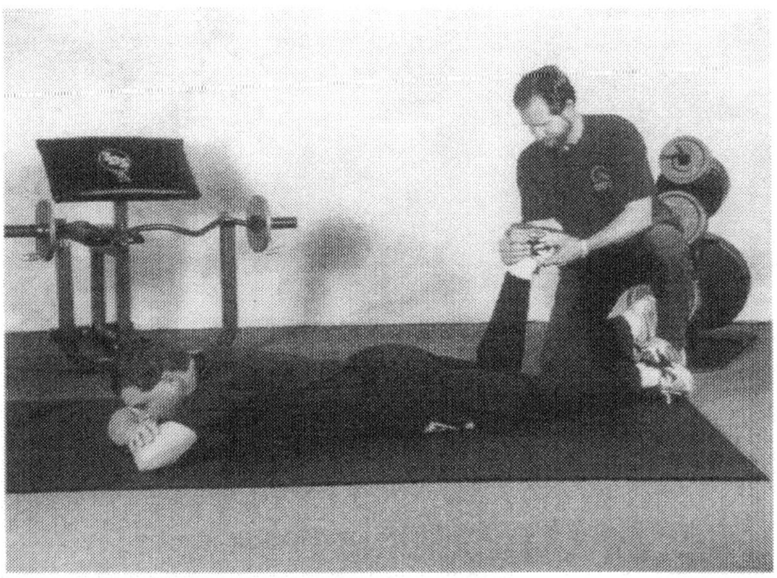

CHEST EXERCISES

1. Barbell Bench Press (strengthens chest, shoulders, and triceps)

Lie on your back on a firm padded bench, feet flat on the floor. Position yourself so that the bar is located directly above your eyes. Grasp the bar in an overhand grip with your hands about 6 inches wider than the width of your shoulders. Your hands should be evenly spaced from the center of the bar.

Push the bar off the support racks until your arms are straight and locked with the bar positioned directly over your chest. Begin inhaling as you slowly lower the bar until it lightly touches your chest midway down your breastbone. The bar should **never** be "bounced" off the rib cage. Begin to exhale and press the bar upwards until your arms are straight and locked. Keep the head, back, and buttocks flat against the bench during the entire exercise.

Spotter: Stands at the lifter's head, assisting only when necessary. When needed, the spotter grasps the bar with both hands using an underhand grip, giving only a minimum amount of assistance so that the lifter can complete a repetition. At the end of the set, the spotter helps guide the bar back to the support racks, being sure the bar is set firmly in the racks before releasing it.

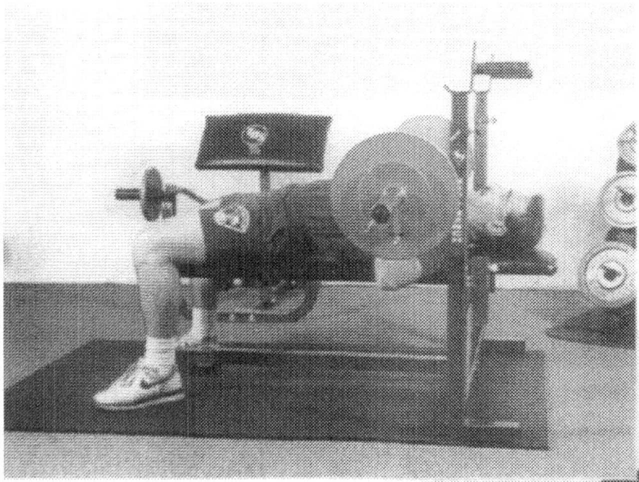

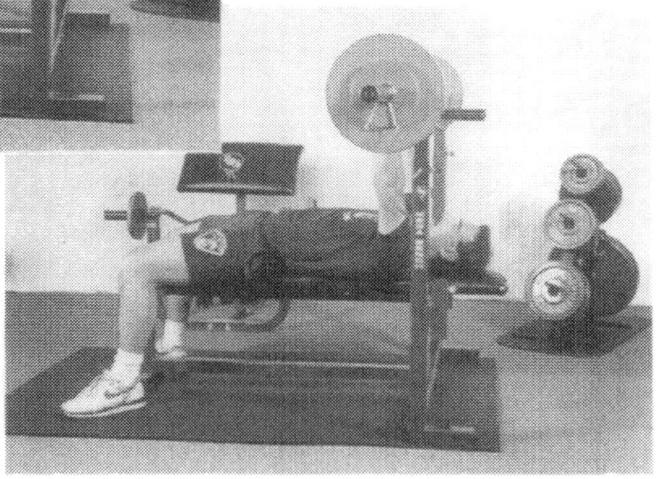

CHEST EXERCISES (continued)

2. <u>Dumbbell Flies</u> (strengthens chest and shoulders)

Lie on your back on a firm padded bench, feet flat on the floor. With your arms straight above your chest, your partner hands you one dumbbell at a time. Hold the dumbbells in each hand over your chest at arms length, palms facing each other. Begin inhaling as you bend your elbows slightly and slowly lower the dumbbells outward to the sides of your chest, following a semicircular path. Begin exhaling and push the dumbbells back upwards, following the same semicircular path, to the starting position. Maintain a slight bend at the elbows (visualize yourself wrapping your arms around a tree).

Spotter: Stands at the lifter's head, assisting lifter only if necessary. When needed, the spotter grasps the outside of the lifter's elbows, giving only a minimum amount of assistance so that the lifter can complete a repetition. At the completion of the set, the spotter should help remove the dumbbells from the lifter's possession and place them aside.

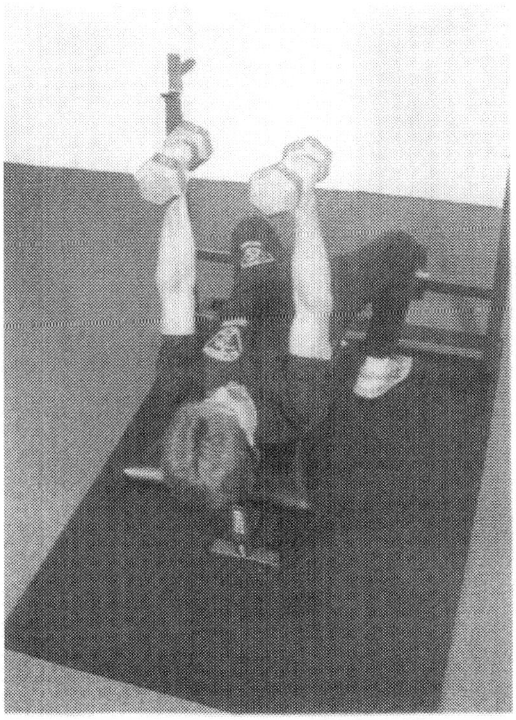

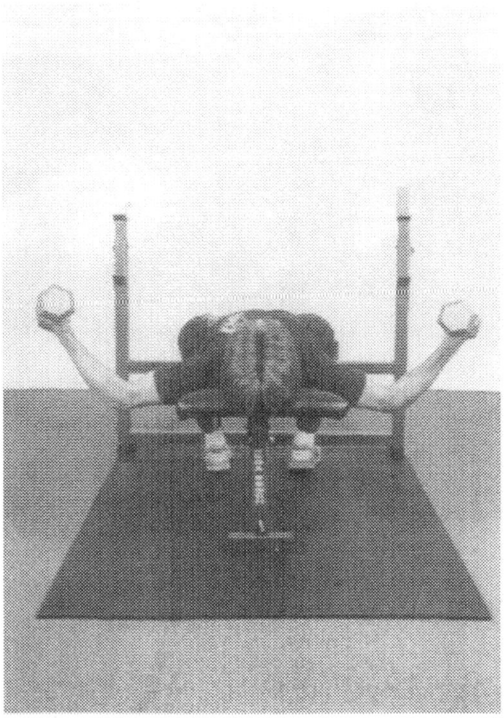

CHEST EXERCISES (continued)

3. <u>Manual Resistance Push-Ups</u> (strengthens chest, shoulders, and triceps)

Perform push-ups (see Chapter 2) while your partner stands over you. Begin the pushup in the "up" position. Keep your body straight and rigid with your arms straight, hands beneath your shoulders. Lower yourself until your chest touches the floor, then return to the starting position. Do not "bounce" your chest off the floor, and maintain straight body posture at all times.

Your partner should apply enough downward force on your shoulder blades to cause muscular exhaustion after about 10 repetitions. As you get stronger, your partner will need to apply more force, both as you are raising your body and while you are lowering it.

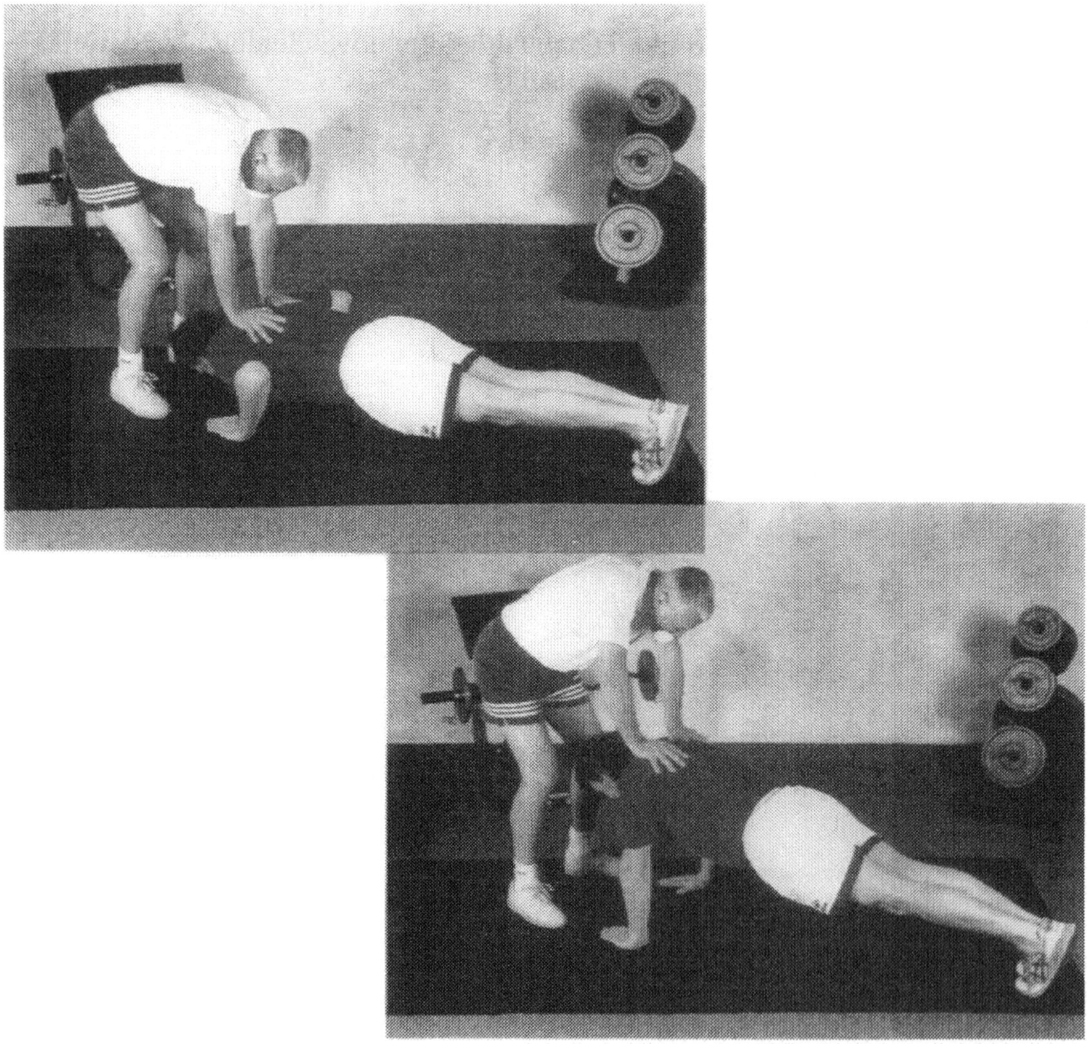

4. <u>Manual Resistance Flies</u> (strengthens chest and shoulders)

Lie on your back, arms out to the side, bent at the elbows with your hands by your ears. Your partner kneels above your head, placing his/her hands on the inside of your elbows. Attempt to bring your elbows together in front of your chest while your partner applies resistance. Pause, and attempt to slowly lower your elbows back to the floor in control while your partner pushes them downward. Your partner should apply enough downward force so that muscular exhaustion occurs after about 10 repetitions.

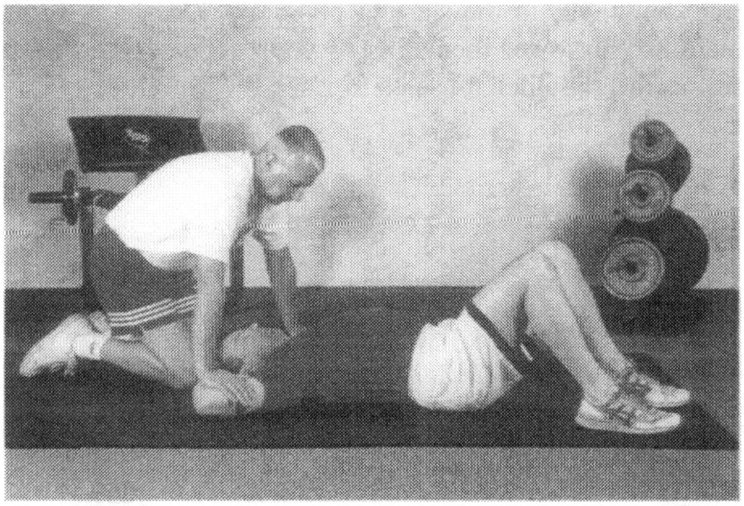

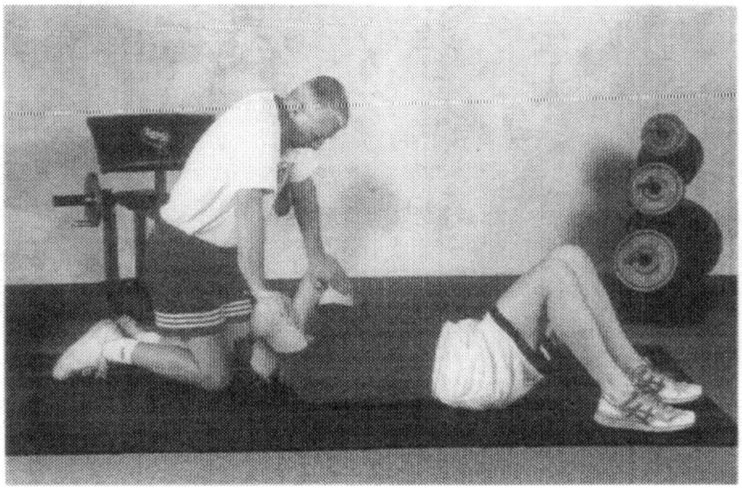

SHOULDER EXERCISES

1. <u>Dumbbell Lateral Raise</u> (strengthens deltoids)

Stand with your feet shoulder width apart. Hold a dumbbell in each hand just in front of your body, palms facing in. Keeping your arms straight at the elbow, lift the dumbbells directly out to your sides, away from your body, to shoulder level. At the peak of the movement, your palms should be facing straight down and your hands should be at the same height as your elbows. The dumbbells should be held level, parallel with the floor. Pause briefly, then slowly lower the dumbbells to the starting position. Exhale as you raise the dumbbells, inhale as you lower them. Keep your upper body still during this movement, forcing the shoulder muscles to raise the weight.

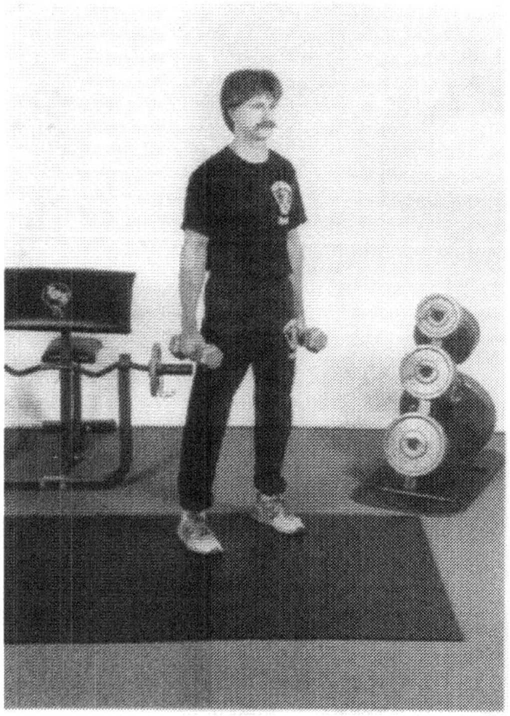

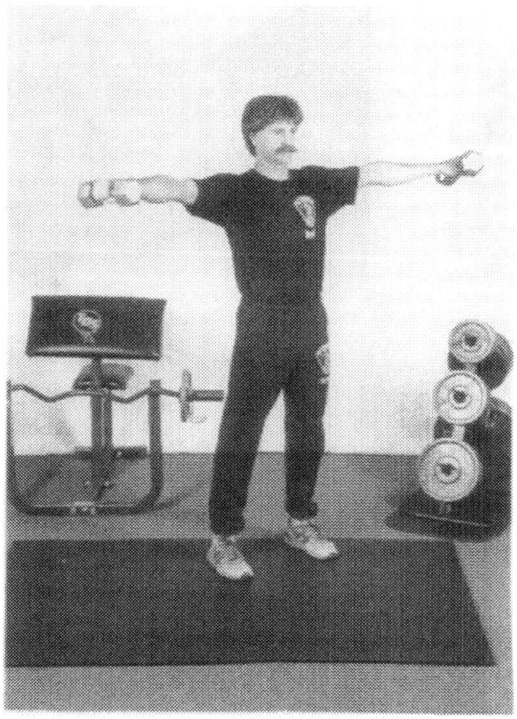

2. <u>Manual Resistance Lateral Raise</u> (strengthens deltoids)

Stand with your arms at your sides. Your partner stands behind you, placing his/her hands on the outside of your elbows. Keeping your arms straight, raise your arms out to the side until they are even with your shoulders while your partner applies resistance at your elbows. Pause, then attempt to slowly lower your arms in control while your partner pushes them downward. Your partner should apply enough downward force so that muscular exhaustion occurs after about 10 repetitions.

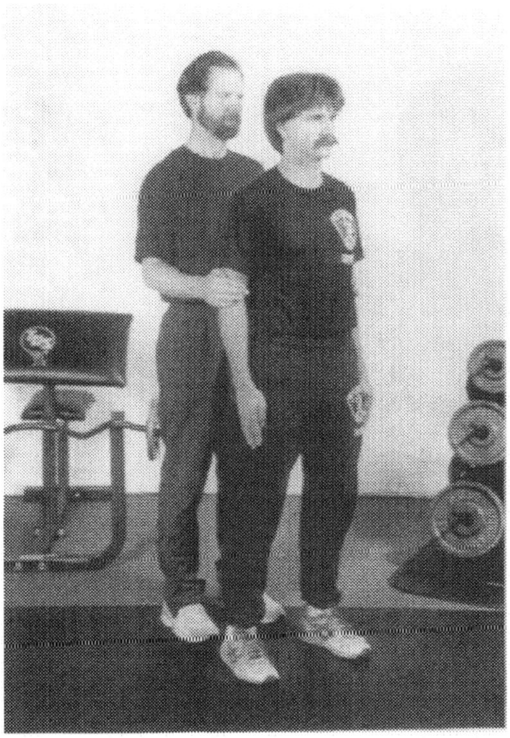

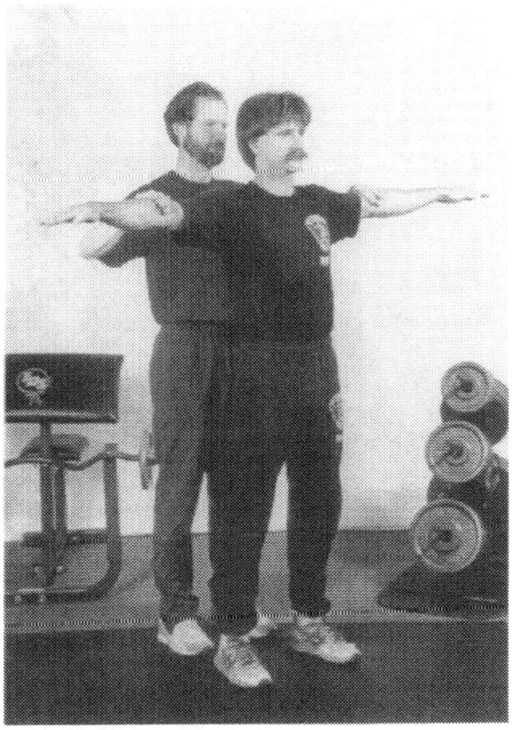

BACK EXERCISES

1. Dumbbell One Arm Rowing (strengthens upper back and biceps)

Approach the foot of a flat exercise bench. Place one knee and the same-side hand on the bench towards the end. Reach down with the opposite hand and grasp a dumbbell lying alongside of bench on the floor. Keeping your head down, back straight, and torso motionless (do not twist at the waist), pull the dumbbell upward in a rowing movement until it lightly contacts your chest. Pause briefly, then slowly lower the dumbbell to the starting position.

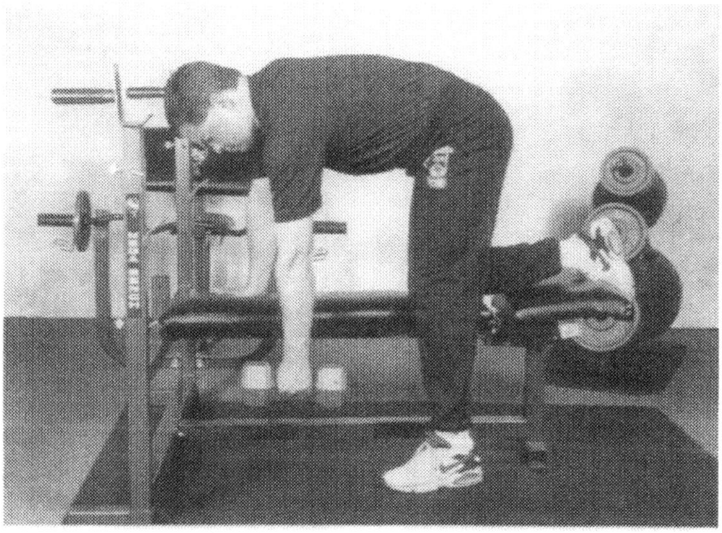

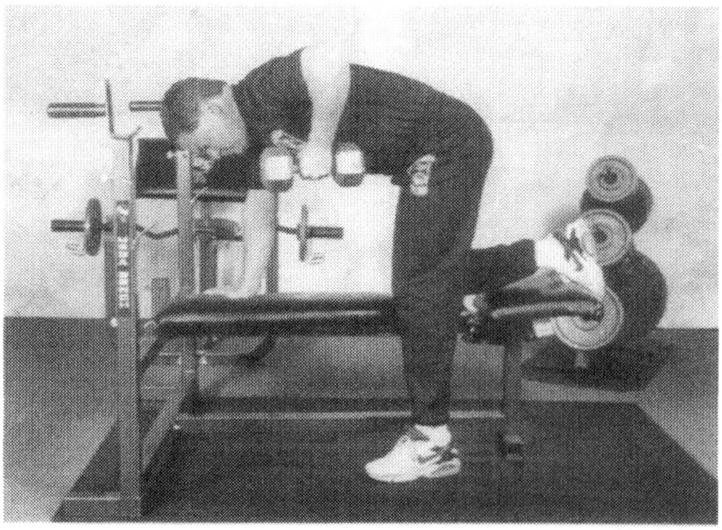

2. <u>Manual Resistance Rowing</u> (strengthens upper back and biceps)

Sit face to face with your partner. Hold a bar or towel in both hands while your partner does the same. Attempt to pull the bar or towel into your lower chest region while your partner applies resistance. Then attempt to slowly return to the starting position in control while your partner continues pulling on the bar or towel. Your partner should apply enough force so that muscular exhaustion occurs after about 10 repetitions.

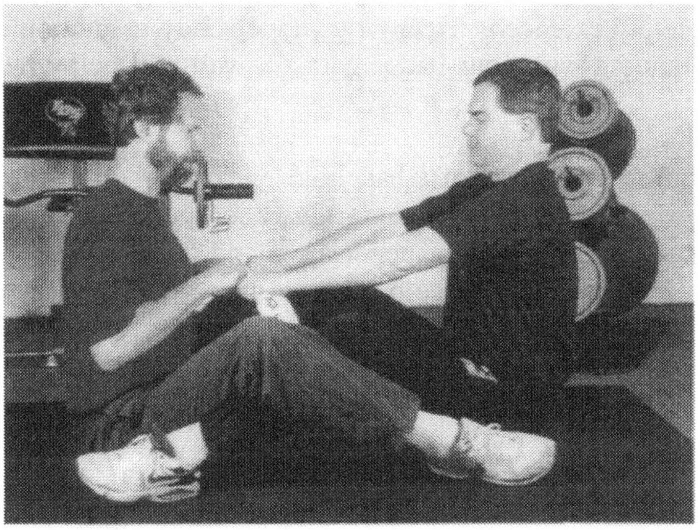

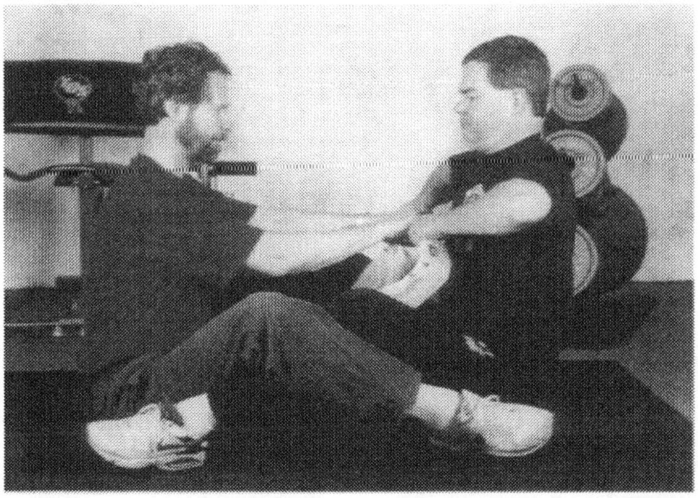

ARM EXERCISES

1. Barbell or Dumbbell Biceps Curl (strengthens front of upper arm)

Stand with your feet shoulder width apart. With arms fully extended, grasp a weighted bar at thigh level with an underhand grip, hands shoulder width apart. Keeping your upper arms vertical and unmoving, bend at the elbows and curl the bar to your shoulders. Pause briefly, then slowly lower the bar until your arms are completely extended. Keep your upper body as motionless as possible throughout. Standing with your back against a wall will help you prevent "cheating."

When using dumbbells instead of a bar, hold one dumbbell in each hand with an underhand grip, arms fully extended. Curl the dumbbells toward your shoulders, being sure to keep your upper arms and torso as stationary as possible. This exercise can also be performed using only one arm at a time, completing an entire set of repetitions before switching arms.

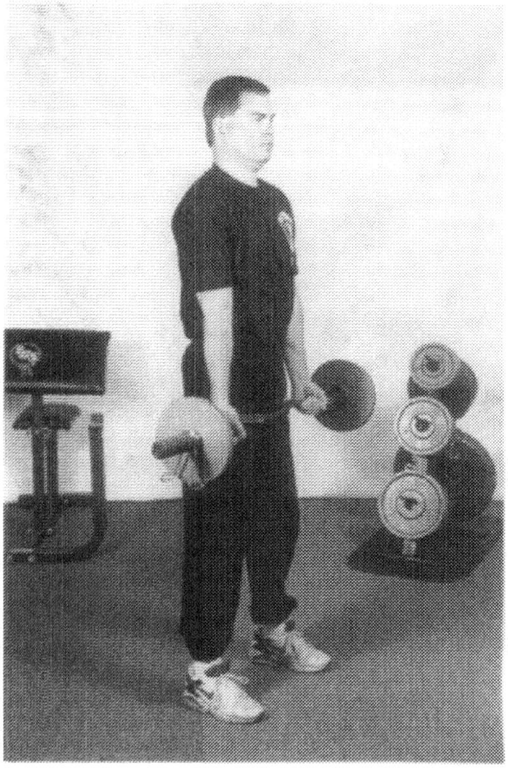

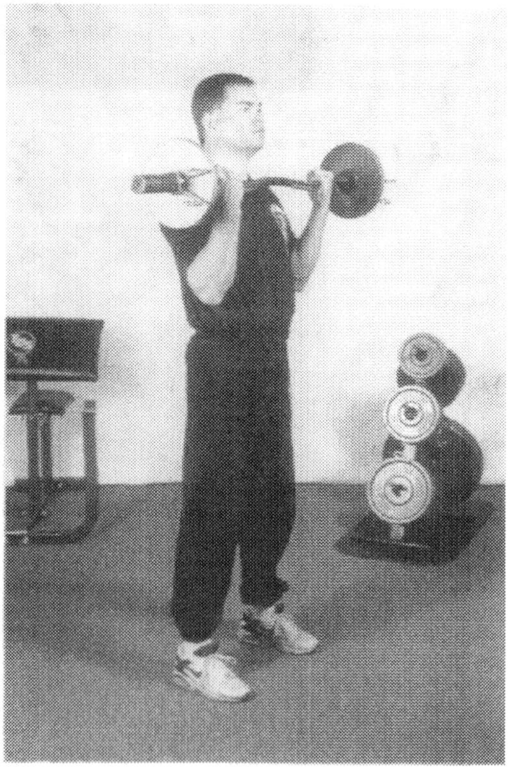

ARM EXERCISES (Continued)

2. <u>Barbell or Dumbbell Triceps Extension</u> (strengthens back of upper arm)

Lie on your back on an exercise bench, feet flat on the floor. Extend your arms straight up and grasp the bar with overhand grip, hands about six inches apart. Keeping your upper arms vertical and unmoving, bend at the elbows and slowly lower the bar until it lightly contacts your forehead. Push the bar upwards by straightening at the elbows, keeping your upper arms as motionless as possible.

When using dumbbells instead of a bar, hold one dumbbell in each hand with your arms extended, palms facing inward. Slowly lower the dumbbells toward your shoulders, to either side of your head, being sure to keep your upper arms as stationary as possible. This exercise can also be performed using only one arm at a time, completing an entire set of repetitions before switching arms.

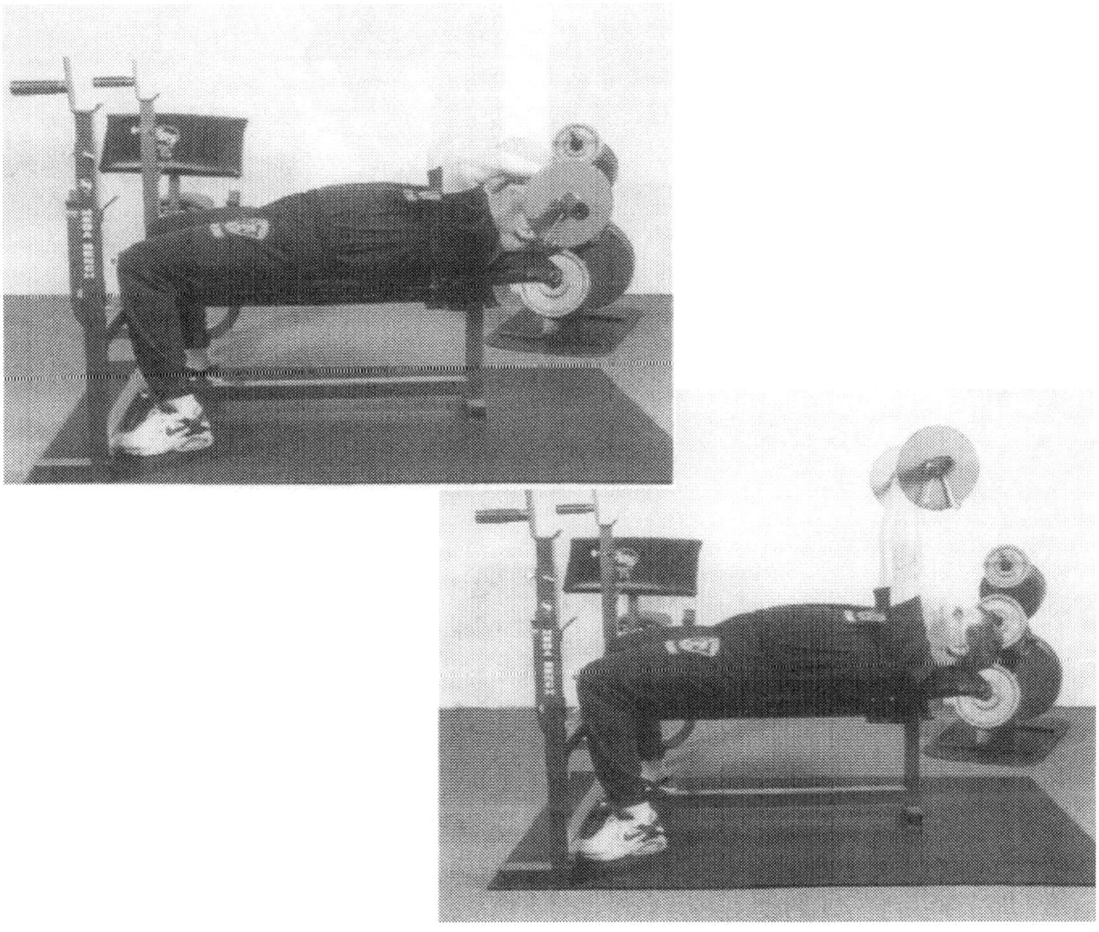

ARM EXERCISES (continued)

3. <u>Manual Resistance Biceps Curl</u> (strengthens front of upper arm)

Lie on your back. Your partner kneels next to you so that his/her knee is directly next to your armpit area. Place the back of your upper arm along the front of your partner's thigh with your arm straight. Your partner stabilizes your arm by placing one hand at your elbow while the other hand grips your wrist. Attempt to bend your arm while your partner applies resistance. Pause, then attempt to slowly return to starting position in control while your partner tries to straighten your arm. Your partner should apply enough resistance so that muscular exhaustion occurs in about 10 repetitions.

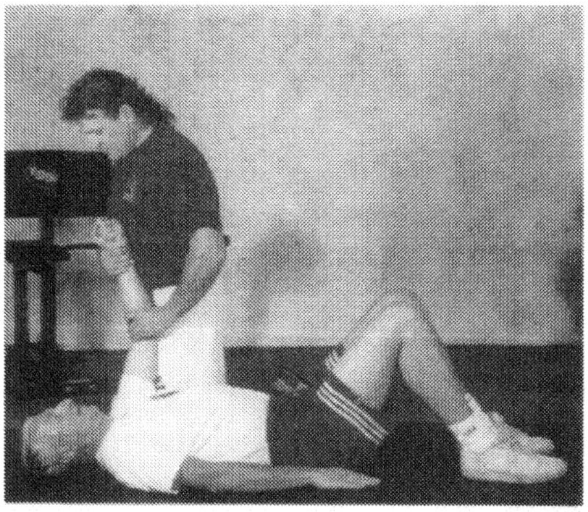

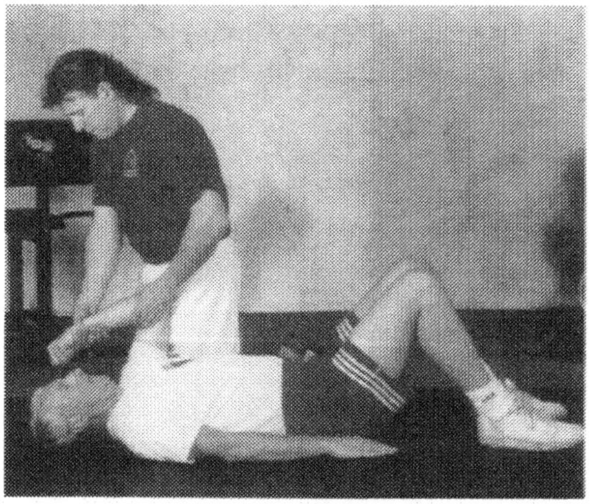

4. Manual Resistance Triceps Extension (strengthens back of upper arms)

Sit on a chair or stool with your partner standing behind you. Grasp the center of a bar or towel in both hands, and bend your arms so that your hands are behind your head. Your partner grasps the ends of the bar or towel and applies resistance while you attempt to straighten your arms overhead. At the top of the movement, pause, then slowly return to the starting position in control while your partner continues to pull downward. Your partner should apply enough resistance so that muscular exhaustion occurs in about 10 repetitions.

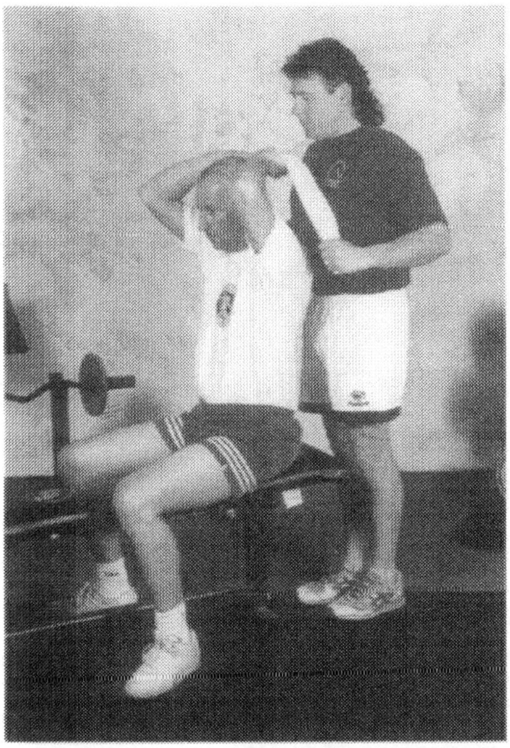

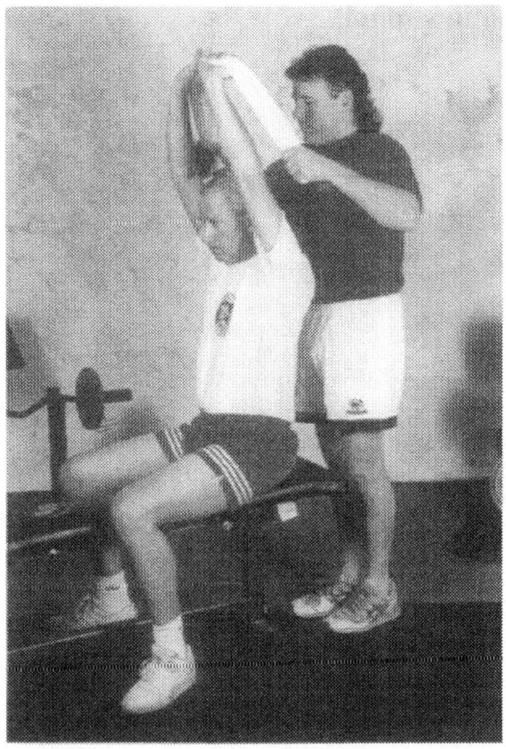

OPTIONAL EXERCISES

1. **<u>Barbell or Dumbbell Shoulder Shrug</u> (strengthens upper back, neck)**

Stand with your feet shoulder width, holding a barbell with an overhand grip in front of you at thigh level, your arms fully extended at the elbow. (A dumbbell held in each hand, palms inward, can be substituted for the barbell). Tilt your head forward slightly. Shrug your shoulders upward, attempting to touch your ears with your shoulders. Pause, then lower your shoulders slowly and in control.

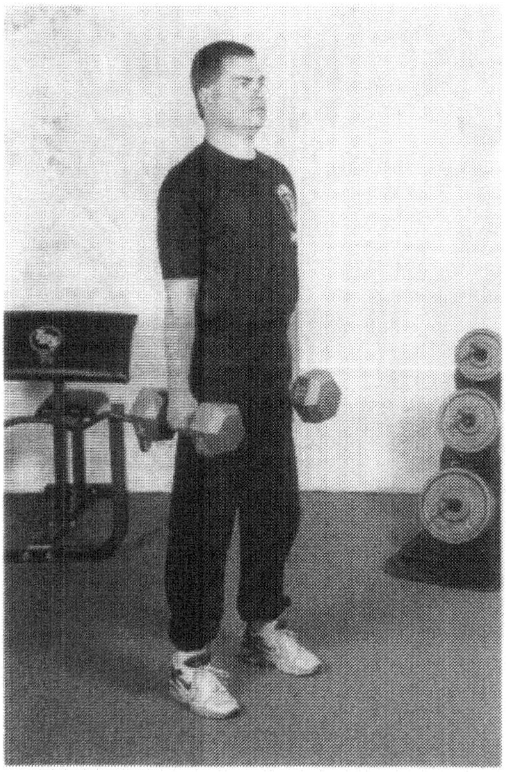

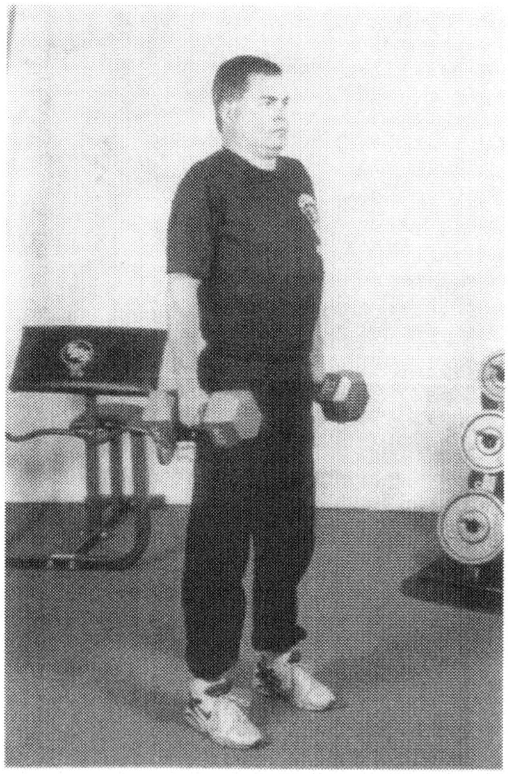

2. Manual Resistance Shoulder Shrug (strengthens upper back, neck)

Stand over your partner, who is lying face up on the floor, and straddle his/her torso. With your arms straight, grasp a bar in front of you at thigh level with an overhand grip. Your partner hangs onto the bar from below. Shrug your shoulders upward, attempting to touch your ears with your shoulders. At the top of the movement, pause, then lower your shoulders slowly and in control. If your partner's weight is too great to perform 10 repetitions, have him/her bend at the knees to lessen the resistance.

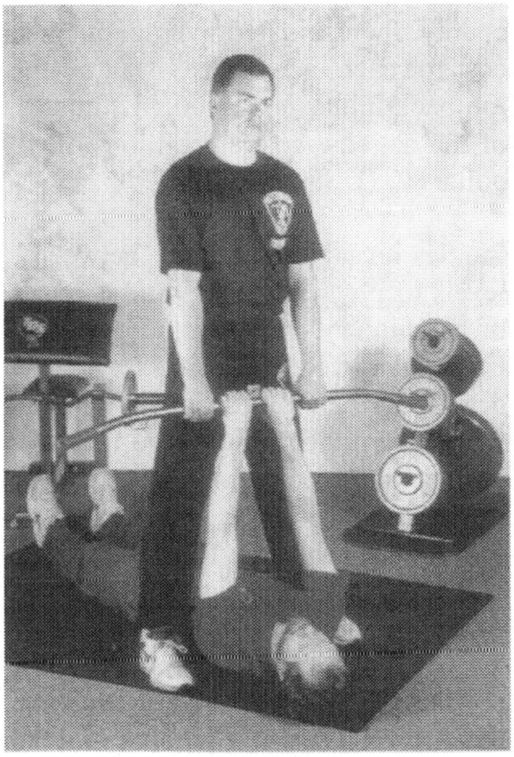

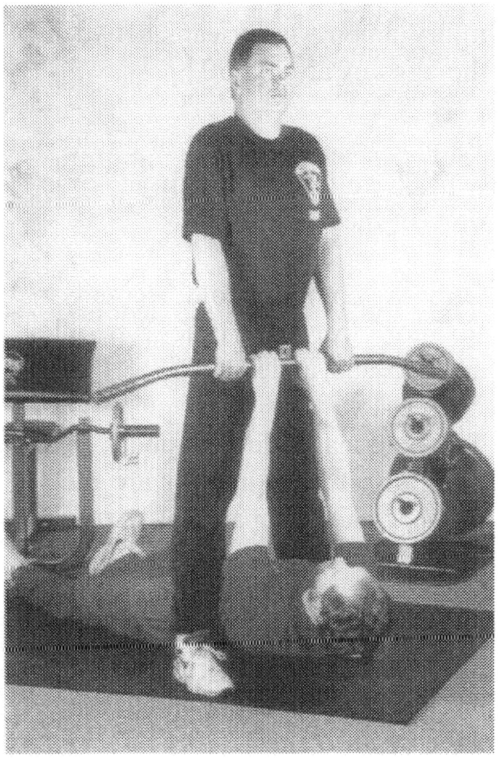

BACK INJURIES AND CARE

Low-back pain is one of the most common problems in our civilization. The following facts document the importance of taking care of your back, and the consequences that many people face because they don't:

- Back injury is the most common injury among Americans between the ages of 25 and 50.
- As many as 80 percent of adults experience low back pain at some time in their lives.
- Only the common cold accounts for more lost work time in people ages 45 and under.
- The National Safety Council reports that back injuries are the number one occupational hazard in the U.S.
- Back injuries are also the number one reason for workers' compensation claims, comprising 22% of all claims.

Back injuries are a particularly important problem for firefighters and rescue workers. According to a document published by the National Fire Protection Association, "back injuries follow heart disease as the second major cause of premature retirement among firefighters....In one county, the estimated average medical cost for each occurrence of an on-the-job back injury is $1,500. Estimates of the national cost are billions of dollars." (USFA 1990)

Studies reveal a direct link between levels of physical fitness and chances of back injury. In one study, firefighters were measured to determine their fitness levels. They were then divided into three fitness groups, and back injuries for each group were recorded. The results showed that both the frequency and cost of back injuries is greater for less fit firefighters. The least fit group had 7.1 percent injuries, the middle group received 3.1 percent injuries, and the most fit only had 0.8 percent injuries. (Cady 1979)

"Three simple factors will allow us to predict which firefighters will develop disabling back injuries. It is almost as though they are accidents waiting to happen. These are obesity, poor endurance of the abdominal muscles, and poor flexibility of the lower back and hamstring muscle group (the muscles in the back of the leg). All of these conditions compound the load on the lower portion of the back or vertebral column."
(Davis and Curtis)

CAUSES OF BACK PAIN

The good news is that low back pain is a symptom, not a disease, and many back injuries are avoidable. Prevention of back injuries is possible by following specific guidelines for lifting and carrying, and by participating in a physical fitness program to maintain adequate strength and flexibility.

Back pain can be divided into five basic areas: mechanical factors, disc injury, muscle dysfunction, traumatic injury, and acquired conditions.

Mechanical Factors

The majority of back injuries are a result of mechanical factors—excessive body weight; poor posture while standing, sitting, walking, driving, and sleeping; and inadequate levels of either strength or flexibility. These factors, plus weak abdominal muscles, create an excessive forward curvature of the lower spine, called "lordosis" or sway back. This condition causes strain and chronic pain in the lower back due to the muscle imbalance created by weak abdominals and tight back muscles. Weight control through regular exercise will decrease the likelihood of these problems.

Disc Injury

Degeneration of the vertebral discs is associated with the aging process. Aging causes the spinal column to lose fluid and supporting back muscles to lose some of their tone. After years of minor wear and tear, a small amount of extra damage may cause part of the disc to protrude (or herniate) from its usual position as a cushion between the vertebrae.

This "slipped" disc may exert pressure on a spinal nerve, causing back pain and radiating pain down the buttocks and leg, a condition known as sciatica. This nerve irritation may also cause numbness, weakness, or a tingling sensation in one or both legs.

Muscle Dysfunction

Although stress is not a direct cause of low back pain, stress-provoked tension may induce muscles to tighten up. The resulting strain on the muscles that support the back can result in pain, stiffness, and even muscle spasms.

Occupational hazards may also contribute to back injury. The repetitive nature of many physical jobs can promote exceptional strength in certain muscles, while others remain underdeveloped. When unused muscles are subjected to unusual or sudden movement, a strain or tear may result that could cause the back to lose vital support.

Traumatic Injury

Traumatic injury from athletics, accidents, falls, or lifting and moving heavy objects are all causes of back problems. Forward bending with a straight back and straight knees is one of the leading causes of lower back pain.

Acquired Conditions

Joint problems may also contribute to back problems. Joints may become stiff or immobile from underuse. Conversely, too much joint movement can cause the surface to become unstable and surrounding ligaments to become damaged or loose. Back muscles that try to compensate for the excessive joint movement may become sore and irritated.

Arthritis and the vertebral fractures that accompany osteoporosis are also causes of back pain. Even though these conditions result naturally through the aging process, they are promoted through a sedentary lifestyle characterized by inadequate levels of physical fitness. Regular exercise will lower the risk and often lessen the pain caused by these conditions.

On rare occasions, infections and tumors may be the cause of back problems. Additionally, the brain can sometimes mistake pain signals from other organs, such as the kidneys or uterus, as originating in the lower back area. This type of pain is known as "referred" pain.

Activity 5-1

RISK FACTORS FOR BACK INJURY

Although some back problems result from uncontrollable factors like age or heredity, most injuries are preventable. The majority of back problems build gradually and progressively through the accumulated effects of poor posture, faulty biomechanics, stress, loss of flexibility, and/or a lack of physical conditioning.

Your predisposition to back problems is directly related to the number of risk factors that apply to you. Take this quick quiz to check your level of risk. Answer "TRUE" or "FALSE" to each statement. The more "TRUE" answers, the greater your risk of back injury.

1. I often do not maintain good posture.	TRUE or FALSE
2. I sit for long periods of time without a break.	TRUE or FALSE
3. I often am required to <u>lift</u> heavy objects.	TRUE or FALSE
4. I often am required to <u>carry</u> heavy objects.	TRUE or FALSE
5. I often do not practice proper techniques for lifting and carrying heavy objects.	TRUE or FALSE
6. I often engage in strenuous physical activity without warming up or stretching.	TRUE or FALSE
7. I am overweight.	TRUE or FALSE
8. I do not stretch and exercise my back on a regular basis.	TRUE or FALSE
9. I do not strengthen my abdominal muscles on a regular basis.	TRUE or FALSE
10. I usually do not think about my back when I begin a task.	TRUE or FALSE

PROPER LIFTING TECHNIQUES

Often it's not how much you lift or carry, but the method you use that is most important. Over 90 percent of all back injuries are not due to a sudden trauma. They are instead the "last straw" of many years of "micro-damage" that accumulates, caused by poor posture, improper body mechanics, and poor lifting techniques. Some tips for proper lifting, whether a heavy box or a piece of paper off the floor, follow.

- Whenever possible, **plan** the lift. Clear the path, minimize slippery conditions, think through options, etc. Brief everyone involved on exactly how to proceed.
- Get as close to the object as possible. Loads held away from the body create 10 times more force on your back than those held close.
- Ideally, place one foot on either side of the object. Maintain a wide, balanced base of support.
- Bend at the knees and lower yourself to grasp the object.
- Test the weight of the object before actually lifting it. **If it seems too heavy, get someone to help you.**
- Keep your head and shoulders up, chin tucked, back arched (torso should never be rounded forward).
- Use the power of your leg muscles to lift the object as you stand up, not the strength of your back. Lift smoothly, don't use an explosive, jerking motion.
- Keep the load as close to your body as you can while standing up.
- Never twist while lifting. Never reach while lifting.
- If possible, push or pull the load across the floor, rather than lifting it. Pushing is preferable to pulling—you can push twice as much as you can pull.
- If you need to turn with the load once you have lifted it, always turn your entire body, starting with your feet so that you face the new direction. Never twist at the waist while holding an object.
- Never lift with your legs straight. Whenever possible, support your torso by placing a hand down, or place a knee up on a supporting surface as you lift.

TAKING CARE OF YOUR BACK

Since back pain is often associated with muscular weakness and inflexibility, exercise is known to prevent most back problems and to speed recovery for the majority of sufferers. The most effective regimen includes stretching and strengthening exercises, coupled with aerobic activities like walking and swimming. Helpful exercises include lower back and abdominal stretches (see Chapter 3), and regular and oblique curl-ups (see the last section).

> "The long-awaited cure for back pain has been discovered. This treatment could relieve the suffering of an estimated 80% to 90% of the American public and save the country between $16 and $50 billion annually....In a word...exercise."
>
> (Klein 1993)

When pain occurs, remember that most episodes improve on their own within three to four weeks, and surgery is usually not necessary. However, you should consult with a medical specialist if you have severe or chronic pain, or you suspect a more serious problem (fracture, tumor, etc.)

For uncomplicated back pain, new guidelines from the Agency for Health Care Policy and Research suggest over-the-counter painkillers and moderate exercise as soon as possible. Extended bed rest can actually weaken muscles and may do more harm than good; no more than two to three days is typically needed.

The study also found that spinal manipulation, usually performed by chiropractors, may be helpful in the early stages. (The most effective chiropractors also emphasize lifestyle modifications and exercise as part of care.) Other treatments—including traction, transcutaneous electrical nerve stimulation, massage, biofeedback, and ultrasound—may give temporary relief, but have not been proven effective for long-term recovery.

Other suggestions from the panel of health care experts include:

- Wear comfortable, low-heeled shoes.
- Place a pillow or rolled-up towel behind the small of the back when driving long distances.
- Place a pillow under the knees when sleeping on your back, or in between your knees when sleeping on your side.
- Use a chair with good lower back support, and rest your feet on a low stool when sitting for long periods.
- Put work surfaces at a comfortable height.

STRENGTH TRAINING PROGRAMS

GENERAL GUIDELINES

The basic criteria for an effective strength training program is the same for everyone. To review, on two to three days per week, a heavy load is lifted repeatedly so that muscle fatigue occurs in approximately 10 repetitions. Different exercises are employed to strengthen all the major muscle groups. This section presents more detailed guidelines for planning your strength training program.

Which Muscle Groups Should Be Exercised?

Your strength training program should include exercises for all the major muscle groups found in the three main segments of the body. These are listed in the adjacent table. Exercises can also be performed for other muscle groups (trapezius, spinal erectors, etc.), if desired. However, a thorough workout for the muscle groups shown is generally adequate for total body strengthening.

Muscle Groups

Upper Body
Chest (Pectorals)
Shoulders (Deltoids)
Back (Latissimus Dorsi)
Arms, front (Biceps)
Arms, rear (Triceps)
Lower Body
Buttocks (Gluteals)
Thighs, front (Quadriceps)
Thighs, rear (Hamstrings)
Calves (Gastrocnemius)
Mid-Section
Stomach (Abdominals)

How Many Different Exercises Should I Perform?

Many different exercises can be used to build strength in any single muscle group. The recent development of specialized exercise machines has added significantly to this array. For example, a partial list of strength training exercises for the chest or pectoral muscles would include:

- Bench press using free weights
- Bench press using machines
- Inclined bench press using free weights
- Inclined bench press using machines
- Declined bench press using free weights
- Declined bench press using machines
- Bent arm flies using dumbbells
- Bent arm flies using machines
- Dips
- Push ups

Quite a few! A similar list can be generated for most muscle groups in the body. Fortunately, it's not necessary to use more than **one** exercise for any muscle group during your workout. As long as you use proper form and enough resistance, performing one-to-three sets of a single exercise will adequately stimulate the building of new muscle tissue. Performing additional sets, or performing another exercise for the same muscle group, will not produce further or faster gains.

Therefore, during any workout, choose one strength training exercise per muscle group. Perform one-to-three sets of that exercise using good form and heavy resistance. Then move on to another muscle group.

How Much Resistance Should I Use?

The amount of resistance you use will vary for different exercises. For example, you need heavier loads to strengthen the large muscles in your legs than you do for the smaller muscles in your arms.

One way to figure out the right resistance for all these different exercises is to determine the number of repetitions you can perform with various weights before muscular fatigue occurs. Obviously, you will be able to perform fewer repetitions with a heavier weight. A load you can lift only eight times (8 rep max) will be heavier than one you can lift 12 times (12 rep max).

Remember, a weight too heavy can cause injury; one too light will not build strength. **The CW-F Program recommends that you use weights you can repeatedly lift between 8 and 12 times before muscular fatigue occurs.** The only way to determine this weight on different exercises is through trial and error, starting with lighter weights and gradually increasing the load.

In What Order Should Exercises Be Performed?

A good rule of thumb is to begin each strength training session with exercises for the larger muscle groups, and finish with smaller muscle groups. Larger muscles contain more muscle fibers, so heavier weights must be used to strengthen them. You need more energy to work larger muscle groups. Hence, large muscles should be worked early in the session when you have the most energy. Later in your workout, you will be somewhat fatigued and less able to expend the energy needed for large muscle groups.

It is also important to realize that some exercises designed primarily for large muscle groups simultaneously use some of the smaller ones. For example, bench presses (for the chest) require the use of shoulders and triceps, and rowing (for the upper back) requires the use of the biceps. Therefore, performing exercises that target these smaller muscles **first** would somewhat fatigue them, reducing your ability to work the larger muscle groups effectively.

STRENGTH TRAINING EXERCISE ROUTINES

Keeping in mind the three main segments of the body (upper body, lower body, and mid-section) and the fact that each muscle group should not be exercised more frequently than every <u>other</u> day, here are some sample exercise "routines" which vary both in the number of exercises performed and the muscle groups exercised during each workout.

The "full body routine" is recommended as the basic workout for most people.

Full Body Routine

In this type of workout, you exercise all major muscle groups during each strength training session. Begin with the largest muscle groups, alternating exercises between upper body and lower body. All muscle groups are exercised three times per week (e.g., Monday, Wednesday, and Saturday):

1. Buttocks
2. Chest
3. Thighs, front
4. Back
5. Thighs, rear
6. Shoulders
7. Calves
8. Arms, front
9. Abdominals
10. Arms, rear

"Split" Routines

This type of workout separates muscle groups so that only half of them are exercised on any given day, while the other half are resting from the previous day's strength training session.

1. Upper Body/Lower Body Split Routine

Workout #1 (Monday, Wednesday, Friday)	Workout #2 (Tuesday, Thursday, Saturday)
Chest	Buttocks
Back	Thighs, front
Shoulders	Thighs, rear
Arms, front	Calves
Arms, rear	Abdominals

2. Extension/Flexion ("Push/Pull") Split Routine

Workout #1 (Monday, Wednesday, Friday)	Workout #2 (Tuesday, Thursday, Saturday)
Buttocks	Hamstrings
Chest	Back
Thighs, front	Abdominals
Shoulders	Arms, front
Calves	
Arms, rear	

Activity 5-2

INDIVIDUAL EXERCISE PLANNING

During the first part of this activity, you will develop a muscular fitness training program designed to meet your specific needs and goals. You will then expand upon the work you did in previous chapters to prepare a **comprehensive** exercise program that addresses flexibility, cardiovascular fitness, and muscular fitness training.

DETERMINING SETS AND RESISTANCE

In this planning approach, the **number of sets** of each exercise you perform during your workout (1, 2, or 3) depends on your fitness goal (bronze, silver, or gold), defined as before. The higher your fitness goal, the more sets you will have to perform to reach it. Since each set takes about 25 minutes (10 major muscle groups, 2½ minutes per exercise), you must also plan for longer or more frequent workouts.

The **amount of resistance** (load or weight) you use is based on your fitness level (1, 2, or 3), determined during the assessment in Chapter 2. If you are at a higher level of fitness, you will use a heavier (lower rep max) weight, and visa versa. This approach recommends that you use between an eight and twelve rep max weight.

Planning Instructions

1. Follow the directions on **Worksheet 1, Part A** to determine how many sets you should perform (1, 2, or 3) and how much resistance you should use (8, 10, or 12 Rep Max) for each strength exercise you perform. Note: warm-up sets are not included.

2. Follow the directions on **Worksheet 1, Part B** to select a strength training exercise routine and to estimate the amount of time each workout will take. Add time for warm-up sets, as appropriate.

Remember, as you follow your strength training program, you'll naturally increase the intensity of your exercise. You do this by adding slightly more weight or resistance to the exercises as the weeks go by.

Activity 5-2 (Cont'd)
WORKSHEET 1

A. MUSCULAR WORKOUT GUIDELINES

In the appropriate spaces, fill in your muscular fitness level from your physical fitness assessment and your personal muscular fitness goal. Then use the table below to estimate the number of sets and the amount of resistance you should use for each exercise in your strength training workout.

1. Muscular Fitness Level (1, 2, or 3) __________

2. Muscular Fitness Goal (Gold, Silver, or Bronze) __________

YOUR FITNESS GOAL	YOUR FITNESS LEVEL		
	Level 1	Level 2	Level 3
Gold	3 Sets, 12 Rep Max	3 Sets, 10 Rep Max	3 Sets, 8 Rep Max
Silver	2 Sets, 12 Rep Max	2 Sets, 10 Rep Max	2 Sets, 8 Rep Max
Bronze	1 Set, 12 Rep Max	1 Set, 10 Rep Max	1 Set, 8 Rep Max

B. ESTIMATING WORKOUT TIME

Select a workout routine (the full body routine is recommended). Then fill in the number of sets from Part A. Finally, estimate how long your workout will take based on the following equation: number of exercises X number of sets X 2½ minutes. Add time for warm-up sets as needed.

EXERCISE ROUTINE	# OF EXERCISES	# OF SETS	ESTIMATED TIME
1. Full Body	10	1	25 min
	10	2	50 min
	10	3	75 min
2. Other			
3. Other			

DEVELOPING A COMPREHENSIVE EXERCISE PLAN

Depending on your exercise program, an aerobic workout should take at least 30 minutes, including warm-up and cool-down. Flexibility exercises, which may be part of the cool-down, generally take from 10-30 minutes. A good strength training routine covering the 10 major muscle groups will take about 25 minutes per set. Your program should include at least three flexibility and cardiovascular workouts and two to three muscular fitness workouts per week.

Given these requirements, many options are available for scheduling the various components of your exercise program. You can complete all three exercise components during the same workout, or spread them out over the day. You can work out on alternate days or on consecutive days (as long as you allow at least one day's rest between muscular strength workouts for the same muscle group). You can skip some days entirely, or use them for recreational sports.

When combining aerobic and strength training elements in one workout, choose which component you want to emphasize most and do that one first. Stretching for flexibility can be performed as a transition between the two workouts or as a cool-down at the end. Some people also prefer doing stretching exercises between strength training exercises.

How you structure your plan is up to you. Consider the time you have available, other commitments, cost of equipment and facilities, convenience, working out with friends, and other factors that might affect your success. Most importantly, figure out what will be the most enjoyable and productive use of the limited time you have available for physical conditioning. Be realistic: if your exercise program is a hassle, chances are you won't stick with it very long.

Planning Instructions

1. Using the first half of each column (P = Planned), transfer the time estimate from **Worksheet 1, Part B** to the "Strength" portions of **Worksheet 2** to establish your own muscular fitness workout plan for the coming weeks.

2. Add time for aerobic and flexibility workouts based on the exercise plans you developed in Chapters 3 and 4.

3. Use the second half of each column (A = Actual) to record the amount of time you spend working out over the next four weeks.

Activity 5-2 (Cont'd)
WORKSHEET 2

DAY OF WEEK	ACTIVITY(IES) SELECTED	WEEK 1		WEEK 2		WEEK 3		WEEK 4	
		P	A	P	A	P	A	P	A
DAY 1 MONDAY	Aerobic								
	Strength								
	Flex/Cool-down								
DAY 2 TUESDAY	Aerobic								
	Strength								
	Flex/Cool-down								
DAY 3 WEDNESDAY	Aerobic								
	Strength								
	Flex/Cool-down								
DAY 4 THURSDAY	Aerobic								
	Strength								
	Flex/Cool-down								
DAY 5 FRIDAY	Aerobic								
	Strength								
	Flex/Cool-down								
DAY 6 SATURDAY	Aerobic								
	Strength								
	Flex/Cool-down								
DAY 7 SUNDAY	Aerobic								
	Strength								
	Flex/Cool-down								

P = Planned A = Actual

CHAPTER SUMMARY

In this chapter, you learned some of the basic principles of strength training, which can be remembered by the acronym *PROGRESS*: progression, resistance, opposing muscle groups, good form, range of motion, exhaustion, sets, and speed of movement. The benefits of different exercises, equipment types, and diet supplements were discussed.

Then you learned proper techniques for common free weight and manual resistance strength training exercises. You examined some of the causes of back pain and ways to prevent and treat it. Finally, you prepared a short-term personal exercise plan that includes muscular fitness, cardiovascular fitness, and flexibility training.

Having completed this chapter, you should now be able to:

- Describe muscular fitness and its role in health and performance.
- Identify and apply eight principles of strength training in muscular fitness exercises.
- Identify common causes of back injuries and basic precautions for avoiding problems.
- Use proper technique in performing various strength training exercises.
- Develop a personal exercise plan for strength training and comprehensive fitness.

BIBLIOGRAPHY

Cady, Lee D., et al, "Strength and Fitness and Subsequent Back Injuries in Firefighters," *Journal of Occupational Medicine*, Vol. 21, No. 4, April 1979.

Davis, Paul O., and Arthur V. Curtis, *The Firefighter's Survival Manual: A Guide to Physical Fitness*, National Fire Protection Association.

Fleck, Steven J., and William J. Kraemer, *Designing Resistance Training Programs*, Champaign: Human Kinetics Books, 1987.

Kendall, Florence, and Elizabeth McCreary, *Muscles: Testing and Function*, Baltimore: Williams and Wilkins, 1983.

Klein, Arthur C., and Dava Sobel, "Put an End to Back Pain," *American Health*, September 1993.

McArdle, W., et al, *Exercise Physiology*, Philadelphia: Lea and Febiger, 1986.

Pollock, Michael L., Jack H. Wilmore, and Samuel M. Fox III, *Health and Fitness Through Physical Activity*, New York: John Wiley & Sons, 1978.

Riley, Daniel P., *Maximum Muscular Fitness*, West Point: Leisure Press, 1982.

Ring, Leonard, "Back Injury Prevention—Awareness Versus Performance," *Professional Safety*, July 1989.

Terribilini, Casey, and Kate Dernocoeur, "Save Your Back: Injury Prevention for EMS Providers," *JEMS*, October 1989.

United States Fire Administration, *Physical Fitness Coordinator's Manual for Fire Departments*, FA-95, September 1990.

Weineck, Jurgen, *Functional Anatomy in Sports*, Chicago: Year Book Medical Publishers, Inc., 1986.

Westcott, Wayne L., *Strength Fitness: Physiological Principles and Training Techniques*, Boston: Allyn and Bacon Inc., 1987.

Wilmore, Jack H., and David L. Costill, *Training for Sport and Activity*, Dubuque: Wm. C. Brown Publishers, 1988.

COMPREHENSIVE WELLNESS FOR FIREFIGHTERS

Chapter 6

Nutrition: Practical Guidelines For Good Health

CHAPTER INTRODUCTION

Certain foods increase your risk of heart attacks, cancer, diabetes, and many other diseases. Others minimize or prevent these same problems. In addition, some foods contain many more calories than others, leading to weight gain and its negative effect on health and performance. In short, <u>what</u> you eat is as important as <u>how much</u> you eat.

In this module, you will learn about nutrition, the science of eating right. The information is summarized in several straightforward dietary guidelines that cover most of what you need know about this complex topic. You will also have the opportunity to think about some different ways of <u>applying</u> the guidelines in your daily life. Finally, you will identify some short-term action steps for improving your own eating behaviors.

Keep in mind that proper nutrition should be viewed as an important part of daily life—the saying "you are what you eat" is not without merit. Therefore, the information presented here is just a starting point in a lifetime of learning and application in this critical component of wellness.

LEARNING OBJECTIVES

After learning the information in this chapter, you will be able to:

- Identify the risks associated with unhealthy eating patterns.
- Explain basic terms and concepts of nutrition.
- Describe dietary guidelines for good health in daily life.
- Discuss different suggestions for developing your own healthful eating style.
- Develop a short-term action plan for improving your nutrition.

BASIC CONCEPTS OF NUTRITION

THE IMPORTANCE OF GOOD NUTRITION

Nutrition and Health

In recent years, scientists have learned that the average American diet can be dangerous to your health. Diet is implicated in one-third of all cancer deaths and a large proportion of heart attacks. In fact, what we eat and drink is now known to be a factor in 6 of the 10 leading causes of death—heart disease, cancer, stroke, diabetes mellitus, chronic liver disease and cirrhosis, and atherosclerosis. Combined, these disorders account for nearly 70 percent of all deaths in the United States. (NAS 1992) The consumption of alcohol also plays a major role in two other leading causes of death—accidents and suicide.

> "For the two out of three adult Americans who do not smoke and do not drink excessively, one personal choice seems to influence long-term health prospects more than any other: what we eat."
>
> Surgeon General

Diet is also a factor in a wide variety of other health problems, including high blood pressure, high blood cholesterol, osteoporosis, gallstones, and dental diseases. Eating too many calories contributes to obesity, which affects about 34 million people in this country.

Excess body fat is of particular importance to firefighters. As noted by the United States Fire Administration:

> *"Besides its adverse cardiovascular effects, excess body fat impedes mobility and heat dissipation and increases the likelihood of orthopedic problems. In addition, research... has shown that obesity significantly limits the performance of firefighters....Relative body fat in excess of 20% has a more deleterious effect on physical performance than has age." (USFA 1990)*

Furthermore, some experts believe that firefighters may have special needs for certain nutrients because of exposure to smoke and other pollutants. (Passwater 1989) Unfortunately, fire chiefs recently surveyed indicated that the nutritional quality of the meals and snacks in their department was somewhere between "poor" and "fair." (Lafferty 1985) Attitudes, however, are rapidly changing as weight standards, performance tests, an emphasis on fitness, and an awareness of health hazards have altered the way the fire service views nutrition.

Practicing Good Nutrition

Although the link between diet and disease is well established, many people are misinformed or confused about nutrition. Others are apathetic or have trouble making the changes necessary to adopt a healthful eating pattern. As a result, the country continues to pay a steep price, both in terms of human suffering and massive health care costs.

One problem is that the science of nutrition is very complex. The huge array of possible food choices, each with different nutritional qualities and health implications, can seem absolutely overwhelming. Much information is unknown, and new studies come out all the time, often conflicting with older reports. Sometimes, even the experts disagree, so how can anyone make sense of it all?

Fortunately, you don't need to know biochemistry to make intelligent decisions about eating. Over the years, a consensus has developed about the requirements of a healthy diet, and this information has been distilled into some fairly simple guidelines for proper nutrition. It's sort of like driving a car: you don't need to understand how the engine works or the physics of internal combustion. You just need know where to buy gas, how much it costs, and how often to fill the tank.

The same is true for nutrition. During this section, you will learn some general rules for healthful eating. You probably know most of them already. You'll also learn ways to implement these guidelines that, for most people, do not involve a great amount of sacrifice. The approach is intentionally kept simple, but all the basic elements of a healthful diet are covered.

The rest is up to you. Making the personal changes needed to incorporate the guidelines into your every-day life requires some commitment, knowledge, and effort. But the results are well worth it!

THE BUILDING BLOCKS OF FOOD

Before proceeding, it's necessary to first define some important terms and concepts. In particular, you need to know the "building blocks" of food and how they are used by the body.

Carbohydrates

Carbohydrates are the cheapest and most efficient source of energy for the body. Two types of carbohydrates exist:

- Simple carbohydrates, also called sugars, can be readily digested and converted directly into energy, or stored in the body as fat.

- Complex carbohydrates, comprised of many sugar molecules hooked together, are concentrated energy sources. The most common form is starches, found in breads, cereals, vegetables, pasta, rice, beans, etc.

One form of complex carbohydrates, called **fiber** or roughage, cannot be digested by the body. However, soluble fiber is believed to lower blood cholesterol levels; insoluble fiber aids in elimination and may be associated with reduced rates of colon cancer.

Fats

Fats, or lipids, are concentrated sources of calories that supply more than twice the energy of carbohydrates. High-fat foods include meats, dairy products, butter and oils, pastries, and nuts. The major components of fats are fatty acids, which fall into two basic categories:

- Saturated fats, found mostly in animal products, which are associated with elevated cholesterol levels and heart disease.

- Unsaturated fats, derived mostly from vegetable sources, which can reduce total cholesterol levels.

Fats store energy, protect and insulate the body, and aid in the absorption of fat-soluble vitamins. They also provide essential fatty acids, needed for growth and development.

Protein

Proteins are used for building, maintaining, repairing, and replacing tissues. The building blocks of protein are amino acids, which can be found in animal or plant sources. If too few calories from carbohydrates and fats are available in the diet, proteins will be used for energy. When excess protein calories are eaten, they are stored as fat.

Vitamins and Minerals

Vitamins are complex organic compounds that function as catalysts to help regulate metabolic processes. Minerals are inorganic compounds that are required in the many chemical reactions that normally occur in the human body, including the formation of tissues and the regulation of physiological processes. Both vitamins and minerals are essential for metabolic balance and energy production. (Exhibits 6-1 and 6-2 describe the function and sources of many important vitamins and minerals.)

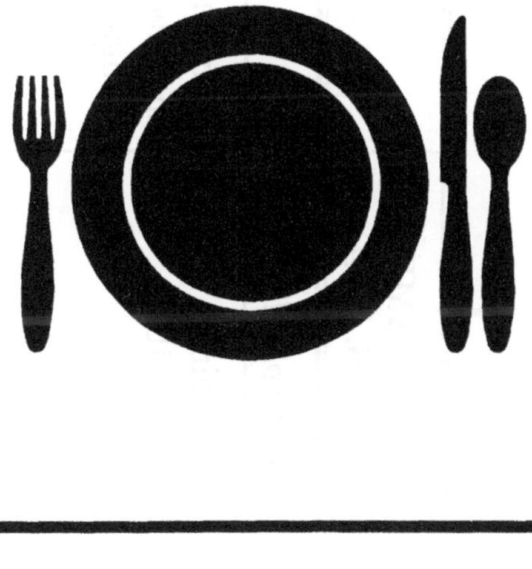

Exhibit 6-1

TABLE OF VITAMINS

VITAMIN (U.S. RDA)	FUNCTIONS	FOOD SOURCES
Fat Soluble Vitamins		
Vitamin A (5,000 IU)	Maintains normal vision and healthy skin and mucous membranes; necessary for normal growth and for reproduction	Liver, butter, whole milk, egg yolks; margarine, skim milk, and certain breakfast cereals fortified with vitamin A; the body also makes vitamin A from carotenoids, compounds present in dark-green leafy vegetables, yellow and orange vegetables, and fruit
Vitamin D (400 IU)	Promotes calcium and phosphorus absorption from the intestines; influences bone growth	Liver, butter, fatty fish, egg yolks; milk fortified with vitamin D
Vitamin E (30 IU)	Antioxidant that prevents cells from being damaged by various biochemical reactions that occur naturally	Best sources are vegetable oils; also found in nuts, seeds, whole grains, and wheat germ
Vitamin K	Aids in blood clotting	Best source is dark-green leafy vegetables; also found in cereals, dairy products, meat, and fruits
Water soluble vitamins		
Vitamin C (60 mg)	Promotes growth of connective tissues; antioxidant	Citrus fruits, tomatoes, broccoli, green peppers, strawberries, melons, cabbage, and leafy green vegetables; vitamin C is destroyed when foods are overcooked or cooked in large amounts of water
Thiamin (Vitamin B_1) (1.5 mg)	Aids in obtaining energy from carbohydrates	Meat, eggs, beans, and whole grains; enriched breads and cereals

VITAMIN (U.S. RDA)	FUNCTIONS	FOOD SOURCES
Riboflavin (Vitamin B_2) (1.7 mg)	Aids in energy production and in many other biochemical processes	Liver, milk, and dark-green leafy vegetables; whole grains and enriched breads and cereals
Niacin (20 mg)	Aids in energy production from fats, proteins, and carbohydrates; aids in manufacture of fatty acids	Grain products, meat, poultry, fish, nuts, and beans
Pyridoxine (Vitamin B_6) (2.0 mg)	Aids in manufacture of amino acids; aids in energy production from protein	Meat, poultry, fish, grain products, and fruits and vegetables
Cobalamin (Vitamin B_{12}) (6 μg)	Aids in DNA synthesis, and in energy production from fatty acids and carbohydrates; aids in production of amino acids	Meat, milk and milk products, and eggs
Folacin (.4 mg)	Aids in manufacture of genetic material in cells; aids in production of amino acids	Dark-green leafy vegetables, liver, and fruits
Biotin (.3 mg)	Aids in energy production	Egg yolks, liver, beans, and nuts
Pantothenic acid (10 mg)	Aids in energy production; aids in the manufacture of fatty acids; participates in many other biochemical processes	Most foods

Exhibit 6-2

TABLE OF MINERALS

MINERALS (U.S. RDA)	FUNCTIONS	FOOD SOURCES
Calcium (1.0 g.)	The most abundant mineral in the body, 99 percent is in bones; also important in muscle function	Dairy products, bones of sardines and canned salmon, dark-green leafy vegetables, and lime-processed tortillas
Chloride	A component of stomach acid; aids in maintaining fluid balance in cells	Table salt, eggs, meat, and milk
Chromium	Works with insulin to promote carbohydrate and fat metabolism	Liver and other organ meats, brewer's yeast, whole grains, and nuts
Copper (2 mg.)	Aids in energy production; aids in absorption of iron from digestive tract; forms dark pigment in hair and skin	Liver, meat, whole grains, and nuts
Fluoride	Strengthens teeth and bones	Some natural waters, fluoridated water, and tea
Iodine (150 μg.)	Part of the thyroid hormones that regulate metabolism	Iodized table salt, ocean seafood, dairy products, and commercially made bread
Iron (18 mg.)	Aids in energy production; helps to carry oxygen in the blood stream and muscles	Meat, poultry, fish, nuts, whole and enriched grain products, and green vegetables
Magnesium (400 mg.)	Is necessary for nerve function, bone formation, and general metabolic processes	Grain products, vegetables, dairy products, fish, meat, and poultry

MINERALS (U.S. RDA)	FUNCTIONS	FOOD SOURCES
Manganese	Aids in regulation of carbohydrate metabolism and in general metabolic processes	Cereals and most other plant foods
Molybdenum	Aids in energy production	Meat, beans, and cereals
Phosphorus (1.0 g.)	Aids in bone formation, general metabolic processes, and energy production and storage	Dairy products, meat, poultry, fish and grain products
Potassium	Necessary to maintain fluid balance in cells, transmit nerve signals, and produce energy	Fruits and vegetables, nuts, grains, and seeds
Selenium	Protects cells against harmful reactions involving oxygen; aids in detoxifying toxic substances	Meat, ocean fish, and wheat
Sodium	Necessary to maintain fluid balance in cells, transmit nerve signals, and relax muscles	Table salt and salt added to food during processing
Zinc (15 mg.)	Necessary for cell reproduction and tissue repair and growth	Oysters and other shellfish, meat, poultry, eggs, hard cheeses, milk, yogurt, beans, nuts, and whole-grain cereals

Water

Water is the primary component of body fluids. In fact, the human body is mostly composed of water—55 to 65 percent for females and 65 to 75 percent for males. This simple compound is crucial for many of the body's most important functions:

♦ Digestion and absorption of food from the gastrointestinal tract, and the elimination of waste products.

♦ Carrying nutrients and oxygen to and from working tissues through the blood and other body fluids.

♦ Dissipating heat through the evaporation of sweat.

♦ Lubricating and cushioning joints and tissues.

♦ Maintaining proper muscle tone and endocrine gland function.

Water is also important for weight control since adequate levels of hydration suppress the appetite naturally and help the body metabolize stored fat. On average, you should drink 6-8 cups of water a day—that's about two quarts.

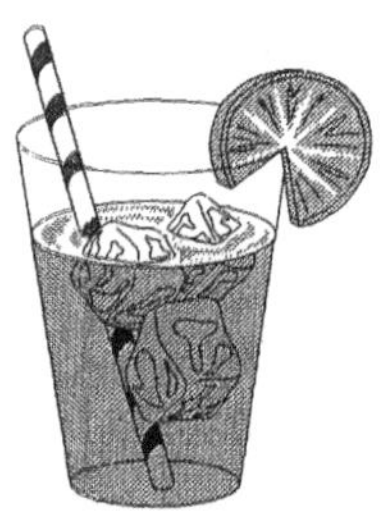

FOOD ENERGY

Foods provide the energy needed to perform the many activities you do each day. The energy in food is measured in kilocalories, or more simply, **calories**.

Most of the energy you need, about two-thirds, is used for metabolism, the basic processes required to sustain life. These include the constant functioning of the heart, kidneys, liver, brain, lungs, muscles, and other organs. The remaining energy is used for physical activity, including all movement for work or play. The more activities you perform, the more energy you need.

"Caloric balance" occurs when the intake of food energy equals the energy expended for metabolism and physical activity. When excess energy is consumed in food, it is stored as fat. Conversely, when more energy is used than consumed, the body burns its internal fat or other sources of stored energy.

Different foods contain different amounts of energy. Carbohydrates are the cheapest and most abundant source, containing 4 calories per gram. Fats are a particularly high source of energy, with 9 calories per gram. The other primary source of food energy is protein, containing 4 calories per gram. Proteins are metabolized for energy during periods of starvation, crash dieting, etc.

DIETARY GUIDELINES FOR GOOD HEALTH

NAS STUDY

A great number of studies have been conducted on the relationships among diet, nutrition, and health. As a result, much has been learned about proper eating. Unfortunately, the volume, diversity, and technical nature of the studies sometimes makes it difficult for non-experts to sort out all the information.

To provide useful advice to the American public, scientists of the Committee on Diet and Health of the Food and Nutrition Board at the National Academy of Sciences (NAS) reviewed thousands of pertinent studies. Their goal was "to determine what dietary constituents, if any, play a role in the occurrence of chronic diseases" and "to recommend dietary changes that would promote longer, healthier lives for the general public of the United States." (NAS 1992)

Based on this effort, the NAS prepared a series of dietary guidelines designed to reduce the risk of developing various diseases and health problems. Several characteristics about these guidelines should be noted:

- Unlike the majority of studies and recommendations, the guidelines address a broad spectrum of chronic diseases. Therefore, they provide a comprehensive framework for healthful eating.

- The guidelines are not the rules of a "diet" but an "eating pattern for life." They can be implemented in many ways, in many different types of cooking styles. They provide "a philosophy of eating" that can guide you as you plan meals, cook, shop, and eat out.

- The guidelines may require you to make some changes in the way you eat, but any changes should be gradual and progressive. There's no need to give up all your favorite foods or switch overnight to new ones.

The three most important NAS dietary guidelines are discussed in detail below. Other guidelines, which have more limited applicability and health implications, are then briefly summarized.

Guideline #1

Reduce total fat intake to 30 percent or less of your total calorie consumption. Reduce saturated fatty acid intake to less than 10 percent of calories. Reduce cholesterol intake to less than 300 milligrams (mg) daily.

Total Fat and Saturated Fats

Americans eat too much fat. Diets high in saturated fats are associated with the buildup of plaque in coronary arteries and heart disease. Diets high in total fats are also linked to some types of cancer, particularly cancer of the colon, prostate, and possibly breast. Finally, high-fat foods contribute to weight gain and obesity.

The NAS guidelines recommend limiting consumption of fat to 30 percent of total calories consumed (versus 36 percent in the average American diet). Saturated fats should be held to 1/3 or less of this amount, or 10 percent of total calories (versus the current 13 percent). **These recommended levels are considered to be upper limits.** Evidence suggests that further reductions may result in even greater health benefits.

Since each gram of fat contains 9 calories, foods high in fat tend to be high in calories, too. How much fat you should eat depends on your energy needs, which are different for everyone. Factors include a person's size, gender, metabolism, and activity level.

Most saturated fats in the American diet come from dairy and meat products. Other sources include certain vegetable oils, particularly coconut and palm oils. A lot of these same foods are also high in total fat. Other high-fat foods include many sweets, other oils, chocolate, nuts and nut butters, avocados, and olives.

To get a rough estimate of your calorie needs and how much fat is appropriate in your diet (in calories and grams), see Exhibits 6-3 and 6-4 on the following pages.

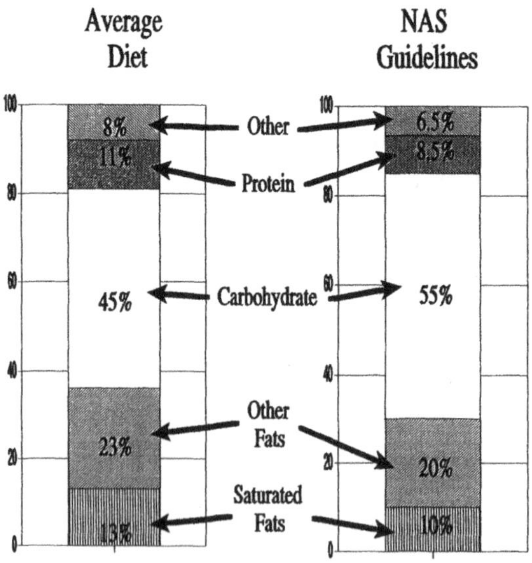

Exhibit 6-3

ENERGY NEEDS IN CALORIES

WEIGHT	MEN			WOMEN		
	A	B	C	A	B	C
80				1,264	1,480	1,688
90				1,302	1,525	1,739
100	1,630	1,900	2,170	1,340	1,570	1,790
110	1,685	1,964	2,243	1,378	1,615	1,841
120	1,740	2,028	2,316	1,416	1,660	1,892
130	1,795	2,092	2,389	1,454	1,705	1,943
140	1,850	2,156	2,462	1,492	1,750	1,994
150	1,905	2,220	2,535	1,530	1,795	2,045
160	1,960	2,284	2,608	1,568	1,840	2,096
170	2,015	2,348	2,681	1,606	1,885	2,147
180	2,070	2,412	2,754	1,644	1,930	2,198
190	2,125	2,476	2,827	1,682	1,975	2,249
200	2,180	2,540	2,900	1,720	2,020	2,300
210	2,235	2,604	2,973	1,758	2,065	2,351
220	2,290	2,668	3,046	1,796	2,110	2,402
230	2,345	2,732	3,119	1,834	2,155	2,453
240	2,400	2,796	3,192	1,872	2,200	2,504
250	2,455	2,860	3,265	1,910	2,245	2,555
260	2,510	2,924	3,338	1,948	2,290	2,606
270	2,565	2,988	3,411	1,986	2,335	2,657
280	2,620	3,052	3,484	2,024	2,380	2,708
290	2,675	3,116	3,557			
300	2,730	3,180	3,630			

Key: A = Little physical activity B = Moderate activity C = Regular exercise or manual labor
Based on formulas provided in *Eat for Life* by the National Academy of Sciences

Exhibit 6-4

RECOMMENDED FAT INTAKE

TOTAL CALORIES	CALORIES FROM FAT	CALORIES FROM SATURATED FAT	GRAMS OF FAT	GRAMS OF SATURATED FAT
1200	360	120	40	13
1300	390	130	43	14
1400	420	140	47	16
1500	450	150	50	17
1600	480	160	53	18
1700	510	170	57	19
1800	540	180	60	20
1900	570	190	63	21
2000	600	200	67	22
2100	630	210	70	23
2200	660	220	73	24
2300	690	230	77	26
2400	720	240	80	27
2500	750	250	83	28
2600	780	260	87	29
2700	810	270	90	30
2800	840	280	93	31
2900	870	290	97	32
3000	900	300	100	33
3100	930	310	103	34
3200	960	320	107	36
3300	990	330	110	37
3400	1,020	340	113	38
3500	1,050	350	117	39

Cholesterol

Cholesterol is a fat-like substance transported in the blood that is used to make hormones, cell membranes, nerve fibers, etc. Although your body needs cholesterol, high levels in the blood (above 200 milligrams per deciliter) have been shown to contribute to atherosclerosis, heart attack, and stroke.

Cholesterol in the body comes from two sources. One source is the foods we eat, so-called dietary cholesterol. The body can also manufacture all the cholesterol it needs from other foods. In particular, a diet high in saturated fat raises blood cholesterol levels in many people. Although most experts believe that dietary cholesterol is less important than saturated fat in causing heart disease, it is recommended that dietary cholesterol be limited to 300 milligrams per day.

WHERE'S THE CHOLESTEROL?
(milligrams)

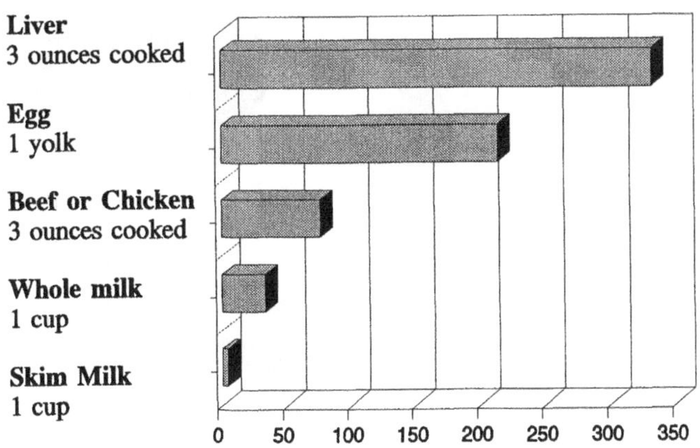

Dietary cholesterol comes only from animal products. The major foods providing dietary cholesterol are meat (particularly organ meats like liver), poultry and shellfish, egg yolks, and dairy products. Approximately 40% of all the cholesterol in the food supply comes from egg yolks.

Reducing Fat and Cholesterol

You can reduce the fat and cholesterol in your diet by limiting the amount of animal products, oils, fried foods, and other fatty foods you eat. One way to do this is to reduce the number or size of portions of these products. Another is to substitute leaner cuts of meat, fish, poultry without skin, and lower-fat dairy products for less healthy alternatives.

You need not be concerned that diets lower in animal products don't provide enough iron, calcium, or other nutrients. The study found that most people can safely reduce fat and cholesterol intake to recommended levels without risk of nutrient deficiency. In addition, low-fat diets can easily provide enough calories for couch potatoes and athletes alike. Even totally vegetarian diets can be completely healthful if an adequate variety of foods is eaten.

Guideline #2

Eat five or more servings of a combination of vegetables and fruits daily, especially green and yellow vegetables and citrus fruits. Increase your intake of starches and other complex carbohydrates by eating six or more servings of a combination of breads, cereals, and legumes. Eat a reasonable amount of protein, maintaining your protein consumption at moderate levels.

Basically, this guideline says to build your diet around vegetables, fruits, and complex carbohydrates, such as rice, pasta, whole grain cereals and breads, dry beans and peas, potatoes, and corn. These foods are good sources of vitamins, minerals, and dietary fiber. In addition, they generally contain less fat and fewer calories, thus helping to prevent heart disease and obesity. Fruits and vegetables, particularly those in the cabbage family (broccoli, cauliflower, brussels sprouts, etc.), may also contain substances that reduce cancer risk.

Five servings of fruits and vegetables and six servings of carbohydrates daily may seem like a lot, but it's really not. What counts as a serving is shown in Exhibit 6-5 on the next page. For example, a bagel for breakfast, a sandwich for lunch, and a cup of rice for dinner includes six servings of carbohydrates. As you can see, it adds up quickly! Where dishes contain portions of different food groups, use the serving sizes as a general guide—it's not necessary to be exact.

Concerning protein, most adults already eat more than they need. Therefore, it is rarely necessary to eat more protein to make up for a lower-fat diet. Consumption of meat and other animal products can be safely reduced, provided that a variety of foods is eaten. One suggestion is to limit meat to 6 ounces per day; a 3-ounce portion of meat is about the size of a deck of cards. Eating less would be even better.

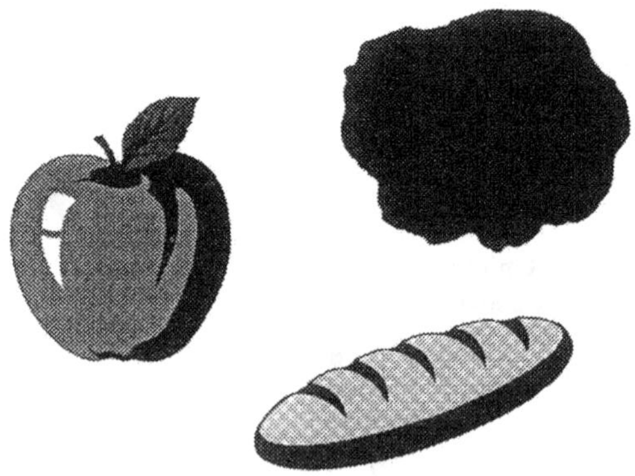

Exhibit 6-5

WHAT COUNTS AS A SERVING?

Bread, Cereal, Rice, and Pasta		
1 slice of bread	1 ounce of ready-to-eat cereal	1/2 cup of cooked cereal, rice, or pasta
Vegetables		
1 cup of raw leafy vegetables	1/2 cup of other vegetables, cooked or chopped raw	3/4 cup of vegetable juice
Fruit		
1 medium apple, banana, or orange	1/2 cup of chopped, cooked, or canned fruit	3/4 cup of fruit juice
Milk, Yogurt, and Cheese		
1 cup of milk or yogurt	1½ ounces of natural cheese	2 ounces of process cheese
Meat, Poultry, Fish, Dry Beans, Eggs, and Nuts		
2-3 ounces of cooked lean meat, poultry, or fish	1-1½ cups of cooked dry beans; 1 egg or 2 tablespoons of peanut butter count as 1 ounce of lean meat	

Source: USDA

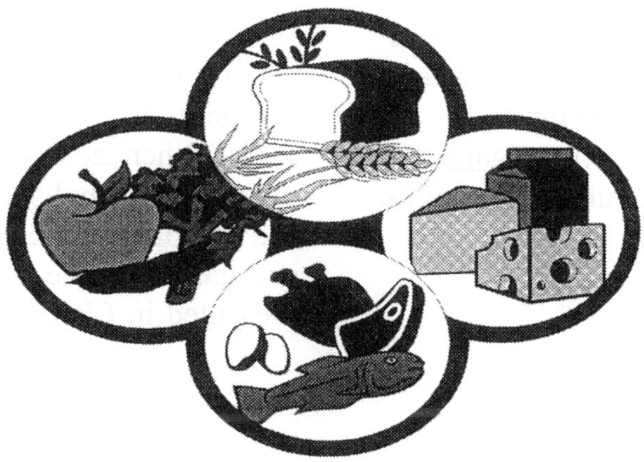

Guideline #3

Balance the amount of food you eat with the amount of exercise you get to maintain appropriate body weight.

Being overweight is associated with high blood pressure, high blood cholesterol, diabetes, heart disease, stroke, some cancers, and gall bladder disease. It also may be a factor in osteoarthritis of the weight-bearing joints. Approximately 34 million adults between the ages of 20 and 74 are overweight. Of these, 12 million are considered obese, often defined as 20 percent or more above desirable body weight. More women are overweight than men.

The basic concept behind balancing food consumption and exercise is relatively simple. If you eat more calories than you need for energy, they are stored as fat. If you do not eat enough calories, stored fat is burned to make up the difference. **To lose body fat, you must either consume fewer calories, increase your level of activity, or do some combination of the two.** According to most research, this latter strategy is the most successful. Alternatively, to gain weight, you need to eat more calories.

In spite of the health risks, average weight in the United States is increasing. Since the amount of calories consumed is actually diminishing, the difference seems to be due to lower levels of activity. Many occupations are now less physically demanding than in generations past, and too few people are exercising. According to a recent survey, about three quarters of Americans get some form of regular exercise—a 1 percent drop in the last few years. Only 33 percent engage in strenuous exercise at least three times a week, down from 37 percent in 1991. (Louis Harris and Associates 1992)

The diet described in Guidelines #1 and #2 above is generally low in fat and calories. For most people, it provides a good foundation for maintaining appropriate body weight. However, in practice, the process of weight management is more complex than simply "calories in and calories out." Other factors—including genetics, metabolism, diet history, and activity patterns—influence weight loss and gain. (More on weight control is presented in Chapter 7.)

Other NAS Guidelines

4. **Drink alcohol moderately or not at all.** Excessive alcohol consumption is associated with a long list of health problems, addiction, increased injuries, and tremendous social and personal costs. Alcoholic beverages also provide many calories (7 per gram) and few nutrients. For these reasons, it is not recommended that you drink alcohol. If you do, limit the amount to two drinks in a single day. Pregnant women should avoid alcoholic beverages entirely.

5. **Limit the amount of salt you eat.** For about half the 60 million people with high blood pressure, salt consumption may be a contributing factor. Since many people don't even know if they have the problem, it is suggested that everyone limit their daily consumption of salt to 6 grams (slightly more than 1 teaspoon), which is equivalent to 2400 milligrams of sodium. For people without high blood pressure or risk factors for developing the disease, a salty diet does not appear to pose a significant problem.

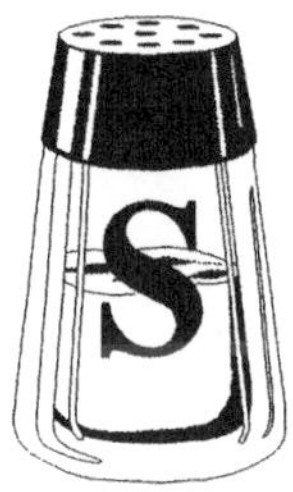

6. **Maintain adequate calcium intake.** Most people can get enough calcium from a well-balanced low-fat diet. Good sources include low-fat or non-fat milk products and dark green vegetables. However, calcium supplements may be advisable for women who have risk factors for osteoporosis, especially after menopause.

7. **Avoid taking dietary supplements in excess or the U.S. Recommended Daily Allowances (U.S. RDAs) in any one day.** Although probably not harmful in normal dosages, diet supplements—extra vitamins or minerals—are not necessary for most people who eat a variety of foods. According to the American Dietetic Association, groups who may benefit from diet supplements include women with excessive menstrual bleeding; women who are pregnant or breastfeeding; people with very low caloric intake and some vegetarians; newborns; and people with certain disorders or diseases. (U.S. RDAs for important vitamins and minerals are listed in Exhibits 6-1 and 6-2.)

8. **Maintain an optimal level of fluoride in your diet.** Drinking fluoridated water decreases tooth decay and cavities, especially in children. In 1988, about 61 percent of the population were served by fluoridated community water systems. In other areas, some schools have fluoridated water supplies. (NCHS 1992) Others should use a dietary fluoride supplement under the direction of a doctor or dentist.

Conclusions

Nutrition is a complex field, with new studies being conducted all the time. These studies provide additional information and verification about the health impacts of various foods and nutrients—antioxidants, cruciferous vegetables, different vitamins and minerals, ethnic cuisines, and so forth. While this information is valuable, the NAS guidelines presented here contain the basic framework for proper nutrition for the vast majority of persons. (People with special needs should consult with a physician, dietitian, or other expert for additional information.)

Implementing these dietary guidelines could provide major health benefits for the nation. Research shows that proper dietary practices could prevent more than 100,000 deaths from heart disease and 160,000 deaths from cancer each year. And millions of other people would be able to live fuller, more productive, and more enjoyable lives. (NAS 1992)

These recommendations should be considered **minimum** requirements for a healthy diet. They are designed to identify "reasonable" changes for the majority of the public instead of an "ideal" diet. Many experts would go even further. For example, a survey of 68 nutrition professionals conducted by *Consumer Reports* concluded that the ideal diet should provide 20-25 percent calories from fat, include seven or more servings of fruits and vegetables a day, and limit red meat to three ounces per week.

These suggestions provide general guidelines for monitoring what you eat. However, the goal is to not become an expert at counting fat and calories, but to make gradual improvements in your diet. To be successful, you need to find ways to apply the guidelines that work for you. That's the subject of the next section.

PRACTICING GOOD NUTRITION

APPLYING THE GUIDELINES

Knowing the basic guidelines for healthful eating is only the beginning. The real key to good nutrition is the ability to apply the dietary guidelines in a way that is practical and enjoyable. For most people, that's easier said than done.

The simplest way to implement the NAS dietary guidelines might be referred to as a "Choose More Often" approach. It doesn't mean giving up everything you like, but choosing more often the following low-fat alternatives:

- **Low-fat meat, poultry, and fish.** Lean cuts of meat trimmed of fat (round tip roast, pork tenderloin, loin lamb chop); poultry without skin; ground turkey; fish, cooked without breading or fat added; canned fish, water-packed and drained; egg whites.

- **Low-fat dairy products.** 1 percent or skim milk, buttermilk; low-fat or non-fat yogurt; 1 percent low-fat or dry curd cottage cheese; lower-fat cheeses (less than 2 grams of fat per ounce); ice milk and sherbet.

- **Dry beans and peas.** All beans, peas, and lentils—the dry forms are higher in protein.

- **Whole grain products.** Breads, bagels, English muffins, and tortillas made from whole wheat, rye bran, and corn flour or meal; whole grain or bran cereals; whole wheat pasta; brown rice and bulgur; low-fat crackers and snack foods (less than 1 gram fat per 1/2 ounce).

- **Fruits and vegetables.** All fruits and vegetables (except avocados and olives), without sauces.

- **Fats and oils high in unsaturated fat.** Vegetable oils (canola, corn, cottonseed, olive) and margarine; "light" mayonnaise and salad dressings.

Exhibit 6-6 lists the saturated fat, total fat, and cholesterol content of many common foods. The list is ranked from low to high saturated fat within each major food category. The products chosen for the chart are meant to be representative of their type. Fat and cholesterol content may vary slightly depending on where the foods are grown, the time of year, and the brand.

Exhibit 6-6

FOOD COMPARISON CHART

FOOD TYPE	Saturated Fat (grams)	Total Fat (grams)	Cholesterol (milligrams)
Meat, Poultry, Fish, and Shellfish (3½ oz.)			
Beef			
Top round, broiled	1.7	5.0	90
Eye of round, roasted	2.0	5.4	69
Sirloin, broiled	2.6	6.8	89
Chuck, arm pot roast, braised	2.8	7.6	101
Short loin, T-bone steak, broiled	4.2	10.4	80
Chuck, blade roast, braised	5.2	13.3	106
Ground lean, broiled	7.2	18.5	87
Salami, about 4 slices	8.4	20.1	60
Pork			
Ham steak, extra lean	1.4	4.2	45
Fresh, tenderloin, roasted	1.7	4.8	93
Shoulder, arm picnic, lean only, roasted	2.4	7.0	48
Fresh, leg, rump half, roasted	3.7	10.7	96
Lamb			
Leg, roasted	2.8	7.7	89
Loin chop, broiled	3.5	9.7	95
Arm chop, braised	5.0	14.1	121
Poultry			
Turkey, fryer-roasters, roasted:			
Light meat without skin	0.4	1.2	86
Light meat with skin	1.3	4.6	95
Dark meat without skin	1.4	4.3	112
Dark meat with skin	2.1	7.1	117
Chicken, broilers, roasted:			
Light meat without skin	1.3	4.5	85
Dark meat without skin	2.7	9.7	93
Light meat with skin	3.0	10.9	84
Dark meat with skin	4.4	15.8	91
Ground turkey	3.8	13.8	69

FOOD TYPE	Saturated Fat (grams)	Total Fat (grams)	Cholesterol (milligrams)
Fish			
Haddock, dry heat	0.2	0.9	74
Halibut, dry heat	0.4	2.9	41
Tuna, dry heat	1.6	6.3	49
Salmon, dry heat	1.9	11.0	87
Shellfish			
Lobster	0.1	0.6	72
Clam, moist heat	0.2	2.0	67
Shrimp, moist heat	0.3	1.1	195
Oyster, moist heat	1.3	5.0	109
Clam, breaded and fried	2.7	11.2	61
Dairy Products			
Milk (8 oz.)			
Skim	0.3	0.4	4
Buttermilk	1.3	2.2	9
Low-fat, 1%	1.6	2.6	10
Low-fat, 2%	2.9	4.7	18
Whole	5.1	8.2	33
Yogurt (4 oz.)			
Plain yogurt, skim	0.1	0.2	2
Plain yogurt	2.4	3.7	14
Soft cheeses (4 oz.)			
Cottage cheese, low-fat	0.7	1.2	5
Cottage cheese, creamed	3.2	5.1	17
Ricotta, part-skim	5.5	8.9	34
Ricotta, whole milk	9.3	14.5	57
Hard cheeses (1 oz.)			
Mozzarella, part-skim	2.9	4.5	16
Mozzarella	3.7	6.1	22
Swiss	5.0	7.8	26
American processed	5.6	8.9	27
Cheddar	6.0	9.4	30
Frozen Desserts (1 cup)			
Sherbet, orange	2.4	3.8	14
Ice milk, vanilla, hard	3.5	5.6	18
Ice cream, vanilla, regular	8.9	14.3	59

FOOD TYPE	Saturated Fat (grams)	Total Fat (grams)	Cholesterol (milligrams)
Eggs			
Egg, white	0	trace	0
Egg, yolk	1.6	5.1	213
Fats and Oils			
Fats and Oils (1 tbsp.)			
Canola oil	1.0	14.0	0
Safflower oil	1.2	13.6	0
Peanut butter, smooth	1.5	7.9	0
Corn oil	1.7	13.6	0
Olive oil	1.8	13.5	0
Margarine, soft tub	2.1	11.4	0
Margarine, stick	2.1	11.4	0
Lard	5.0	12.8	12
Butter	7.1	10.8	31
Nuts and Seeds (1 oz.)			
Almonds	1.4	14.8	0
Pecans	1.5	19.2	0
Sunflower seeds	1.5	14.1	0
English walnuts	1.6	17.6	0
Pistachios	1.7	13.7	0
Peanuts	1.9	13.8	0
Brazil nuts, dried	4.6	18.8	0
Breads, Cereals, Pasta, Rice, and Dry Peas and Beans			
Breads			
Corn tortilla, 1	0.1	1.0	0
English muffin, 1	0.3	1.0	0
Bagel, 1	0.3	2.0	0
Whole wheat bread, 1 slice	0.4	1.0	0
Hamburger bun, 1	0.5	2.0	trace
Croissant, 1	3.5	12.0	13
Cereals (1 cup)			
Corn flakes	trace	0.1	-
Oatmeal, cooked	0.4	2.4	-
Granola	5.8	33.1	-
Pasta (1 cup)			
Spaghetti, cooked	0.1	0.9	0
Chow mein noodles	2.0	13.8	5

FOOD TYPE	Saturated Fat (grams)	Total Fat (grams)	Cholesterol (milligrams)
Rice (1 cup cooked)			
White, long-grain	0.2	0.6	0
Dry peas and beans (1 cup canned)			
Kidney beans	0.1	0.8	0
Garbanzo beans	0.3	2.7	0
Fruits and Vegetables (3½ oz.)			
Fruit, raw			
Peach, 1	0.01	0.08	0
Orange, 1	0.02	0.16	0
Apple, 1	0.08	0.49	0
Banana, 1	0.21	0.55	0
Avocado, California, 1	4.48	29.99	0
Vegetable, cooked			
Carrot, ½ cup	0.03	0.14	0
Broccoli, ½ cup	0.03	0.22	0
Potato, 1	0.05	0.20	0
Corn, ½ cup	0.16	1.05	0
Sweet and Snacks			
Popcorn, air-popped, 1 cup	trace	0	trace
Angel food cake, 1/12 cake	trace	trace	0
Vanilla wafers, 5	0.9	3.3	12
Fig bars, 4	1.0	4.0	27
Potato chips, 1 oz.	2.6	10.1	0
Pound cake, 1/17 cake	3.0	5.0	64
Chocolate chip cookies, 4	3.9	11.0	18

Adapted from: National Institute of Health, Facts About Cholesterol, October 1990.

READING FOOD LABELS

Perhaps the most powerful tool you have in making sound nutritional choices is food labels, found on most items you buy at the grocery store. The new system of labeling is a step in the right direction, helping consumers cut through the confusing ingredient lists and promotional hype on much food packaging.

The labels require manufacturers to standardize portions, limit health claims, and print a chart of nutrients for all packaged foods. The system also formally defines the use of common terms, such as "fat free" (less than 0.5 gram of fat per serving), "low fat" (3 grams of fat or less per serving), and "lean" (less than 10 grams of fat, 4 grams of saturated fat, and 95 milligrams of cholesterol per serving).

When reading labels, look first at the serving size. If you generally eat more than this amount, you need to increase the calorie and nutrient values proportionally (and visa versa). You may also need to adjust the data listed under the "% Daily Value" column—those shown are for a 2,000 calorie per day diet; your needs may be different (see Exhibit 6-3).

Nutrition Facts

Serving Size ½ cup (114g)
Servings Per Container 4

Amount Per Serving	
Calories 90	Calories from Fat 30
	% Daily Value
Total Fat 3g	**5%**
Saturated Fat 0g	**0%**
Cholesterol 0mg	**0%**
Sodium 300 mg	**13%**
Total Carbohydrate 13g	**4%**
Dietary Fiber 3g	**12%**
Sugars 3g	
Protein 3g	

Vitamin A	80%	*	Vitamin C	60%
Calcium	4%	*	Iron	4%

* Percent Daily Values are based on a 2,000 calorie diet. Your daily values may be higher or lower depending on your calorie needs:

	Calories	2,000	2,500
Total Fat	Less than	65g	80g
Sat Fat	Less than	20g	25g
Cholesterol	Less than	300mg	300mg
Sodium	Less than	2,400mg	2,400mg
Total Carbohydrate		300g	375g
Fiber		25g	30g

Calories per gram:
Fat 9 • Carbohydrate 4 • Protein 4

Several bits of information on the nutritional label are helpful for watching your fat intake. First, look at the calories from fat and compare this amount with total calories. Since the dietary guidelines recommend limiting fat to 30% of total daily calories, individual foods that exceed this percentage will probably fall into the "choose less often" category. Also consider the grams of total fat and saturated fat per serving, and decide if you want to expend this amount of your daily "allowance" on this one food (see Exhibit 6-4 to estimate your recommended fat intake). You should do the same with total calories.

Other information is listed on nutrients that the Food and Drug Administration identifies as important to health, calculated as follows:

- Cholesterol, less than 300 milligrams per day
- Sodium, less than 2,400 milligrams daily
- Carbohydrate, 60% or more of calories
- Protein, 10% of calories
- Vitamins and minerals, 100% each day, based on USRDAs (see Exhibits 6-1 and 6-2).

FINDING YOUR STYLE

Learning the NAS nutrition guidelines and the nutrient content of individual foods is critical for improving your diet. But to make long-term progress, you also need to find a healthful eating style that's right for you.

The style you adopt should be enjoyable—you don't need to give up good taste or feel deprived for good nutrition. Furthermore, whatever style you adopt must be made part of your daily routine. That means following this healthful approach "most of the time," particularly at home and at work. Then you can make exceptions as needed for special occasions, and still stay within the nutrition guidelines.

Fortunately, the options for preparing nutritious foods are virtually limitless. The key to finding your style is a willingness to experiment and an openness to new food experiences. When you discover an enjoyable dish, add it to your list of options; if you don't like it, try something else next time.

The difficulty, of course, is that we've all grown up to like certain kinds of foods, and it's difficult to change. Certain situations present overwhelming temptations. Family and friends may contribute to the problem. Often, healthful alternatives are inconvenient, more expensive, or simply not available.

Since everyone is different, you need to think through your own unique situation. Some general suggestions for finding and implementing a healthful eating style follow:

- Try to think of change as an adventure, a chance to learn and to gain new experiences. Be positive—you probably will find many new foods to enjoy.
- Try ethnic foods. Some cuisines from other cultures are healthful and very flavorful. (Restaurants, however, often prepare these dishes for American tastes, adding much more fat and salt.)
- Experiment with vegetarian main courses or meat substitutes. Also, try the new low fat or no fat versions of foods. (However, beware of items like the "lean" burger at fast-food restaurants, which usually have added cheese and mayonnaise-based sauce.)
- Get in the habit of planning meals before you shop. Many excellent healthful cookbooks are available to help guide your selections.
- Be polite but firm at supermarkets and restaurants—you have the right to get what you want.

More on changing eating behaviors is covered in Chapter 8 on weight control.

Activity 6-1

NUTRITION PLANNING

During this activity, you will have an opportunity to identify times when practicing good nutrition is particularly difficult for you. Then you will select a limited number of small changes to make over the next three to six weeks to improve your eating patterns. Remember: change should occur gradually over time; otherwise, most people have a tendency to slip back to old habits or give up entirely.

The number and type of actions you pick is up to you. However, it is important to be specific so that you clearly define your objectives. Also, be realistic: choose actions that you are **willing** and **able** to accomplish. Don't set yourself up for disappointment!

ACTIVITY INSTRUCTIONS

1. Brainstorm a list of common situations (locations, events, circumstances, people, etc.) when you find it difficult to eat well. Write your responses below. (Hint: don't try to analyze the list at this point, just write down the most important ones.)

2. Keeping these situations in mind, fill out the action plan on the next page. As the changes you identify become easier, consider adding others until you reach your long-term goal. In the future, review the plan occasionally and update it as necessary.

Activity 6-1 (Continued)

WORKSHEET

1. Given what you have learned in this chapter, how would you rate the nutritional quality of your own diet (circle one)?

GOOD FAIR POOR

2. Based on your answer to Question 1, select specific steps you will take in each of the three categories below. (If "good," choose at least one action in each category; if "poor," select two actions; if "fair," select one to two actions.)

A. Eating less fat and cholesterol

1. ______________________________

2. ______________________________

3. ______________________________

B. Eating more fruit, vegetables, and complex carbohydrates

1. ______________________________

2. ______________________________

3. ______________________________

C. Controlling situations that encourage poor nutrition

1. ______________________________

2. ______________________________

3. ______________________________

3. Review your action plan and revise it until you feel comfortable with it. Then sign and date it below.

____

Signature and Date

CHAPTER SUMMARY

During this module, you learned how the building blocks of food are used by the body. Guidelines for nutrition developed by the National Academy of Sciences were examined, with a particular emphasis on 1) reducing consumption of fat and cholesterol, 2) increasing servings of fruits, vegetables, and complex carbohydrates, and 3) maintaining proper body weight through diet and exercise.

Then you reviewed some methods for applying the NAS guidelines to your daily life, including a "choose more often" approach to nutrition and a brief review of food labels. Finally, you thought about situations in your own life when eating well is difficult, and identified some specific steps you will take in the near future to improve your eating habits.

Having completed this chapter, you should now be able to:

- Identify the risks associated with unhealthy eating patterns.
- Explain basic terms and concepts of nutrition.
- Describe dietary guidelines for good health in daily life.
- Discuss different suggestions for developing your own healthful eating style.
- Develop a short-term action plan for improving your nutrition.

BIBLIOGRAPHY

American Cancer Society, *Eating Smart*, 1987.

Consumers Union, "Are You Eating Right," *Consumer Reports*, October 1992.

Lafferty, Libby, and Maureen Dillard, "Keep the Fat Out of the Fire," *Fire Chief Magazine*, June 1985.

Louis Harris and Associates, Inc., *The Baxter Survey of American Health Habits*, Study No. 923009, December 1992.

National Academy of Sciences, *Eat for Life*, Washington, D.C.: National Academy Press, 1992.

National Center for Health Statistics, *Health, United States*, Hyattsville, Maryland: Public Health Service, 1992.

Nugent, Mark R., "The Nutritional Overhaul: A Plan You Can Live With," *Firehouse*, July 1993.

Passwater, Dick, "Eating Right," *Firehouse*, June 1989.

President's Council on Physical Fitness and Sports, *Exercise and Weight Control*, Pamphlet.

Sloan, Elizabeth Schaff, "Herb Tea for the Tillerman," *9-1-1 Magazine*, May/June 1990.

United States Department of Agriculture, *Dietary Guidelines for Americans*, November 1990.

United States Department of Agriculture, *The Food Guide Pyramid*, Home and Garden Bulletin Number 252.

United States Department of Health and Human Services, *Diet, Nutrition & Cancer Prevention: The Good News*, NIH Publication No 87-2878, September 1987.

United States Fire Administration, *Physical Fitness Coordinator's Manual For Fire Departments*, September 1990.

University of California at Berkeley, "The New Thinking About Fats," *Wellness Letter*, September 1993.

COMPREHENSIVE WELLNESS FOR FIREFIGHTERS

Chapter 7

Body Composition and Weight Control

CHAPTER INTRODUCTION

Previous chapters of this book emphasized the first three components of physical fitness: flexibility, cardiovascular fitness, and muscular fitness. The fourth and equally important component of physical fitness is **body composition**, defined as the ratio of the body's lean and fat tissues. In other words, body composition measures the percentage of a person's weight that is composed of fat.

Excess fat can directly affect your health, physical fitness, and ability to perform as a firefighter or emergency rescue worker. For this reason, attaining a healthy body weight and maintaining it over your lifetime should be a goal of every member of the fire service.

In this chapter, you will learn some of the basic principles of weight management. What works and what doesn't work for most people is discussed. You will then have an opportunity to take a look at some of your own eating behaviors. Based on this analysis, you will identify personal strategies for controlling your diet and weight. Finally, you will prepare a short-term action plan for weight management.

LEARNING OBJECTIVES

After learning the information in this chapter, you will be able to:

- Define body composition and identify healthy and unhealthy levels of body fat.
- Discuss general principles of weight gain, loss, and maintenance.
- Identify effective and ineffective strategies for weight loss based on current research.
- Analyze your own eating behaviors and identify possible areas for improvement.
- Determine personal strategies and establish short-term goals for weight management.

BODY COMPOSITION AND HEALTH

The excessive accumulation of body fat is one of the most important risk factors for the development of cardiovascular disease. It is also a powerful predictor of many other diseases, including diabetes and certain forms of cancer. Furthermore, excess weight places an enormous strain on joints and muscles, eventually leading to musculoskeletal injuries, especially involving the lower back and knees. In short, high levels of body fat lead to a host of problems that tend to shorten life expectancy and decrease the pleasure of living.

The 1990 National Health Interview Survey reported that approximately 26 percent of both men and women over 18 years of age are overweight. As shown below, more women than men are overweight, and percentages tend to go up with age.

Percent of population overweight (1976-1980)

Age	Male	Female
20-24	12.1	11.4
25-34	20.4	20.0
35-44	28.9	27.0
45-54	31.1	32.5
55-64	28.1	37.0
65-74	25.2	38.5

Source: NCHS 1992

Reductions in the percentage of men who are overweight after age 55 is likely due to the overall reduction of overweight males in the general population through heart disease and related ailments.

WEIGHT CONTROL AND THE FIRE SERVICE

The fire service is not immune to these national trends. "On the average, most firefighters could stand to lose approximately 10 pounds of fat....Firefighters tend to add close to 20 extra pounds of fat to their frame over the span of their careers. The recommended trend would be to hold body fat constant." (USFA 1990)

Excess weight among firefighters contributes to early death from heart attack, the leading cause of incident fatalities. The added stress on muscles and bones also puts overweight firefighters at an increased risk for sprains, strains, and back injuries that already are common occupational injuries. And each extra pound of fat translates into a progressive reduction in cardiovascular fitness and performance in critical job tasks. For these reasons, many departments enforce rigorous weight control standards for fire suppression and rescue workers.

BODY COMPOSITION

In the past, people concerned about health, fitness, and job performance focused a great deal on total body weight. "Height/Weight Charts" were devised to provide some guidance on supposedly "healthy" body weights. The question of what composed this weight did not receive much attention.

However, two people of the same height and weight may have very different amounts of fat and muscle. Nowadays, it is well accepted that an individual's weight is not as important as his/her body composition. That's because the proportion of weight that is fat is a much better indicator of health than just weight alone.

Fat Storage

As you remember from the last chapter, fat is primarily a mechanism for the storage of food energy. After eating, fat is transported through the blood stream until it reaches one of the body's millions of fat cells. The body stores the fat when excess calories taken in through food and drink are not needed for metabolism or physical activity.

Basically, there are two kinds of fat:

- Essential Fat, which surrounds the brain, nervous system, and other internal organs. On average, essential fat comprises about 3% of total body weight for males and 9% for females. The higher percentage for females accounts for breast and reproductive tissue.

- Storage Fat—Storage fat is the result of unused calories. When needed, it is available to provide an abundant source of fuel and energy for movement and various physiologic processes.

Gaining fat is either the result of too little exercise and activity, too many calories in the diet, or a combination of both. Losing fat implies the opposite. "Caloric balance" is achieved when the number of calories in the daily diet approximately equals the number of calories expended.

An "ideal" level of body fat is an amount that provides adequate fuel stores, does not place a significant burden on other body systems, and is associated with optimal health and fitness. In males, an ideal level of body fat is generally considered to be between 10% and 15%; for females, it's between 17% and 23%. Exhibit 7-1 on the next page shows standard body composition categories for men and women.

Exhibit 7-1

BODY COMPOSITION CATEGORIES

Category	Males	Females
Obesity	Over 25%	Over 30%
Overfat	20-25%	26-30%
Healthy	16-19%	23-25%
Ideal	Under 16%	Under 23%

Location of Body Fat

Recent research indicates that the location of fat on the body may be even more important than the total amount a person carries. "Above the waist" fat (android pattern) is typical of males, while "below the waist" fat (gynoid pattern) is typical of females. However, either pattern can be found in members of both sexes.

Fat located above the hips—so called intra-abdominal fat—appears to pose a much greater risk for heart disease than that deposited in the gluteals and thighs. This may be one reason why women, who on average have more fat than men, exhibit a lower incidence of heart problems.

Many experts now advocate broadening the concept of body composition to include the location of fat. One way to estimate this factor is by dividing your waist size by your hip size, as determined through circumference measurements. People whose waist is larger than their hips have a "waist-to-hip ratio" greater than 1; those whose waist is smaller than their hips have a ratio less than one. According to the Food and Drug Administration, ratios above 0.8 for women and 0.95 for men indicate a high risk of weight-related health problems.

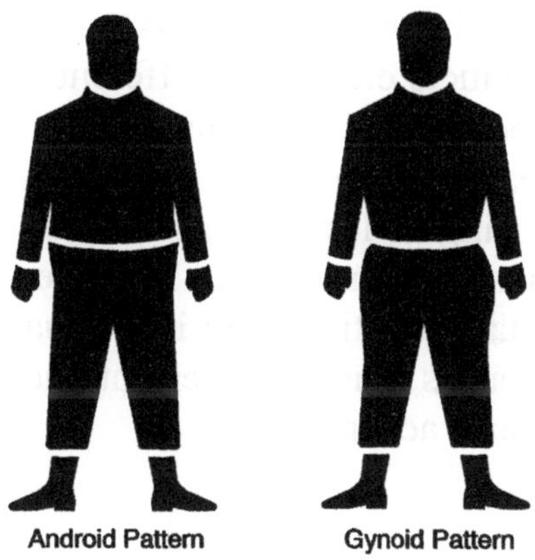

Measuring Body Composition

Experts are continually searching for more practical and inexpensive ways to assess body composition. Right now, the most common methods include skinfold measurement, bioelectrical impedance analysis, and underwater weighing. These methods are reviewed briefly below. (Otis 1991 and Kravitz 1992)

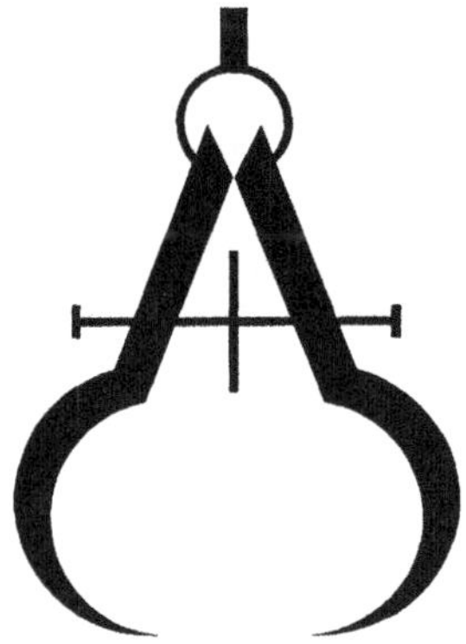

Underwater (hydrostatic) weighing compares a person's weight in air with his/her weight submerged in water. Since fat is more buoyant than dense muscle and bone, leaner people (all else being equal) weigh more underwater. Underwater weighing is relatively accurate and widely used, although the procedure may be somewhat more expensive than other methods. The margin of error is between 2 and 3.5 percent.

Bioelectrical impedance analysis measures the current flow between electrodes placed on the skin. Body fat estimates are based on the principle that fat tissue contains less water, and so conducts electricity differently than lean body mass. The process is safe and painless, and its popularity is increasing as less expensive equipment options are introduced. However, external conditions and individual differences must be taken into account to ensure accuracy.

Skinfold measurements are the least expensive and most common method of measuring body fat. This approach involves pinching skin and fat between calipers at several different sites on the body to measure thickness. Age- and gender-specific calculations can then be used to estimate total body fat, based on subcutaneous fat. The margin of error, which is largely dependent on the skill of the measurer, is typically is between 2 and 5 percent.

Other methods used to estimate body composition include circumference or diameter measures taken at various sites on the body, near-infrared spectrophotometry, ultrasound analysis, magnetic resonance imagery, and proton absorptionmetry. All of these methods show some promise, although accuracy, equipment requirements, and costs vary significantly.

In summary, a range of methods exist to assess body composition, each with advantages and disadvantages. Simple techniques are generally available through health clubs and personal trainers, sometimes for free or a small fee. Others methods are available through hospitals, industrial medicine facilities, or other experts. None are 100 percent accurate, so most people should choose a method based on cost, convenience, and related factors.

WEIGHT GAIN AND LOSS

Dieting has become a national obsession. Data from the 1990 National Health Interview Survey shows that 46 percent of overweight men and 61 percent of overweight women tried to lose weight in 1990. Unfortunately, most of these attempts were unsuccessful in the long run. A study last May by the National Institutes of Health found that 90 percent of dieters regain almost all their weight within five years, most within a year or two.

PRINCIPLES OF WEIGHT GAIN AND LOSS

Number of Fat Cells

Excess calories are stored in fat cells. As these cells hold more and more fat, they swell in size. Conversely, when fat is released from the cells into the bloodstream for energy, the fat cells shrink again. But they never shrink so much that they go away completely. When low in fat, the cells are merely waiting to store fat again the next time excess calories are available.

In general, the number of fat cells in the body is determined by genetics. However, there is now convincing evidence that this number does not necessarily stay constant throughout life. When fat cells reach a critically large size, they can divide into more fat cells!

Extra fat cells in the body mean more fat receptacles and an increased ability of the body to store fat. Once the number of fat cells has increased, there are more of them that will never go away. Since people with a high number of fat cells have a harder time losing fat, periods of obesity tend to make future weight loss even more difficult.

Metabolism

The daily processes inside your body that sustain life are collectively referred to as your "metabolism." These include the constant functioning of the heart, kidneys, liver, brain, lungs, digestive tract, muscles, and other organs. Such processes consume thousands of calories every day.

Metabolic rates of individuals are primarily determined by two factors: the functioning of the thyroid gland, and the amount of a person's lean body mass. The functioning of the thyroid gland is largely a product of your genes. Certain chemicals and hormones can affect this gland, but such manipulations should occur only in the case of documented disease, and only under the direct supervision of a physician.

For example, some weight control programs have actually used synthetic thyroid hormone to boost metabolism. The drug works well, but it puts the body into a hyper-metabolic state, where side effects include racing heart, insomnia, and hair loss. It can also cause a slowing of normal metabolism once the drug is discontinued, meaning that fat is regained easily.

Muscles are the real "engines" of the body, potentially burning thousands of calories each day. As a result, people with a high degree of lean body mass tend to have higher metabolic rates, which help to maintain a stable body weight without much dieting.

This principle provides another good reason to incorporate daily physical activity into your lifestyle. Without it, muscles begin to shrink, resulting in a gradual loss of lean body mass. Strength training is particularly effective for increasing muscle mass, thus gradually raising the body's metabolic rate. Aerobic exercise, for at least 20-30 minutes, 3-5 times a week, also helps reduce body fat and increase metabolic rate.

Rapid Weight Loss

Some people try to lose weight quickly, usually by fasting or drastically reducing their caloric intake. Many common diet plans advocate this strategy, a process sometimes referred to as "crash dieting."

In this situation, the body attempts to preserve itself as it would in times of famine or starvation. Its natural response or defense mechanism is to conserve calories. Life processes slow down so that the overall metabolic rate is reduced. Fat cells become increasingly resistant to giving up the fat molecules they contain. With prolonged caloric deprivation, they actually adapt to become even more efficient in the storage of fat. **This slower burning of calories and more efficient fat storage combine to make weight loss even harder.**

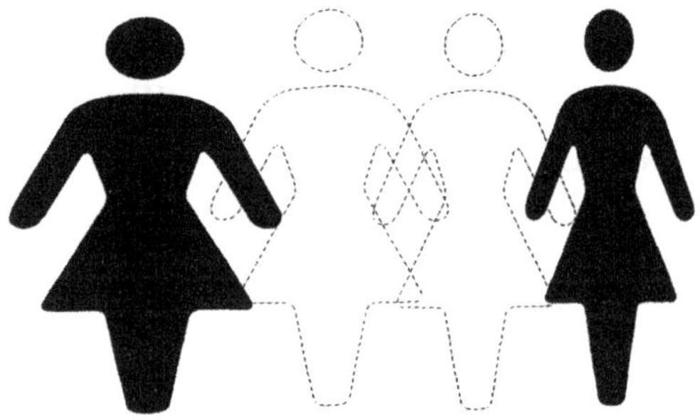

In addition, since less fat is available for fuel, stored glycogen within muscle tissue is burned instead. This process releases large amounts of water. Hence, when someone loses weight rapidly, much of the "weight" lost is only fluid, primarily from muscle tissue. Since fat contains very little water, this fluid loss doesn't have much impact on stored fat.

"Yo-Yo Dieting"

Many people, including firefighters and rescue workers, are "yo-yo dieters" whose weight fluctuates dramatically. Weight gain and loss may occur several times during the same year. These persons approach weight loss as a short-term, all-out effort, usually involving fasting or crash dieting. After a brief period of weight loss, they revert to their old habits of excessive eating or too little activity, and they begin to gain weight again...until they decide it's time for another crash diet.

What really happens during "yo-yo dieting?" In the crash diet phase, when they think they are losing fat, they're mostly losing fluid (from their muscles and lean body mass, primarily). Their fat cells don't shrink much at all, but they do improve their fat storage efficiency. After the diet is over, more fat is stored and the fat cells swell to even greater size. Eventually, those fat cells may divide into more fat cells, with each new cell having the same capacity as the original one. This pattern repeats itself with each new cycle.

The end result of yo-yo dieting is too often someone who gradually gains more and more fat. **In fact, a history of weight loss and gain actually makes losing weight more difficult in the future.**

Weight and Genetics

The number of fat cells you are born with, their location, and your metabolic rate are all largely determined by genetics. So may be the body's efficiency at storing fat. In fact, the link between weight and genetics is so strong that many experts now postulate the existence of "obesity genes" which strongly predispose certain people to being overweight.

Many experts also believe that everyone has an established "set point" for weight. If anything is done to change weight from this set point—either up or down—the body makes adjustments to restore fat content to the predetermined level. Unfortunately, this set point appears to go higher after sustained weight gain, but the reverse may not be true.

Besides genetics, factors like childhood eating patterns and dieting history, both of which affect future weight loss efforts, are effectively beyond our control. For these reasons, it may sometimes seem like the "deck is stacked" against certain people and real weight management is not possible.

However, becoming obese due to an actual medical disorder is not all that common. In the vast majority of cases, gaining fat is a result of long-term lifestyle habits that involve eating more calories than are expended through physical activity. **This process can be reversed over time**, although some people may have to work at it much harder than others.

WHAT WORKS

Fortunately, you already know a lot about what works for weight management, since proper nutrition and exercise are key factors. Reducing the amount of high-fat foods you eat and increasing servings of fruits, vegetables, and carbohydrates—the components of a nutritious diet—also reduce calories. Raising the metabolic rate through exercise burns off even more calories, thus contributing to total weight loss. Exercise also may temporarily suppress the appetite.

According to most research, this "combination" strategy—diet and exercise—is the most successful. The key is making these changes a part of your everyday lifestyle.

Reducing Caloric Intake

As long as someone burns more calories than they take in, they will continue to gradually lose body fat. In order to lose one pound of fat, the body must burn an excess of 3500 calories. Since this is a lot of calories to burn on any given day, most experts recommend that losing weight be approached gradually.

Realistic goals include a moderate reduction of calories combined with a moderate increase in activity so that an excess of 500 to 1000 calories are burned in any given day. Over a week, this translates to an excess caloric expenditure of 3500 to 7000 calories, or a loss of between one to two pounds of fat.

Focusing on Fats

One of the best and simplest ways to watch calories while simultaneously emphasizing good nutrition is to monitor fat intake. Although fat gives flavor and consistency to food, each gram of fat contains 9 calories, so most foods high in fat are also high in calories. Switching to lower-fat alternatives allows you to enjoy larger portions for the same "price" in calories.

In addition, some research indicates that the amount of fat in your diet may actually be more important for causing weight gain than other calories you consume. This is because calories from fat are used differently by the body. Fat is immediately stored in fat cells, while calories from carbohydrates are used for fuel until all the body's energy needs are met.

As a result, focusing on fats can be an effective weight control strategy. Even if you don't need to lose weight, the approach is useful for limiting the risk of heart disease, cancer, and other illnesses. However, don't be fooled: fat intake is only one factor in weight control. You will not lose weight by cutting out fats if you continue to eat too many calories from other sources.

Exhibit 7-2 shows the grams of fat in a representative serving of many common high-fat foods. Compare these amounts with your own daily fat allowance that you determined in Chapter 6, *Nutrition: Practical Guidelines for Good Health.*

Exhibit 7-2

FAT CONTENT OF SELECTED FOODS
(Grams)

Butter, Oils

Butter, margarine (1 tbsp)	12
Mayonnaise, regular (1 tbsp)	11
Salad dressing, regular (1 tbsp)	7
Vegetable oil (1 tbsp)	14
Bacon fat or lard (1 tbsp)	10

Pastries

Croissant (1 large)	12
Doughnut (1 medium)	11
Danish (1 medium)	13
Muffin (1 medium)	9

Dairy Products

Cream cheese (1 oz).	10
Sour cream (2 tbsp)	6
Whole milk (1 cup)	8
Heavy cream (¼ cup)	22
Half and half (¼ cup)	7
Natural cheddar cheese (1½ oz).	14
Process cheese (2 oz).	18
Whole milk yogurt (1 cup)	8

Sweets, Desserts

Cake, frosted (⅛ average)	26
Brownies (1 medium)	15
Pie, fruit, 2-crust (⅛ 8" pie)	14
Whipped cream (¼ cup)	11
Ice cream, regular (1 cup)	14
Chocolate bar (2¼ oz.)	20

Meat, Eggs, Nuts

Chicken, with skin, fried (3 oz).	13
Cold cuts (2½ oz).	21
Ground beef, lean, cooked (3 oz).	16
Bacon (3 slices)	21
Sausages (2 oz.—1 link)	22
Porterhouse steak (10 oz. serving)	89
Pork spareribs (7 oz. serving)	77
Eggs (2 large)	12
Peanut butter (2 tbsp)	16
Nuts (⅓ cup)	22

Vegetables

Avocado (¼ whole)	9
Olives (4)	5

Fast Foods

Cheeseburger (1)	14
Double hamburger on roll (1)	54
Ham and cheese sandwich (1)	20
Tuna submarine (6" sandwich)	28
Pepperoni pizza (2 slices)	24
Taco (2)	26
French fries (21—small order)	16
Onion rings (6)	22
Chocolate milk shake (1)	14
Potatoes, scalloped (1 cup)	8
Potato salad (1 cup)	16
Canned cream soups (1 cup)	6-10
Chips: potato, taco (1 oz.)	12
Crackers (10)	10

Increasing Physical Activity

Many people try to lose weight by dieting alone. For folks who are only slightly overweight, this approach may work. However, for people with a long-standing weight problem, dieting alone usually proves to be a partial and temporary solution at best. As noted previously, severely limiting calories is generally not an effective strategy for permanent weight loss. Unless new diet and eating behaviors become a fairly permanent fixture in a person's life, any pounds lost tend to be gradually regained once the diet is ended.

If you are truly serious about losing weight and keeping it off, it is essential to consider the other side of the coin—calorie expenditure. Becoming more active and burning more calories on a daily basis allows for less drastic measures with respect to dieting. Sometimes, no change in eating patterns is needed at all!

Keep in mind that more calories are burned the longer, more frequently, and more intensely you are active. Regular exercise also helps to prevent a reduction in your underlying metabolic rate. Your metabolism increases during the activity, and it remains elevated for several hours after the activity is over!

Exhibit 7-3 shows the amount of calories burned in various types of activities. Remember, all activities needn't be formally planned or structured. As somebody once said: "Don't sit when you can stand; don't stand when you can walk; and don't walk when you can move even faster." Simple techniques—like walking when possible instead of driving, taking stairs instead of elevators, and parking as far as possible from stores and other businesses—can make a big difference over time.

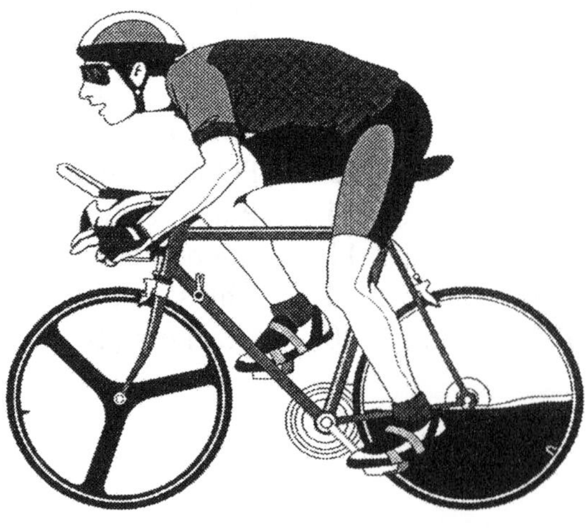

Exhibit 7-3

ENERGY REQUIREMENTS OF VARIOUS ACTIVITIES
(Calories per hour, based on a 150-pound man)

Rest and Light Activity

Lying down, sleeping	80
Sitting	100
Driving a car	120
Standing	140
Domestic work	180

Moderate Activity

Bicycling (5.5 mph)	210
Walking (2.5 mph)	210
Gardening	220
Canoeing (2.5 mph)	230
Golf	250
Lawn mowing (power)	250
Bowling	270
Lawn mowing (hand)	270
Fencing	300
Rowboating (2.5 mph)	300
Swimming (.25 mph)	300
Walking (3.75 mph)	300
Badminton	350
Horseback riding (trotting)	350
Square dancing	350
Volleyball	350
Roller skating	350

Vigorous Activity

Table tennis	360
Ditch digging (shovel)	400
Ice skating (10 mph)	400
Wood chopping/sawing	400
Tennis	420
Water skiing	480
Hill climbing (100 feet/hour)	490
Skiing (10 mph)	600
Squash, handball, racquetball	600
Cycling (13 mph)	660
Scull rowing (race)	840
Running (10 mph)	900

Source: USFA 1990

The Lifestyle Factor

Almost everyone can temporarily lose weight and reduce his/her amount of body fat. However, if the weight gradually returns to previous levels, then the person is really no better off. The real measure of success in losing weight is keeping it off.

Many weight loss programs are successful for short-term weight loss. However, follow-up with former program participants shows that almost all of them, within a year or two, re-gain the weight they had lost. Many even gain more weight than they had before.

Approaching weight loss as a brief, short-term project usually results in long-term failure. Since previous eating and activity behaviors probably created the problem in the first place, temporary changes won't solve it! Resuming old habits once the weight loss goal is achieved means that fat will accumulate once again. And this time, weight loss may be even more difficult.

The key to success is becoming committed to the goal of losing fat and not letting yourself regain it. All of the critical factors of caloric balance—calories consumed, foods and drinks chosen, and activity levels—are under your voluntary control. Each person needs to consider his/her own unique situation, and take the steps necessary to maintain an appropriate body weight. It may be difficult, but it can be done!

Other General Tips

- Keep in mind that it's usually easier to prevent gaining weight than to take off the excess pounds. Try to address any unwanted weight gain as early as possible.
- **Keep track of what you eat.** Most people who are overweight underestimate how much food they really take in. To find out, read food labels and maintain a simple food diary at least long enough to understand your eating habits and daily fat and calorie intake. Exhibit 7-4 on the next page is a sample food record form.
- **Allow some flexibility in your diet plan.** Leave room for some of your favorite foods and for special occasions. To do this, balance your diet over the course of a week. For example, if you know you will be going to a restaurant that serves rich food, "bank" some calories now for later.
- **Experiment with new foods and cooking techniques** to find ones you like. Try low-fat products and some ethnic cuisines. Avoid fried foods whenever possible; bake, broil, or roast instead.
- **Adopt new eating styles gradually.** The focus is on permanent changes in lifestyle, so pick a limited number of actions and implement them over time. Then choose a few others. Remember, rapid weight loss is counterproductive.

Exhibit 7-4

THREE-DAY FOOD RECORD

Name: ______________________________ Date Beginning: ____/____/____

Meal, Time, Place	**Day 1**	**Day 2**	**Day 3**
Breakfast _____ a.m. ________________			
Snack _____ a.m. ________________			
Lunch _____ ________________			
Snack _____ p.m. ________________			
Dinner _____ p.m. ________________			
Snack _____ p.m. ________________			
Servings/Day			
Carbohydrates	________	________	________
Meat/Fish (3 oz.)	________	________	________
Vegetables	________	________	________
Fruits	________	________	________
Dairy Products	________	________	________
Water	________	________	________
Sweets	________	________	________
Alcohol	________	________	________
Nutrient Totals			
Calories	________	________	________
Fats (grams)	________	________	________
Sat. Fats (grams)	________	________	________

WHAT DOESN'T WORK

Americans spend an estimated $30 billion a year on all types of diet programs and products. Since as few as 5 percent of dieters are successful in long-term weight reduction, most people obviously aren't getting much for their investment.

> "Losing weight may not be effortless, but it doesn't have to be complicated. To achieve long-term results, it's best to avoid quick-fix schemes and complex regimens. Focus instead on making changes to your life's daily routine."
>
> FDA

One reason for this problem is that many people are looking for a short-cut or simple solution to their weight problems. Unfortunately, **any claims that you can lose weight effortlessly are false**. For dieters, this statement provides some bad news and some good news. The bad news is that very many programs and products on the market don't work; the good news is that you don't have to buy them.

Fad Diets—According to the Food and Drug Administration (FDA), fad diets, often emphasizing one or more types of food (grapefruit, rice, high protein, etc.), rarely have any permanent effect. Most prove difficult to sustain over time, and some may be deficient in nutrients. In addition, rapid weight loss can trigger the yo-yo syndrome and future difficulties in losing or maintaining weight.

Very-Low-Calorie Diets—Modified fasting, supported by various diet formulas and nutrient supplements, severely restricts calorie intake, often to as low as 400-800 calories per day. Although many people lose weight under these programs, the American Dietetic Association (ADA) notes that very-low-calorie diets have poor long-term results: most dieters regain over half the weight lost in the program. The ADA states that these diets should be undertaken "only with the supervision of a multi-disciplinary health team that includes monitoring by a physician and nutrition counseling by a registered dietitian."

"Spot Reducing"—Some people buy creams and lotions or perform special exercises for certain "problem areas" where fat accumulates. As an example, they perform hundreds of sit-ups to reduce fat around the waist line. This strategy doesn't work. When you burn fat, you lose it gradually from all over your body, not just one place. No matter how you exercise, you cannot select the areas from which fat will be lost. (You can, however, disproportionately strengthen and tone the muscles in one area.)

Appetite Suppressants—Studies have shown that prescription appetite suppressants can help people lose weight. However, these drugs do not teach you how to change your behavior, and they can have serious side effects and the potential for addiction. Their use should be limited to 8-12 weeks under the direction of a physician.

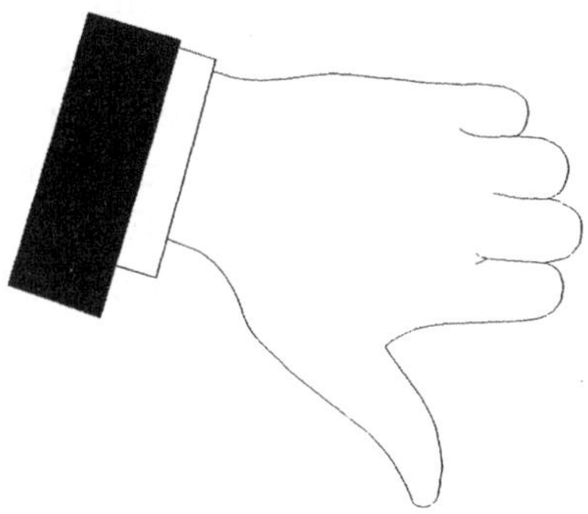

Most over-the-counter medications, on the other hand, have not been proven effective in weight loss, and some may pose health risks. The use of over 100 common ingredients in these products, such as alcohol and caffeine, was banned by the FDA in 1991.

Phony Products and Gadgets—A wide variety of products marketed as weight-loss aids have not been proven to be safe or effective. At a minimum, they are a waste of money. Some examples include diet patches, "fat blockers," "starch blockers," "magnet" diet pills, electrical muscle stimulators, and even "appetite suppressing eyeglasses" and "weight-loss earrings."

"Sweating It Off"—As noted previously, much of the weight lost during excessive exercise is fluid, primarily from muscle tissue. However, fat tissue contains very little water, so losing fluid doesn't have much impact on reducing fat stores. Therefore, it is useless (and potentially dangerous) for someone to attempt to "sweat off" fat by using rubber suits and belts, saunas, or steam rooms.

Activity 7-1

ANALYZING YOUR EATING BEHAVIORS

Although many people know what to eat, sometimes other behaviors and habits get in the way of success. This activity is designed to help you analyze your own eating behaviors. Fortunately, most of these behaviors are controllable. Once you are aware of them, you can begin to identify strategies that will help you lose weight. (Note: you may want to keep a food diary for at least several days before completing this activity.)

Instructions

Various eating behaviors are listed in Worksheet 1 below and on the next page. For each one, decide whether you demonstrate that behavior OFTEN, SOMETIMES, or RARELY. Then circle the corresponding point value in the appropriate column. When you are finished, total up the scores on Worksheet 2, which follows. More explanation is provided in the next section.

Worksheet 1

EATING BEHAVIOR QUESTIONNAIRE

	Eating Behaviors	Often	Some-times	Rarely
1.	I eat when I am in a bad mood.	3	2	1
2.	I eat while I am watching TV	3	2	1
3.	I lose control of how much I eat.	3	2	1
4.	I can't say "NO" to my favorite foods.	3	2	1
5.	I lose weight to please others.	3	2	1
6.	I eat in the living room or family room.	3	2	1
7.	I finish my food quickly.	3	2	1
8.	I get hungry when others are eating.	3	2	1
9.	If my weight goes up, I break my diet.	3	2	1
10.	I don't eat three regular meals each day.	3	2	1

	Eating Behaviors	Often	Some-times	Rarely
11.	I eat when I am happy.	3	2	1
12.	I eat while I am driving.	3	2	1
13.	I can't stop eating favorite foods once I start.	3	2	1
14.	I have difficulty refusing food that is offered to me.	3	2	1
15.	I need outside motivation to lose weight.	3	2	1
16.	I eat in the bedroom.	3	2	1
17.	I tend to gulp my food.	3	2	1
18.	The sight and smell of food makes me hungry.	3	2	1
19.	I can't stick to a diet long enough to reach my goal.	3	2	1
20.	I skip meals when I'm busy.	3	2	1
21.	I eat when I am bored.	3	2	1
22.	I eat while I am reading or studying.	3	2	1
23.	When I get discouraged, I start eating and can't stop.	3	2	1
24.	I can be "talked into" breaking my diet.	3	2	1
25.	I don't know how to get my diet started.	3	2	1
26.	I eat at my desk or work area.	3	2	1
27.	I eat without tasting the flavor of my food.	3	2	1
28.	I eat because the clock says it is mealtime.	3	2.	1
29.	The longer I diet, the lower my willpower.	3	2	1
30.	I eat the same amount whether I'm active or not.	3	2	1

Activity 7-1 (Cont'd)

WORKSHEET 2

Instructions

1. Fill in your score for each question below. Then add up your scores for each group of questions (A-J). Your total score for each category should be between 3 and 9.
2. If your score in any one category is between 7 and 9, circle the corresponding letter (A-J) on the worksheet. Then proceed to the explanation on the next page.

A		B		C		D		E	
1.	_____	2.	_____	3.	_____	4.	_____	5.	_____
11.	_____	12.	_____	13.	_____	14.	_____	15.	_____
21.	_____	22.	_____	23.	_____	24.	_____	25.	_____
Total	_____	**Total**	_____	**Total**	_____	**Total**	_____	**Total**	_____
F		**G**		**H**		**I**		**J**	
6.	_____	7.	_____	8.	_____	9.	_____	10.	_____
16.	_____	17.	_____	18.	_____	19.	_____	20.	_____
26.	_____	27.	_____	28.	_____	29.	_____	30.	_____
Total	_____	**Total**	_____	**Total**	_____	**Total**	_____	**Total**	_____

Activity 7-1 (Cont'd)

In this activity, you examined your own eating behaviors in 10 important categories (Sections A through J on Worksheet 2). These behavioral categories can be summarized as follows:

A: **Feelings and moods**—Do they affect your eating behaviors?

B: **Other activities**—Do they influence how much you eat?

C: **Binges and "snack attacks"**—Are you in control of your cravings?

D: **Assertiveness**—Can you say "no" to food?

E: **Motivation**—What things get you going?

F: **Location**—Does where you eat make a difference?

G: **Eating too fast**—Why is rapid eating a potential problem?

H: **Real hunger**—Can you tell the difference?

I: **Willpower**—What things <u>keep</u> you going?

J: **Food/energy balance**—Do your eating patterns match your needs?

Use the key below to evaluate your score in each category. A high score in any area may indicate a potential obstacle to your weight loss goals.

3-4 Your eating behaviors in this category are good.

5-6 Your eating behaviors in this category may benefit from some changes.

7-9 You would definitely benefit from some changes to your eating behaviors in this category.

The next section contains information, suggestions, and strategies to help you implement change in each of these 10 categories. Since higher scores in a specific area indicate a greater potential for problems, you may wish to pay particular attention to those categories that you circled on the worksheet (i.e., with a score of 7-9).

STRATEGIES FOR SUCCESS

SECTION A: FEELINGS AND MOODS

Do you eat because you are happy, sad, or perhaps bored? Research indicates a strong relationship between peoples' feelings and their eating behaviors. Everyone eats sometimes when they aren't really hungry—at a party to celebrate, at work due to frustration or social pressure, or in the evening because of boredom, loneliness, or as a way to relax. This behavior may be OK if you know what you are doing and don't do it too often. But when food begins to be the "solution" to life's challenges, the pattern may contribute to weight gain.

If your emotions lead to eating on a regular basis, you need to learn how to identify those feelings, and then cope with them in ways other than eating. This skill is crucial because it is almost impossible to lose weight if you can't separate hunger from emotions. Since dieting is stressful, you also need to find other outlets for these feelings.

Many of the suggestions referred to in later sections will help you if you are an "emotional" eater. Eating less, eating slower, eating without doing anything else, eating in a designated place, and recognizing true hunger will all help. However, it's important that true "emotional" eaters learn to:

1. **Identify their feelings**
2. **Disassociate those feelings from eating**
3. **Substitute other activities for eating**

Physical activity can be particularly helpful for changing your mood or your awareness of hunger. The list below gives some suggestions for alternative activities; think of others that work for you.

- Take a walk.
- Do aerobic or strength training.
- Conduct a flexibility routine.
- Play a sport or other game.
- Call a friend or write a letter.
- Do some work around the house.
- Take up a hobby.
- Read a book or magazine.
- Change your environment—get out of the house if necessary.
- Write down your feelings.
- Practice self-talk—review your goals, and visualize how you will look and feel on your goal date.
- Try deep breathing or relaxation techniques (see Chapter 9).

Although activity can help, awareness is the real key for dealing with your emotions. Write down the reasons for your feelings and ways you might address them. Where possible, avoid situations that cause negative feelings, or find ways to make them better. More on personal change and growth is covered in Chapter 10.

SECTION B: OTHER ACTIVITIES

What you do while eating can be as important as your feelings at the time. If you eat while watching television, driving, or working, you are most likely to eat more than you want or need, and much more than you think you are eating.

Research indicates that overweight people who eat while doing other activities have a difficult time remembering what and how much they have eaten. They may be using other "activities" to hide their eating, and often don't even remember eating at all. The food they have eaten doesn't satisfy their hunger, so they may feel hungry a short time afterwards.

Television poses a particular danger to many people. Not only does it take the focus away from actual eating, it also provides an incredible source of environmental hunger (see Section H). Studies indicate that when adults and children consistently eat meals in front of the television, they soon become hungry as soon as the television is turned on, even if they have recently finished a meal or snack. This is also true for eating while driving, reading, and even talking on the phone. It seems that when people eat during any activity long enough, it becomes a strong habit to do both at the same time.

It is also significant to note that many overweight people often eat while standing, walking, or lying down. This may be because these positions relate to some other activity that is taking place while eating. Although your body position or activities do not make you gain weight, they keep your attention away from eating.

The following suggestions may help you focus on eating as a single activity:

1. Don't do anything else while you eat, like reading or watching television.
2. Plan enough time for meals, and figure out ways to avoid distractions.
3. Designate a specific eating place.
4. Keep all food in the kitchen, not the living room, bedroom, etc.
5. Don't keep snacks in your car, or in your desk or work space.
6. Always eat in a seated position.
7. Try to avoid too many "business lunches" or social eating situations.
8. Plan your meals, and think of them as special occasions or events.

SECTION C: BINGES AND SNACK ATTACKS

Binges and excessive snacking are strongly related to other eating problems. The first step is to identify your emotions (see Section A). Then review Section I on willpower before trying the following strategies.

1. Identify the problem.

Most bingers are "foodaholics" who may be psychologically addicted to food for some reason. Emotional eating becomes a binge when the automatic response to eat is too strong to stop. The key is replacing the reliance on food.

Individuals lose control for different reasons, including feelings of fatigue, boredom, depression, deprivation, stress, and failure. For some people, bingeing occurs only at certain times of the day, in certain locations, or on certain days of the week or holidays. For others, the trigger may be problem situations or events.

Think of three things that may have caused you to binge in the past.

a. ______________________________

b. ______________________________

c. ______________________________

2. Review the consequences.

A binge usually makes you feel worse when it's over. Once you fulfill an emotional need by eating, anger, guilt, and depression may follow. Think about the consequences: are you willing to pay the price? Ask yourself the following types of questions:

- Is this worth making myself physically uncomfortable or even sick from eating?
- Is it worth the anger or guilt I'll feel?
- Is it worth risking a week with no weight loss, or pushing back my goal date?
- Is it worth the extra exercise or dieting I'll have to do?
- Will it affect my future motivation, willpower, or confidence?
- Am I really hungry?

List three reasons why you don't want to give in to the desire to binge.

a. ______________________________

b. ______________________________

c. ______________________________

3. **Plan ahead**.

While you are in control and highly motivated, plan ahead for ways to avoid a binge. Make a list of things to do instead, stressing pleasurable activities to replace the satisfaction of the binge. In addition to those listed in Section A, the following ideas may help:

- Schedule specific times for your meals, and plan for healthful snacks, if necessary.
- Find a "diet buddy," someone to support you and get you over a binge impulse.
- Watch your alcohol consumption, which can lower inhibitions and self-constraint.
- Don't buy foods that are hard for you to resist, or drive past tempting food "stops."
- Stay away from non-supportive family, friends, and colleagues.
- Keep food out of sight, inside cabinets whenever possible. Use opaque containers on counter tops.

List three activities that you might use to prevent or stop a binge.

a. ______________________________

b. ______________________________

c. ______________________________

4. **Improve the behavior**.

You can make a binge "better" by making it smaller or changing the food. Make it smaller by mentally allowing yourself only a limited portion. Savor the food by tasting, smelling, and eating slowly, allowing the texture of the food to satisfy your craving. You may also be able to improve your binge by substituting a lower-calorie or no-fat version of the same food or other healthful snacks.

Use a timer or watch the clock to better control snack attacks. When you get hungry, wait at least five minutes before doing anything. If you still must eat, have a small portion, and then wait again.

What foods do you usually binge on?

____

____

____

What better foods could be substituted?

____

____

____

How can you limit your portion?

____

____

____

How can you increase the food's satisfaction?

____

____

____

SECTION D: ASSERTIVENESS

An entire chapter could be devoted to assertiveness, which is as important in everyday life as it is in weight control. If your answers in Activity 7-1 indicate that you need some assistance in this area, the following information will get you started.

Assertiveness is a skill that takes practice. It should not be confused with aggression. Assertive people know how to do what is right for them without feeling guilty. They know how to identify and achieve their real goals, while remaining sensitive to the needs and feelings of others.

You can't be assertive until you determine what you really want. What are your priorities? Do you want to lose weight or have ice cream for dessert? Do you want to eat pizza or fit into those pants by a certain date? Only YOU can decide what is most important. Then you need to care enough about yourself to follow through. Remember, you can be your own best friend or worst enemy.

Once you start being assertive, it gets easier with practice. The habit becomes natural, and people around you will begin to believe that you really mean what you say. If you have spent a lifetime saying no, then eating anyway, it may take time for others to realize that this time you are really serious about losing weight.

Assertiveness often tends to be situational. Many people can say no to themselves and to immediate family members at home, but get into trouble at work or in social situations. Try the following if you find yourself in an "assertiveness slump":

Out to Dinner

1. This is your dinner, you are paying for it, and you deserve to have what you want. The waiter or waitress is there to serve you, not the opposite.

2. You have the right to question the menu, ask how food is prepared, and ask for foods to be fixed to suit your weight loss plan. It's no different than being on a restricted medical diet—being overweight is a health risk!

3. If the food comes out wrong, send it back. Would you buy a suit that was altered incorrectly? Don't allow other's mistakes to sabotage your goals.

On the Job

1. Announce your intentions and ask co-workers to be sensitive to your goals. You will learn quickly who are your "friends" and who is the "enemy." Since others are watching, this approach also provides some motivation and accountability.

2. Stay away from the food. If you know there are donuts in a certain place, don't make it worse by going there if you don't have to. Assertiveness only goes so far.

3. Try to get others to join you in eating better. If that doesn't work, bring your own food.

At a Friend's Party or Dinner

1. Practice "defensive eating." Have some fruit or raw vegetables just before you go. This approach may make it easier to skip the rich hors d'oeuvres or to eat less at dinner.

2. Tell your hosts before you go or before they start serving that you need to watch your weight. Then, eliminate certain things (e.g., drinks, soups, dessert), or perhaps ask for smaller portions.

3. If they insist, keep refusing politely. They may think you don't mean it, and that you really want them to talk you into eating. Flatter their cooking—tell them how wonderful it looks and how much you look forward to reaching your goals so you can have some next time.

Remember, your assertiveness may be a threat to some people, especially overweight non-dieters. They may feel guilty and perhaps even angry that you are being successful and they are not. Don't be fooled into thinking that you are being aggressive, or that you are responsible for hurting their feelings.

After Each Situation

1. Evaluate the results—were they what you expected? What you hoped? If not, think how you could have approached the situation differently, and resolve to do better the next time.

2. If the results were good, congratulate yourself. Stop and think, "Wow! That was good. I didn't think I could do that!" Practice mentally "patting yourself on the back" to keep you going.

3. Reward yourself by, for example, putting a quarter in a jar every time you successfully assert yourself. Save the money for something special when you reach your goal.

4. Remind yourself that you are one step closer to your goal. Just keep saying "no," and remember:

    - Don't be judgmental or threatening.
    - Don't feel guilty.
    - Be polite, firm, and friendly, but don't back down.

SECTION E: MOTIVATION

Motivation is the key to successfully changing behaviors. If you had a high score in this section, you may need assistance in defining your reasons for losing weight. Why are you doing it? What do you hope to gain? Will the result be worth the effort?

Internal Motivation

The evidence seems to indicate that weight loss requires internal motivation, the type that comes from within, to increase your chance for long-term success. You have to want to lose weight because you care about yourself and you know it's important, not because someone else thinks you should.

Internal motivation may be based on changing your appearance, improving your health, or securing and keeping a job. It is rarely the result of a single factor—most people are motivated by a variety of incentives. Whatever the reason, you want it for yourself.

External motivation, on the other hand, results from outside factors, such as special events, wanting to impress someone, temporary job requirements, etc. Since most external events or situations tend to be transitory, so does the power of the motivation. After the event is over (the class reunion) or the situation changes (the relationship breaks up), the power of the motivation disappears.

Setting Goals

The first step in developing motivation is establishing your goal. You must know where you are going, how much effort it will take, and when you will get there. Losing weight should not be ambiguous or haphazard. The more clearly you can visualize the end result, the more motivated you will be to get started.

Set a goal that is realistic and obtainable within a reasonable amount of time. Don't plan to lose more than two pounds a week. Thus, a 20-pound weight loss will take a minimum of ten weeks. That's only 70 days! Aren't you motivated already?

If your long-term goal requires a large weight loss, divide it into several short-term goals. It's difficult to achieve a goal that doesn't seem obtainable. If you're more than 20 pounds overweight, plan to lose the first 10 pounds, then the next 10, and so forth.

Use the formula below to start planning:

My current weight is ______ lbs.
My long-term goal is ______ lbs.
The difference is ______ lbs.

My short-term target date (three months or less) is ___/___/___.

My short-term goal (one to two pounds per week) is ______ lbs.

At this rate, I should reach my long-term goal by ___/___/___.

SECTION F: LOCATION

The questions in this section refer to where you regularly eat. If you eat mostly in the living room or family room, in the bedroom, or at your desk or work place, this habit may contribute to eating behaviors that promote weight gain and inhibit successful weight maintenance.

Experts suggest that you eat in the same place for all meals and snacks. Although it may be difficult to follow this guideline all the time, the rationale has merit. When you make eating a separate and distinct activity from the rest of your day, you attain greater physical satisfaction and more emotional fulfillment from eating. It is also easier to monitor the amounts of food you eat.

Our busy lifestyles contribute to hurried meals that often lack meaning or significance. Consider trying to make your meals special and memorable. Designate your kitchen or dining room as the meal place instead of the TV room. Research also shows that using place mats, special plates and silverware, even candlelight, contributes toward making meals special events. This pattern may, in turn, be related to less between-meal snacking during the day.

When you eat away from home—at work or in restaurants—you have less control over the environment. In these situations, the most important factor is the type of food that's served. Choose restaurants that have healthful alternatives on the menu. At the station, try to promote the acceptance of nutritional meals, and assist in planning, shopping, and food preparation. If all else fails, bring your own food.

It may seem insignificant, but the experts suggest that most of the battles involved in weight control end up as "psychological warfare." Besides these suggestions, follow the guidelines in Section B on eliminating other activities while eating, Section G on adjusting your speed of eating during meals, and Section H on recognizing hunger.

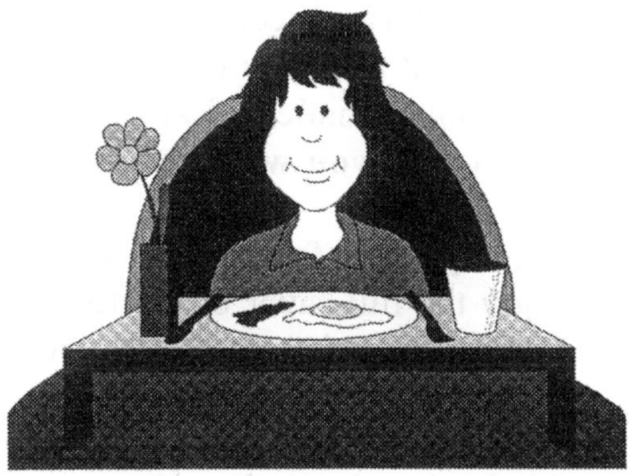

SECTION G: EATING TOO FAST

The questions in this section asked if you eat quickly, if you tend to gulp your food, and if you eat without tasting your food. All of these patterns are related to the speed in which you eat.

Unfortunately, hectic lifestyles affect all of us, and mealtimes often suffer because they take time away from busy schedules. It's common to rush meals, substitute real meals with "fast food," and eat meals on the run between activities. However, you can't make your body rush the eating and digestive processes. There are several reasons:

1. Fast eating does not allow the hunger control mechanism in the hypothalamus gland (appestat) enough time to shut off the hunger drive. Your body takes about twenty minutes to realize it's full. Eating fast does not allow enough time for this to occur, so you eat more food than you need to feel physically satisfied. **Eat more slowly and you will eat less.**

2. When you eat fast, you do not enjoy the full savor of the food. Hurried ingestion decreases your awareness of eating, and acts to limit the olfactory senses. In turn, this habit reduces the pleasure and satisfaction derived from eating. **Eat more slowly and you will enjoy your food more.**

3. Eating fast can cause indigestion, and also a "bloated" feeling that makes you eat more. **Eat more slowly for better health.**

4. Fast eating means you will finish before everyone else. This may cause you to go for second helpings that you don't really need or want, just so you won't have to sit and watch others still eating. **Eat more slowly and you won't feel "left out" of the meal.**

All the above factors apply to both meals and snacks. You have to teach yourself to eat more slowly by practicing the behavior. Some tips that might help:

- Use a timer—take at least 20 minutes for meals.
- Take smaller bites—put less on your fork or spoon.
- Put your utensils down between bites.
- Cut your food into smaller pieces, or cut and eat one piece at a time.
- Take sips of water between bites.
- Listen to slow music or converse while eating.
- Switch your eating hands.

SECTION H: "REAL" HUNGER?

All of us eat when we are hungry, and sometimes when we aren't. The question is, when you feel hunger, is it "REAL"? Do you eat because the clock says it's mealtime, or because the sight or smell of food and others eating makes you hungry? It's important to identify the type of hunger you're feeling, and to eat only when it is "real" hunger.

Legitimate hunger occurs after 3-4 hours without eating anything (including snacks). This process may occur sooner if the last meal did not include the proper balance of food. Too much sugar or carbohydrates can cause excessive feelings of hunger. Skipping meals also contributes to a false sense of hunger.

To maintain a proper metabolic balance, it is essential that food be taken on a regular basis throughout the day. Unfortunately, many of us eat unbalanced meals, skip meals, substitute snacks as meals, and eat at irregular times. Those patterns do not allow the body to respond to real hunger, often leading to weight gain or difficulty losing weight.

The ability to differentiate between real hunger and other types is the key to proper eating behaviors in this area. Other major categories of hunger include the following:

Emotional Hunger—This type of hunger is a major problem for many people who are overweight. It is discussed in detail in Section A.

Scheduled Hunger—This type of hunger has to do with the internal "clock" that programs us to become hungry at the times when we normally eat meals. Scheduled hunger is like an alarm going off in your head—your stomach is signaled to expect food even though you don't really need to eat. This can become a problem when your schedule is thrown off. The hunger you feel at mealtime may not be real, and can even occur with a full stomach. It's easy to see how this type of hunger could pose a problem for firefighters and rescue workers with their irregular schedules.

Environmental Hunger—This type of hunger is influenced by things around you: television, advertisements, other people, foods, etc. Your sensitivity to food may be so high that all you have to do is hear a food mentioned and you "have to have it."

Environmental hunger can be a real problem for people trying to lose or maintain their weight. The sections on motivation, willpower, assertiveness, eating locations, and other activities will all be helpful if you are a victim of environmental hunger. You may need to stay away from these situations as much as possible while you are trying to lose weight, and then limit your exposure to them afterwards.

SECTION I: WILLPOWER

If motivation defines what you need to get started, **willpower is what keeps you going to reach your goal**. When you have difficulty sticking to a weight management program, there are tricks to help increase your willpower, and strategies to avoid "falling off the wagon." If you slip, there are ways to get back on right away so you don't lose too much time or gain back any weight.

Has the following scenario ever happened to you? You begin a weight loss program highly motivated and doing great. After a few weeks or even less, the novelty begins to diminish, the pounds come off more slowly, and feelings of deprivation set in. Your resistance begins to wear thin, you become more vulnerable to outside family and environment influences, and you begin to make careless food choices. The carelessness gets worse, the weight comes off even more slowly, you get more discouraged, and you eventually quit.

If this has happened to you, you need to plan ahead so it doesn't happen again. Be prepared to keep yourself strong. Use suggestions from the following list to maintain your willpower, and to get back on track as quickly as possible if you fall.

1. Review your goals often. Note your goal date on the calendar, and mark off each day when it's over. Plan ahead—look forward instead of back. Remember that changing your eating patterns will get easier with time. Use self-talk to keep yourself going. Think positive. Congratulate yourself on good days. Don't be too hard on yourself if it wasn't a great day. Tomorrow will be better!

2. Keep a food diary. Writing down what you eat is the best way to stay accountable and to avoid making careless decisions. Review your diary at the end of each week. Plan ahead for the following week. Some people like to plan ahead each day for exactly what they will eat. This is especially helpful if you need to "bank" calories for a special event.

3. Weigh only yourself once or twice a week, at the same time of day, on the same scale. Your weight may differ by a few pounds during the day, and scales vary a few pounds from one another. Even when you don't cheat, your weight may temporarily fluctuate upwards for various reasons. Many people cannot mentally withstand a weight gain, even a small one, at this stage. Prevent this "willpower killer" by only weighing in at very specific times on the same scale. This also prevents blaming a weight gain on the wrong reasons.

4. If you fall off the wagon, jump back on immediately. Don't fall into the trap that you have to wait until the next day, or even until the next "Monday" to start again. Evaluate what happened—beginning, middle, and end—and plan ahead to avoid the same mistake.

Failures during past weight control efforts may have conditioned you to use anger and guilt to prevent success. Your subconscious mind may even be predicting failure and encouraging you to get there. Remember, you abandoned your earlier efforts because of old behaviors, not current ones. Unfortunately, your past eating behaviors are much stronger than your new ones. Successful change will take patience and time.

5. When your willpower is low, don't give in! Do whatever it takes to stay strong:

- Stay away from people who continually tempt you to eat.
- Avoid places that get you into trouble.
- Change or modify your activities to avoid things that make you lose control.

The problem may be television, alcohol, the "weekend," or a change in your normal routine or daily schedule. People also are known to seek out tempting situations when they are feeling deprived from weight control efforts. They "accidentally" end up around food and then use the situation as an excuse to eat. But most people know what gets them into trouble before it happens. Use your prior experience to benefit your future success. This time **can** be different.

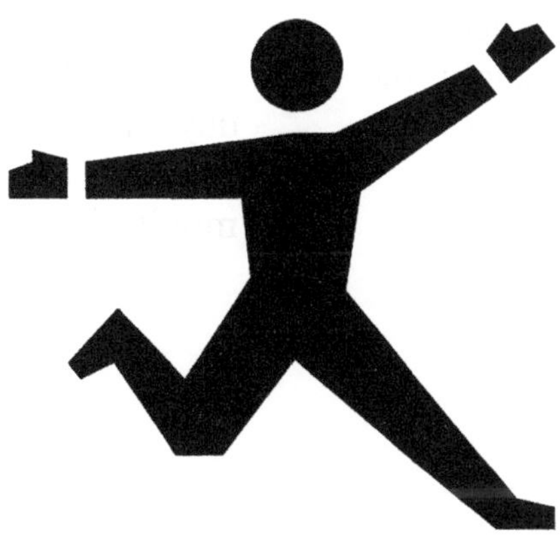

SECTION J: FOOD/ENERGY BALANCE

Proper diet planning is an important component of weight control. **In order to reach and maintain ideal body weight, the amount and types of food you eat must balance your energy needs.** Your food intake should also promote a healthy metabolic system through nutritionally balanced meals, at regular intervals throughout the day.

Skipping meals actually tends to shut down your metabolism, preventing your body from efficiently burning calories. Skipping meals can also eventually lead to overeating or poor food choices. Whenever your body is short-changed on nutritional needs, it will usually crave foods that are high in sugars or fats.

Whatever you eat during a meal supplies the fuel you will use to perform activities after the meal. The absorption of food peaks about seven hours after eating. Since dinner is traditionally the largest meal of the day, most people eat the most food for the activity that requires the least energy—sleeping. Unfortunately, the energy your body does not use is stored as fat.

Most people develop an established pattern of mealtimes that fits their lifestyle. However, this pattern may not provide the body with fuel at the time it is needed. Furthermore, the size and balance of meals can contribute to people being overweight.

People trying to lose weight, and those who have difficulty maintaining their weight, should seriously consider basing their food intake on their planned activity patterns. In other words, they should eat more before active periods, and less when they plan to be sedentary. This means that eating patterns will vary according to personal needs and even daily changes in activities and schedules.

The following section provides seven different strategies for you to consider. Each represents a daily eating pattern—breakfast, lunch, and dinner—reflecting based on the amount you eat at each meal. Each pattern has different effects on energy levels, metabolism, and fat storage.

Identify which strategy is most similar to your own eating behaviors. Then compare this pattern with your energy needs (activity levels) during a typical day. If they don't match, consider adopting another eating pattern and monitoring its effect for a while.

1. For many people, this traditional eating pattern—small breakfast, medium lunch, large dinner—is probably the least desirable from a weight loss standpoint.

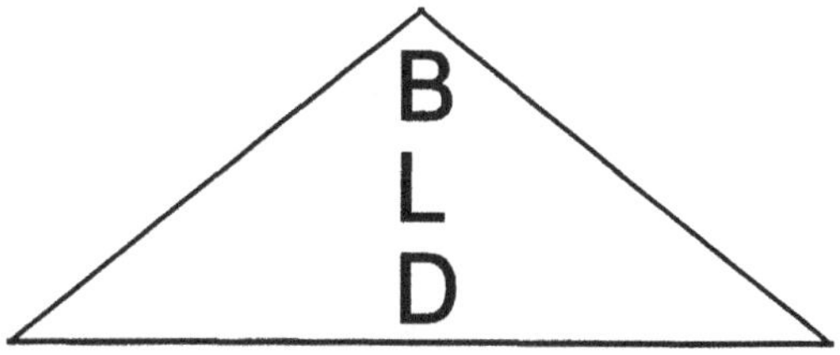

2. This pattern is effective if you have a stable level of activity throughout the day. Meals should be the same size and nutritionally balanced to minimize the desire for snacks.

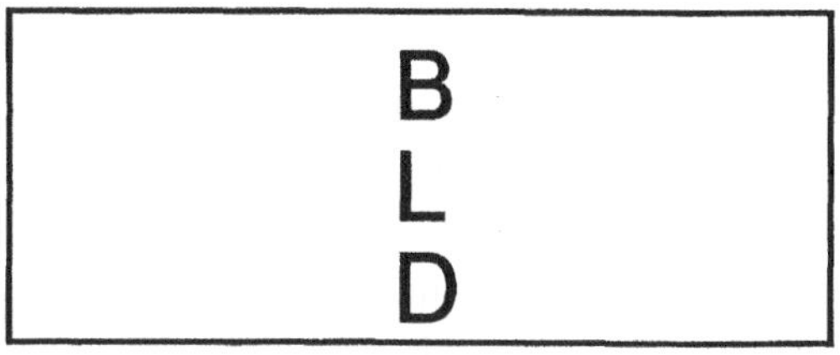

3. This plan eliminates late heavy meals, although early eating may set a pattern of indulgence the rest of the day. The pattern is ideal for early exercisers to increase daily vitality.

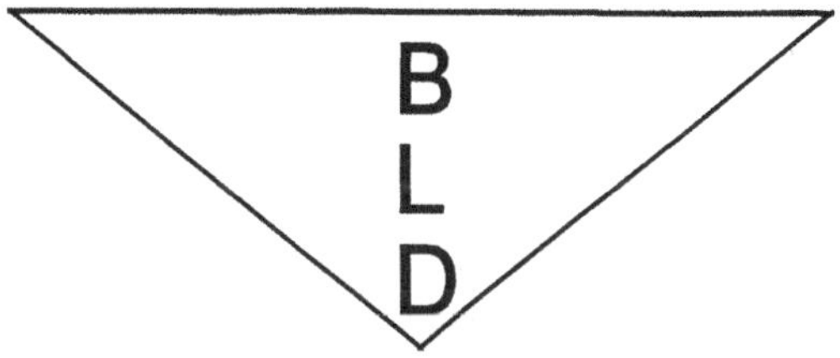

4. This pattern is for those with highest activity between 11 a.m. and 4 p.m. A small breakfast allows for a substantial lunch. A large dinner is not necessary if no late activity is planned.

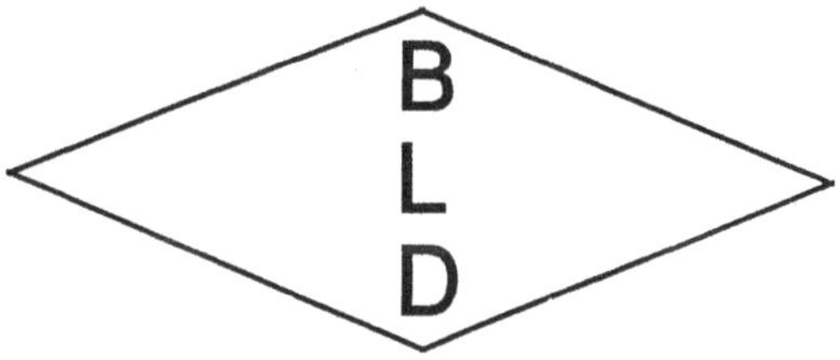

5. This pattern suits those who have high daily activity requirements after dinner. Again, a small breakfast allows more calories for the energy-expending times of the day.

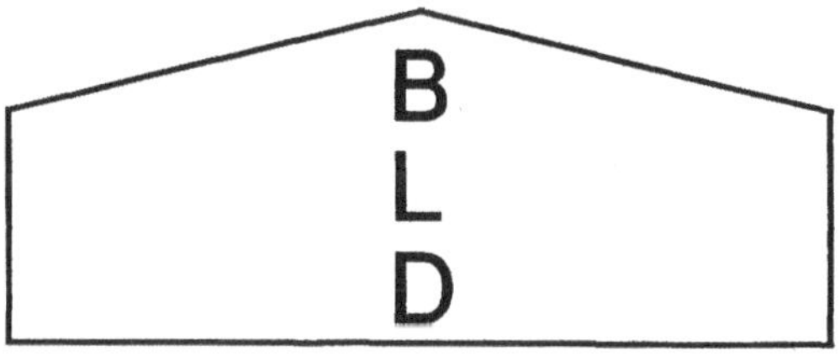

6. This pattern suits those with high activity levels early in the day. If these people skip early meals, they will be ravenous for dinner, followed by low energy expenditure.

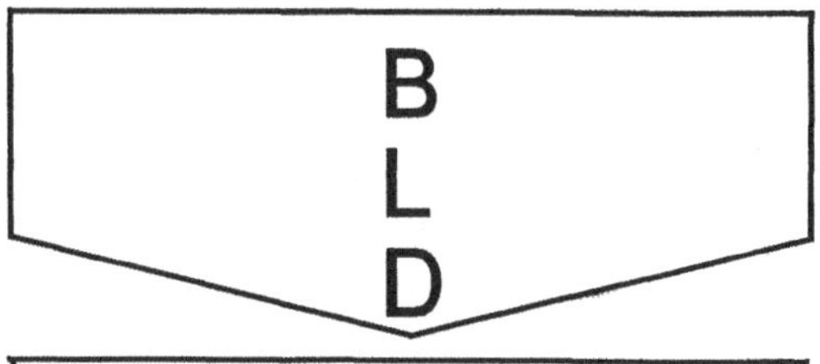

7. Eating a light lunch may be ideal for someone who needs low energy throughout the afternoon, as long as the meals are properly balanced.

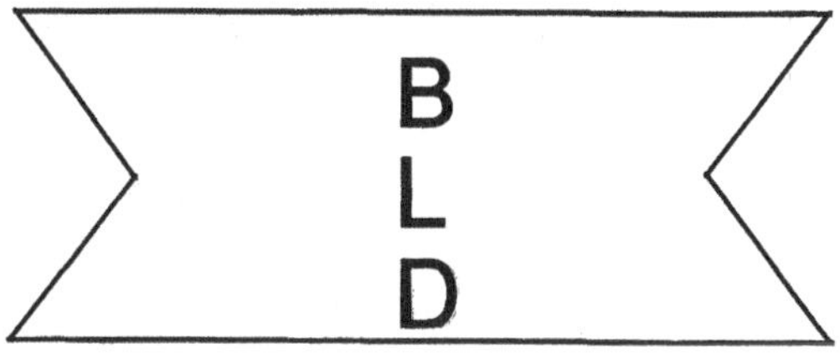

Key: B = Breakfast, L = Lunch, D = Dinner

Activity 7-2

PERSONAL WEIGHT MANAGEMENT

Losing stored body fat should only be accomplished gradually. Remember, 3500 calories must be expended over and above your food intake in order to shed each pound of fat. Thus, for most people, it is unrealistic to expect to lose more than one to two pounds of fat in any given week.

Losing body fat should be approached as an ongoing, long-term project that requires patience, dedication, and discipline. After all, it takes a long time to gain fat; it also takes a long time to lose it.

During this activity, you will apply what you have learned to develop a short-term personal action plan for weight management. The plan should be updated occasionally until you reach your weight loss goal.

Instructions

1. On **Worksheet 1**, fill in your weight, body mass index, and body composition assessment level (1-3) from the physical fitness assessment you completed in Chapter 2.

2. Estimate your ideal or target weight—your long-term goal. Be realistic: take into account genetic factors, your personal happiness, and other considerations.

3. Write down why you want to lose weight. Visualize yourself at your target weight and list some of the benefits.

4. Identify short-term weight loss goals (target weight in pounds) for the next one-month, three-month, and six-month periods. **Remember: going too fast can be counterproductive.**

5. Based on your body composition assessment level, choose a few short-term objectives that you will accomplish in the coming month. (Sample objectives are listed on the attached checklist; identify others based on your own eating behaviors—see Activity 7-1).

- Level 1: Choose at least three objectives
- Level 2: Choose at least two objectives
- Level 3: Choose at least one objective

6. Make change gradual and progressive—as you accomplish some objectives and others become easier, add new ones for months 2-3 and months 4-6. Monitor your progress over the next six months, and revise the plan as necessary.

Activity 7-2 (Continued)
WORKSHEET 1

1. Current weight ________ Body mass index ________ Assessment level _______

2. Estimated ideal/target weight (long-term goal) ________

3. Reasons for losing weight:

____

____

____

4. Short-term weight loss goals (target weight) and objectives:

Month 1	Months 2-3	Months 3-6
Goal: __________ lbs. **Objectives**: ♦ ♦ ♦ ♦	**Goal**: __________ lbs. **Objectives**: ♦ ♦ ♦ ♦	**Goal**: __________ lbs. **Objectives**: ♦ ♦ ♦ ♦

Activity 7-2 (Continued)

CHECKLIST OF WEIGHT CONTROL OBJECTIVES

- ☐ Read food labels
- ☐ Maintain a food diary, and monitor fat or calorie intake
- ☐ Increase exercise by ________ calories/day
- ☐ Eliminate the following food(s):
  - Doughnuts and other pastries during the day
  - Desserts
  - Potato chips, taco chips, etc.
  -
  -
- ☐ Use the following food alternatives:
  - Low fat/non-fat margarine, cream cheese, sour cream, etc.
  - Low fat/non-fat salad dressings
  - Lower calorie beverages (soft drinks, beer, etc.)
  -
  -
- ☐ Avoid the following (types of) restaurants:
  - Fast food restaurants
  - All-you-can-eat buffets
  - Steak houses, barbecue restaurants, etc.
  -
  -
- ☐ Substitute the following activities when you're hungry:
  - Go for a walk
  - Exercise: aerobic, flexibility, strength training
  - Work around the house or practice a hobby
  -
  -
- ☐ Avoid or change the following types of problem situations:
  - Eating in restaurants or at friends' houses
  - Meals at the department
  -
  -
- ☐ Other helpful eating behaviors:
  - Eat more slowly
  - Eat breakfast every day
  -
  -

CHAPTER SUMMARY

In this chapter, you learned some of the basic concepts and principles of weight management. You first defined body composition, and examined what current research shows works and what doesn't work for losing and maintaining weight. You then analyzed your own eating behaviors to identify possible areas for improvement. Strategies and tips for controlling your diet and weight in each of 10 different eating behavior categories were reviewed. Finally, you prepared a short-term action plan for weight management.

Having completed this chapter, you should now be able to:

- ♦ Define body composition and identify healthy and unhealthy levels of body fat.
- ♦ Discuss general principles of weight gain, loss, and maintenance.
- ♦ Identify effective and ineffective strategies for weight loss based on current research.
- ♦ Analyze your own eating behaviors and identify possible areas for improvement.
- ♦ Determine personal strategies and establish short-term goals for weight management.

BIBLIOGRAPHY

Consumers Union, "Losing Weight: What Works. What Doesn't." *Consumer Reports*, June 1993.

Department of Agriculture, Human Nutrition Information Service, *Calories & Weight: The USDA Pocket Guide*, Agriculture Information Bulletin 364.

Federal Trade Commission, *The Facts About Weight Loss*, Flyer.

Food and Drug Administration, "An FDA Guide to Dieting," *FDA Consumer Reprint.*

Food and Drug Administration, "Modified Fast: A Sometime Solution to a Weighty Problem," *FDA Consumer Reprint.*

Kravitz, Len, M.A., and Vivian H. Heyward, Ph.D., "Getting a Grip on Body Composition," *IDEA Today*, April 1992.

Melillo, Wendy, "Keeping It Off," *Washington Post Health*, March 9, 1993.

National Academy of Sciences, *Eat for Life*, Washington, D.C.: National Academy Press, 1992.

National Center for Health Statistics, *Health, United States*, Hyattsville, Maryland: Public Health Service, 1992.

Otis, Carol L., M.D., and Roger Goldingay, "Measuring Body Fat," *Shape*, January 1991.

President's Council on Physical Fitness and Sports, *Exercise and Weight Control*, Pamphlet.

Ubell, Earl, "Will a Diet Help You?" *Parade Magazine*, March 14, 1993.

United States Fire Administration, *Physical Fitness Coordinator's Manual For Fire Departments*, September 1990.

COMPREHENSIVE WELLNESS FOR FIREFIGHTERS

Chapter 8

Substance Abuse: Alcohol, Drugs, and Tobacco

CHAPTER INTRODUCTION

It has been estimated that up to 19% of the adult population in this country suffers from alcohol abuse, other drug abuse, or mental disorders (IAFF 1992). About one of every four people also smoke tobacco, ignoring the overwhelming evidence on this habit's disastrous health effects. The result is untold and unnecessary suffering and death, and billions of dollars in medical costs and lost productivity.

In this chapter, you will learn about the health impacts of substance abuse, both on emergency services personnel and the total population. First, the nature of substance abuse in general is discussed. Then the insidious dangers of alcoholism and drug addiction are examined in more detail. A assessment tool is provided to help you evaluate your own potential for dependency on alcohol and drugs.

In the next section, the facts about cigarette and smokeless tobacco usage are reviewed. Guidelines for quitting are presented. Finally, you think about your own role in the area of substance abuse prevention, both on and off the job.

A detailed description of methods and techniques for quitting or limiting the use of these substances is beyond the scope of this book. Individuals who wish to learn more are encouraged to take advantage of the many sources of information and assistance that can be found within their department and the community.

LEARNING OBJECTIVES

After learning the information in this chapter, you will be able to:

- Define substance abuse and related terms.
- Identify health risks associated with alcohol, drug, and tobacco abuse.
- Assess your own dependency on alcohol and drugs.
- Discuss your role and the department's role in substance abuse prevention.
- Identify sources of information, counseling, and treatment.

SUBSTANCE ABUSE

Substance abuse is an epidemic in this country, affecting the health and well-being of millions of Americans. Alcohol is a factor in eight of the 10 leading causes of death. Use of illegal drugs, such as heroin and cocaine, results in severe mental and physical problems, huge social costs, and untold suffering for those caught in the web of addiction. Cigarette smoking is the leading health risk in the country, killing hundreds of thousands of people each year from heart disease, lung cancer, and an array of other ailments. And all of these problems are completely preventable!

However, the problem is not limited to tobacco, alcohol, and drugs. As defined by the U.S. Fire Administration (USFA), **substance abuse is the use of <u>any</u> substance for non-medical reasons to affect the body, mind, or behavior.** Using this definition, many other substances are abused in our society, including caffeine, prescription and non-prescription medications, and even household solvents. In fact, almost any substance, including food, can be abused, leading to adverse health effects and other negative consequences.

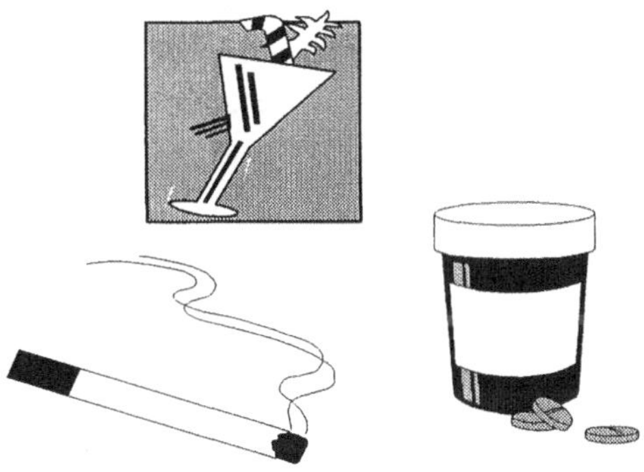

WHAT IS SUBSTANCE ABUSE?

The definition of substance abuse is highly subjective. What is considered a problem by one person may be viewed by another as acceptable behavior. Criteria sometimes used to define whether use of a substance constitutes "abuse" include:

- Impact on health and wellness, both on the user and on others
- Legality
- Personal religious and moral beliefs
- Dependency, either physical or psychological

<u>Physical dependence</u> occurs when a user can't quit without suffering withdrawal symptoms. <u>Psychological dependence</u>, which can be even more difficult to treat, refers to the user's intense craving or compulsion to use the substance.

The bottom line is that nobody can tell you the definition of substance abuse. You have to decide for yourself, and the implications of the decision can be enormous—for you, your family, friends, and co-workers. This chapter is designed to provide some basic information to help you make this important lifestyle choice.

> **"Substance abuse is public health enemy number one in America. The scourge of drug abuse is colorblind, gender-neutral, and oblivious to class status. It is devastating to our health care system."**
> **Joseph A Califano, Jr.**

WHO ARE THE VICTIMS?

A great majority of adults in this country have at least experimented with alcohol or drugs. About half of them will abuse these products at one time or another. Although most people are able to control their usage, about 10% will eventually become addicted, meaning that the substance now controls them. The result is habitual and compulsive use that significantly affects the quality and course of their lives.

Chemical dependency should be viewed as a physiological and psychological disease. Some people—such as children of addicts and children of emotionally disturbed, abusive parents—are more likely to suffer from the problem, but no one is immune. Contrary to some myths, substance abuse crosses all economic, geographic, and cultural lines. And it can happen quickly, often after only one or two experiences with certain powerful drugs.

Unfortunately, no matter what your beliefs and personal habits, you are a victim of substance abuse in this country. Almost everyone knows someone whose life has been damaged or destroyed, perhaps irreparably, through addiction of one form or another. We all pay the cost of increased crime, accidents, and lost productivity at work. Furthermore, a recent study shows that one fifth of the money Medicare spends on hospital care results from substance abuse. This figure translates to about $200 billion a year for all U.S. health care expenditures.

ALCOHOL

ALCOHOL CONSUMPTION

About six in ten adults drink alcoholic beverages, a decline of about 6% over the last decade. Per capita consumption of alcohol (in gallons) has also declined, as shown below. 1988 average consumption figures equate to about 530 drinks for every person over 14 in the country. (Each drink is equivalent to a 12-ounce bottle of beer, a 5-ounce glass of wine, or 1½ ounces of whiskey or other spirits.)

Year	*Gallons*
1978	2.71
1980	2.76
1982	2.72
1984	2.65
1986	2.58
1988	2.49

Source: NCHS 1992

Although average consumption has gone down somewhat, the proportion of problem drinkers among adults 18 and over has remained about the same—roughly 10 percent. According to the National Institute on Alcohol Abuse and Alcoholism, there were about 9.5 million alcoholics in the United States in 1985. Approximately 10 percent of all beginning drinkers become addicted.

THE EFFECTS OF ALCOHOL

Since no digestion is needed, alcohol rapidly enters the blood stream and circulates to all parts of the body. Its effect varies depending on the personality of the user, volume consumed, speed of drinking, body size, amount of food eaten, and other factors. Possible reactions include:

- Happiness, talkativeness
- Relaxation, loss of inhibitions
- Slower brain function and reflexes
- Slurred speech, clumsiness, staggering
- Excitation, erratic behavior
- Confusion, disorientation
- Fear, anger, aggression
- Stupor, unconsciousness

Individual responses vary because alcohol is a powerful mood-altering drug that affects people differently and often in unpredictable ways. It depresses the central nervous system, slowing thought processes, reflexes, and other physical skills. And it is highly addictive, causing both physical and psychological dependency.

HEALTH IMPACTS

Alcohol is also a powerful irritant to the body's organs and tissues. This characteristic contributes to the negative health impacts of chronic alcohol abuse, which include:

- Cancers of the liver, stomach, colon, larynx, esophagus, and breast
- Damage to the brain, pancreas, and kidneys
- High blood pressure, heart attacks, and strokes
- Alcoholic hepatitis and cirrhosis of the liver
- Stomach and duodenal ulcers, colitis, and colon problems
- Lowered immunity to pneumonia and other infections
- Impotence and infertility
- Birth defects and Fetal Alcohol Syndrome (FAS), which causes retardation, small head size, and limb abnormalities
- Premature aging
- Acute withdrawal symptoms and hallucinations
- Many other disorders, such as sleep disturbances, muscle cramps, and edema

In addition to harmful health effects, alcohol continues to be a leading cause of death due to motor vehicle and other types of accidents (for example, falls, fires, drowning, skimobile, and aircraft). It is also often a factor in crimes and violence, resulting in millions of arrests each year. Some studies show that more than 25 percent of hospital emergency room admissions are alcohol-related.

Drunkenness is involved in one-third to one-half of all traffic deaths, 69 percent of drownings, 47 percent of industrial accidents, 70 percent of fatal falls, half of all homicides, and one-third of all suicides. Up to 83 percent of all fire fatalities and 62 percent of all fire burns involved alcohol use at the time of the accident; 53 percent of the fatalities and 23 percent of the burn victims were alcoholics.

The implications of these statistics are all too clear for emergency services personnel.

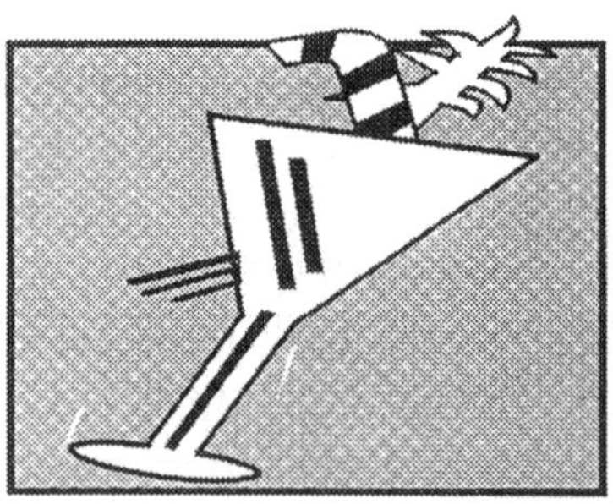

OTHER COSTS

Unfortunately, the toll for alcohol abuse cannot be measured simply in terms of death, disease, and injury statistics. Drinking is a major factor in many divorces, family difficulties, and job problems. It is estimated that an alcohol-related problem strikes one of every four American homes. (IAFF 1992)

By one calculation, alcohol abuse costs the United States $89.5 billion a year, of which $54.7 billion is absorbed by business. (Fitzgerald 1989) According to the National Council on Alcoholism, alcoholics average two-to-three times the absentee rate of other employees. They also have two to four times more on-the-job accidents, and three times more sickness and accident benefit claims.

USE AND ABUSE OF ALCOHOL

Alcohol is enjoyed in moderation as a beverage by millions of adults, and it is abused by millions of others, resulting in huge health and social costs. This dual nature of alcohol leads to a mixed reaction by society—both positive and negative—and mixed signals for individual consumers. The use of alcohol is actively promoted, but the negative impacts of abuse are recognized as a serious health and social problem. No wonder people are confused!

Moderate drinking may not be a significant cause for concern, but it must be remembered that alcoholism is a disease that occurs in stages. Unfortunately, the process of moving from social drinker to psychological dependence to chronic alcoholism is subtle and insidious. For this reason, persons who suspect that they may be losing control of their drinking habits—e.g., drinking too much or for the wrong reasons—are strongly advised to examine their lifestyles and seek help if necessary.

"Alcohol is wondrously dangerous. It causes more sickness, more deaths, more accidents, more lost time, more spoiled work, more social and family disruption, and more crime than all the other drugs put together. And it can, and has, cost loss of life in firefighting. Clouded judgments and fumbled movements are no match for the ever-changing conditions of the fireground."

(McVernon 1984)

Activity 8-1

ARE YOU DEPENDENT ON ALCOHOL?

The following questions can help you determine whether you are chemically dependent on alcohol. Answer each question as truthfully as possible. Then look over your answers. **Only you can decide if you have a problem.**

	Yes	No
1. Has your job performance ever suffered because of drinking?	( )	( )
2. Do you ever drink alone?	( )	( )
3. Do you have the urge to drink at a certain time (e.g., when you wake up, after work, after an incident, etc.)?	( )	( )
4. Do you ever feel guilty, remorseful, defensive, or ashamed about drinking?	( )	( )
5. Do you sometimes feel you need to drink to have a good time or "fit in"?	( )	( )
6. Has your drinking ever caused problems in your home life?	( )	( )
7. Do you ever drink while at work or on duty?	( )	( )
8. Do you think a lot about drinking?	( )	( )
9. Has drinking ever caused you financial difficulties?	( )	( )
10. Are relatives or close friends sometimes upset with your drinking?	( )	( )
11. Does drinking ever affect your sleeping or eating patterns?	( )	( )
12. Do you ever drink to overcome shyness or to build up your self-confidence?	( )	( )
13. Do you ever lie about how much you drink?	( )	( )
14. Have you ever lost time or taken time off from work because of drinking?	( )	( )
15. Has your drinking ever made you careless about your family responsibilities?	( )	( )
16. Do you ever drink to escape from worries, stress, trouble, or emotional pain?	( )	( )
17. Has drinking ever caused you legal or medical problems?	( )	( )
18. Do you avoid people or places that do not approve of drinking?	( )	( )
19. Have you ever had a loss of memory or other strong negative reaction (overdose) as a result of drinking?	( )	( )
20. Is the amount or frequency of your drinking increasing?	( )	( )

LEGAL AND ILLEGAL DRUGS

DRUG USE IN THE UNITED STATES

The proportion of young adults 18-25 years of age reporting frequent use of illegal drugs other than alcohol over the last decade has declined markedly for marijuana and stayed roughly the same for other drugs (see below).

Year	*Marijuana*	*Other Drugs*
1977	19%	0.8%
1979	22	2.4
1982	16	2.3
1985	11	1.8
1988	7	1.3
1990	5	0.6

Source: NCHS 1992

The *National Household Survey on Drug Abuse, 1985* indicated that 37 percent of the population age 12 or older have tried illicit drugs, and 12 percent (23 million people) could be classified as current users. After marijuana, cocaine use ranked second with 3 percent of the population; abuse of other drugs typically fell in the 0.5-1.5 percent range.

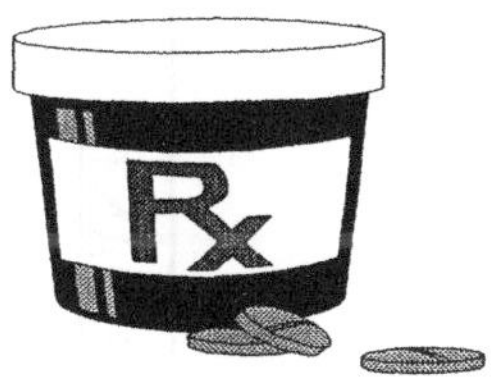

Some experts believe the "five percent rule" should be assumed: in any group, five percent of the personnel are probably involved with illegal drugs. Percentages for certain populations (e.g., young males, urban residents) are even higher.

CATEGORIES OF DRUGS

According to USFA, the large variety of abused drugs can be grouped according to the major effects produced. These substances, which are summarized in Exhibit 8-1, include:

- Cannabis (marijuana, hashish)—alters mood and perception.
- Stimulants (amphetamines, cocaine, "crack")—speed up the action of the central nervous system.
- Depressants (barbiturates, tranquilizers, methaqualone)—relax the central nervous system.
- Hallucinogens (LSD, PCP, etc.)—temporarily distort reality.
- Narcotics (heroin, morphine, codeine, opium)—lower the perception of pain.
- Deliriants (aerosols, paint thinner, etc.)—cause mental confusion.

Exhibit 8-1

DRUGS AND THEIR EFFECTS

GENERIC TYPE	DRUG NAME	EARLY EFFECTS	LATE ADVERSE EFFECTS
CANNABIS Alters mood and perception	MARIJUANA Grass, Pot, Weed HASHISH Hash	Euphoria, relaxed inhibitions Intoxication (2-3 hours) Impaired memory, perception, and judgment Impaired fine motor skills (4-24 hours) Anxiety, panic reactions	Damage to respiratory system Increased lung cancer risk Permanent damage to memory and immune system Psychological dependence Effect on reproductive system and maturation processes
STIMULANTS Speed up central nervous system	COCAINE Coke, Snow, Flake CRACK FREEBASE	Euphoria (1/2 hour) Increased alertness Increased heart rate, blood pressure Depression and confusion Occasionally hallucinations Possibility of overdose and death, especially with crack and freebase	Chronic depression Hallucinations and psychosis Damage to nasal membranes and lungs Tolerance and physical dependence
	AMPHETAMINES Speed, Uppers Bennies, Pep pills	Rapidly developing "high" (hours) Excitation, extreme talkativeness, tremors Persecutory delusions and hallucinations possible Confusion, anxiety, and sleep problems possible	Brain damage Skin disorders, malnutrition, and ulcers Tolerance and psychological addiction Liver and cardiovascular disease Psychiatric problems
DEPRESSANTS Slow down central nervous system	BARBITURATES Goofballs, Downers TRANQUILIZERS Valium, Seconal METHAQUALONE Quads, Soapers, Ludes	Calming effects, drowsiness, sleep Confusion and poor coordination Slurred speech, staggering gait, uncertain reflexes Poor judgment With overdose, death possible (especially dangerous in combination with alcohol)	Physical and psychological dependence Tolerance Physical withdrawal symptoms: anxiety, insomnia, tremors, delirium Possible birth defects Possible convulsions and death

Exhibit 8-1 (Continued)

GENERIC TYPE	DRUG NAME	EARLY EFFECTS	LATE ADVERSE EFFECTS
HALLUCIN-OGENS Temporarily distort reality	LYSERGIC ACID DIETHYLAMIDE LSD, Acid MESCALINE PSILOCYBIN	Illusions and hallucinations Poor perception of time and distance Wild swings in sensations and feelings "Bad trips" with panic, confusion, anxiety, loss of control Impaired memory, attention span, and thought processes	"Flashbacks" giving prior effects without renewed drug use Neuroses, character disorders Brain damage, psychosis Tolerance Possible birth defects
	PHENCYCLIDINE PCP, Angel Dust	Feelings of strength, power, and invulnerability Sometimes anger and rage Depression, hallucinations, confusion, irrational behavior With overdose, convulsions, coma, and death possible	Tolerance Memory loss, speech difficulties Impaired motor skills Depression, mood disorders Accidents and injuries Paranoia, agitation, withdrawal
OPIATES (NARCOTICS) Reduce perception of pain	HEROIN MORPHINE CODEINE OPIUM	Relaxation and euphoria (hours) Swings from alertness to drowsiness Restlessness, nausea, and vomiting Lethargy, apathy, poor judgment, loss of control With overdose, unconsciousness, convulsions, coma, and death	Heart and lung damage Hepatitis and AIDS from injection Physical and psychological addiction Severe withdrawal symptoms Heart and lung abnormalities Skin infections, ulcers, and abscesses Tolerance
DELIRIANTS and INHALANTS Cause mental confusion	SOLVENTS, AEROSOLS ANESTHETICS OTHERS	Mild stimulation, euphoria Impaired judgment, confusion, panic Loss of coordination Nausea and vomiting Drowsiness, stupor, unconsciousness With overdose, heart failure and death	Damage to nervous system, liver, kidneys, blood, and bone marrow Weight loss, electrolyte imbalance and muscle fatigue Tolerance Physical dependence

Source: USFA 1988

DRUG EFFECTS

As shown in Exhibit 8-1, the health effects associated with drug abuse differ depending on the substance chosen and the method of intake. Typically, drugs convey some initial pleasurable effects—a "high" or feeling of euphoria, relaxation, increased alertness, etc. Because they affect the brain, drugs can also alter perceptions, impair motor skills, and change emotions, sometimes drastically.

In the long run, drug use can lead to physical and psychological addiction and a vast array of physical, mental, and social problems. Furthermore, abuse of drugs is a factor in accidents, injuries, and lost productivity, both on and off the job. As a result, illicit drug use cost the United States $58.3 billion in 1988. (National Council on Alcoholism and Drug Dependence, Inc.)

TYPES OF USERS

According to USFA, users can be classified along a continuous range of drug involvement, as follows:

- Experimental user—motivated by peer or social pressures to try a drug once or twice
- Casual or recreational user—occasionally involved in drug use, usually in social settings
- Circumstantial user—uses drug to cope with a specific problem situation or condition
- Intensified user—has developed a long-term, patterned use of drugs at least once daily
- Compulsive user—virtually every aspect of life revolves around obtaining, maintaining, and using a supply of the drug

As noted by USFA, "rehabilitation can arrest the tendency towards heavier drug abuse and can, in most cases, lead the individual to a drug-free existence. In the absence of rehabilitation, most drug dependent users will eventually slide into a terminal state where death will usually result from excessive drug use (overdose), accidents, or illness related to drug abuse."

Since denial is a common characteristic of drug abuse, most users don't know where they fall on the scale. Therefore, the keys to successful rehabilitation are 1) recognizing that you have a problem, and 2) seeking the professional help needed to address it.

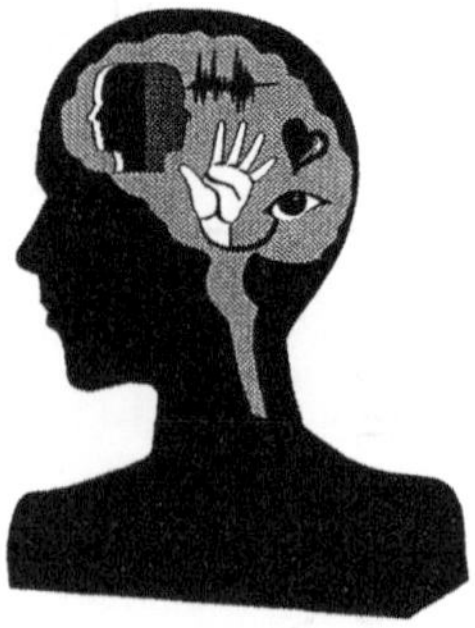

Activity 8-2

ARE YOU DEPENDENT ON DRUGS?

The following questions, like those in Activity 8-1, can help you decide whether you are dependent on drugs. As before, answer each question, then look over your answers. The total number of "yes" answers is less important than how you feel about yourself and how drugs have affected your life.

	Yes	No
1. Has your job performance ever suffered because of taking drugs?	( )	( )
2. Do you ever take drugs alone?	( )	( )
3. Do you have the urge to take drugs at a certain time (e.g., when you wake up, after work, after an incident, etc.)?	( )	( )
4. Do you ever feel guilty, remorseful, defensive, or ashamed about drug use?	( )	( )
5. Do you sometimes feel you need to drink to have a good time or "fit in"?	( )	( )
6. Has your drug use ever caused problems in your home life?	( )	( )
7. Do you ever take drugs while at work or on duty?	( )	( )
8. Do you think a lot about taking drugs?	( )	( )
9. Has taking drugs ever caused you financial difficulties?	( )	( )
10. Are relatives or close friends sometimes upset with your taking drugs?	( )	( )
11. Does taking drugs ever affect your sleeping or eating patterns?	( )	( )
12. Do you ever take drugs to overcome shyness or to build up your confidence?	( )	( )
13. Do you ever lie about how much you take drugs?	( )	( )
14. Have you ever lost time or taken time off from work because of drugs?	( )	( )
15. Has drug use ever made you careless about your family responsibilities?	( )	( )
16. Do you ever take drugs to escape worries, stress, trouble, or emotional pain?	( )	( )
17. Has taking drugs ever caused you legal or medical problems?	( )	( )
18. Do you avoid people or places that do not approve of taking drugs?	( )	( )
19. Have you ever had a loss of memory or other strong negative reaction (overdose) as a result of taking drugs?	( )	( )
20. Is the amount or frequency of your drug use increasing?	( )	( )

ALCOHOL, DRUGS, AND THE FIRE SERVICE

ABUSE BY FIRE/RESCUE PERSONNEL

Firefighters and rescue personnel confront the same pressures as members of the general public—family problems, financial difficulties, and health concerns to name a few. In addition, they face high levels of stress on the job. Special pressures include:

- Fear of injury or death
- Long periods of intense activity, or conversely, inactivity
- Traumatic incident stress (seeing victims or co-workers hurt)
- Boring, repetitive tasks (e.g., vehicle maintenance)
- Physical stressors (noise, heat, cold, toxic environments)
- Performance evaluations, annual physicals, training, etc.
- Long shifts, excessive time away from family
- Lack of appreciation

Communicating these problems or seeking assistance is particularly difficult for many fire and rescue personnel. In addition, co-workers sometimes unknowingly encourage the situation by allowing members with problems avoid detection. For all these reasons, some experts feel that the fire service environment may actually be somewhat conducive to the abuse of alcohol and drugs.

Although comprehensive data are not readily available, substance abuse exists in fire departments like anywhere else. As noted by USFA: **"The fragmentary data and professional judgment suggest that the prevalence of current drug abusers is probably in the range of 1% to 10% of the firefighters, depending upon the policies of the department, the age distribution of the firefighters, and the local environment. It is likely that most of these abusers will be from the younger age groups. It is also likely that most of the abusers will have a light to moderate problem."**

USFA concludes it is "reasonable to assume that drug abuse is as prevalent among new employees as it is among the same age groups in the local work force. In fact, considering the stress, occasional horror, and image problems, the firefighter may be even more susceptible than the average worker to alcohol and drug abuse." (USFA 1988)

The IAFF reports that the fire service experiences approximately twice the national average of people addicted to drugs and alcohol. According to another expert, "at least 75 percent of all fire/rescue service members have used dangerous substances (alcohol and drugs) at one time or another. Further research reveals that 30 percent or more of those users could be considered abusers." (Estepp 1985)

IMPACT ON FIRE SERVICE

In addition to the health implications for individual workers—the department's most valuable resource—alcohol and drugs impair performance and behavior, leading to major organizational problems:

- Degraded capability to respond to emergencies
- Increased accident rates, injuries, and deaths
- More interpersonal strife, employee complaints, disciplinary actions, and arbitrations
- Increased absenteeism and health benefit claims
- Increased public complaints and diminished public trust
- Higher departmental administrative costs
- More liability lawsuits

Simple manual tasks and repetitive work are less affected than work requiring complex decision processes or coping skills. Unfortunately, "firefighters face many situations where coping skills are essential. In addition to driving fire equipment in response to an emergency, firefighters can face a constantly changing set of dangers at the scene of the emergency. For the firefighter's own protection and the protection of others at the scene, the firefighter must be able to recognize emerging dangers, make a timely response, and have the strength and ability to sustain that response." (USFA 1988)

> "It needs to be realized that firefighting, rescue, and the delivery of emergency medical services has to be provided by individuals that are free and unimpaired by dangerous substances. This is a dangerous occupation that requires sound logical decisions and the ability to react quickly to protect the public, fellow firefighters, and oneself. Substance abuse hinders and curtails the functions to think and react at this critical level."
>
> (Meister 1990)

To counteract the problem, fire departments have the responsibility to establish and enforce substance abuse policies, to include education, detection, intervention, rehabilitation, and disciplinary action. The goal of the program should be to restore the individual to a healthy and fully productive life. If help is refused and job performance continues to deteriorate, department guidelines must be followed to address the problem, to include suspension or termination after other measures have failed.

EMPLOYEE ASSISTANCE PROGRAMS

Early detection and treatment can typically lead to high rates of recovery and rehabilitation of alcohol and drug abusers, including a return to full capability in the workplace. Some specific forms of treatment include individual counseling, psychotherapy, family therapy or counseling, encounter group therapy, detoxification, and aftercare.

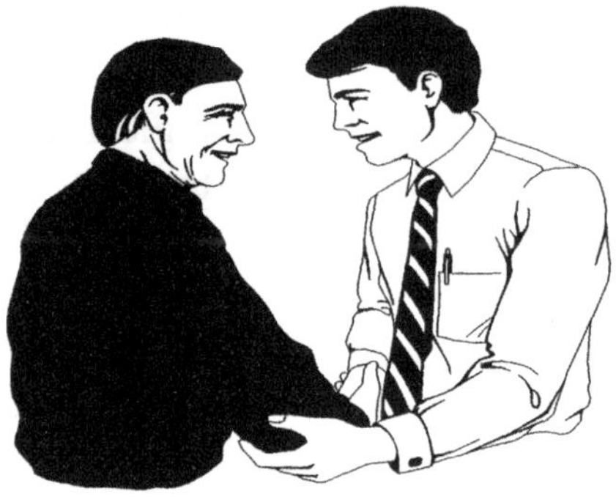

Fire departments often assist in this process by establishing Employee Assistance Programs (EAPs) for their members. As defined by the Employee Assistance Professionals Association, an EAP is "a worksite-based program designed to assist in the identification and resolution of productivity problems associated with employees impaired by personal concerns, including, but not limited to: health, marital, family, financial, alcohol, drug, legal, emotional, stress, or other personal concerns that may adversely affect employee job performance." Some fire and rescue departments also include infection control, gambling addiction, career/vocational guidance, and health promotion (physical fitness, nutrition, weight control, smoking cessation, etc.) under the EAP.

Studies show that 60% to 80% of individuals counseled through an EAP return to fully productive status in the workplace. Departments also benefit—for every dollar invested in an EAP, employers save $5 to $16 through "decreased use of medical and insurance benefits, savings in worker's compensation claims, fewer grievances and arbitrations, less absenteeism, less use of management time with troubled employees, less employee turnover, and less personnel replacement costs....Benefits of the EAP are also expressed through the improved morale of the workforce and the rehabilitation of a valuable trained and experienced worker." (IAFF 1992)

As a result, the National Fire Protection Association *Standard on Fire Department Occupational Safety and Health Program* (NFPA 1500) states that "the fire department shall provide a Member Assistance Program that identifies and assists members and their immediate families with substance abuse, stress, and personal problems that adversely affect fire department work performance. The assistance program shall refer members and their immediate families, as appropriate, to the proper health care services for the purpose of restoring job performance to expected levels, as well as for the restoration of better health."

TOBACCO: THE NUMBER ONE HEALTH HAZARD

TOBACCO USE IN THE U.S.

Approximately 26 percent of the American population 25 years of age or older smoked in 1990—about 50 million people. Among men, about 28 percent smoked; among women, the percentage was about 23. As shown by the figures below, the proportion of people who smoke has been steadily and dramatically declining for the last decade:

Year	*Percent*
1979	33.5
1980	33.2
1983	32.1
1985	30.1
1987	28.8
1990	25.5

Source: NCHS 1992

About 12 million people use smokeless tobacco (chewing tobacco, snuff), and consumption is growing. For example, the use of moist snuff has risen about 40 percent over the last 20 years. Almost all users are males, about one in four under the age of 21.

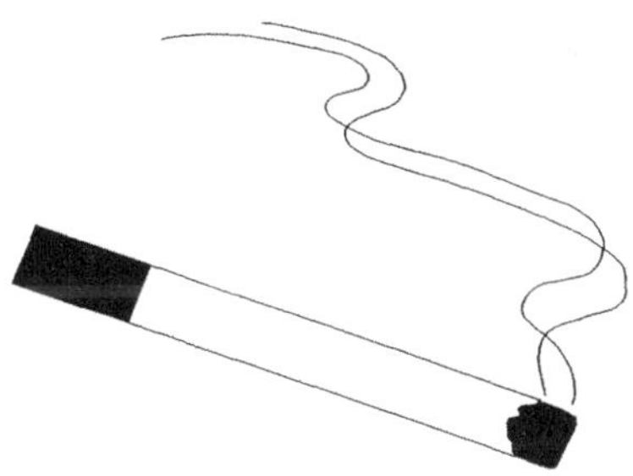

CIGARETTE SMOKING

According to the Department of Health and Human Services, "cigarette smoking has been identified as the largest risk factor for mortality in the United States. Over 400,000 lives are lost each year from smoking, primarily from lung cancer, cardiovascular disease, and chronic obstructive lung disease. The adverse effects of cigarette smoking on pregnancy and infant health are also well documented."

That's about 1,100 lives lost each day, or one of every five deaths in the United States! Smokers age 35 or older increase their risk of death from many major causes, including (DHHS 1990):

- Lung cancer—12 times risk
- Chronic obstructive pulmonary disease—10 times risk
- Larynx (voice box) cancer—10 times risk
- Mouth cancer—6 times risk
- Coronary heart disease—2 times risk
- Stroke—2 times risk

The risk depends to some extent on the amount you smoke. According to the American Cancer Society, **heavy smokers are actually 24 times more likely to die of lung cancer than nonsmokers.** Men who smoke less than one half pack per day have a death rate about 30 percent higher than nonsmokers; one-to-two packs a day, about 100 percent higher; and two-or-more packs a day, 140 percent higher.

In addition, tobacco contains hundreds of poisons and thousands of chemicals which contribute to other health problems, including phlebitis, cavities and gum disease, peptic ulcers, cancer of the urinary bladder, and birth defects. The risk even extends to non-smoking family members. Spouses of smokers are estimated to have twice the risk of lung cancer, and children of smokers are hospitalized for bronchitis, pneumonia, and lower respiratory tract infections at twice the rate of other children. (DHHS 1990)

> "Smoking costs the nation $65 billion per year in health-care costs and lost productivity—that's $262 per American per year."
> American Lung Assn.

SMOKELESS TOBACCO

You don't have to smoke tobacco to experience its harmful effects. Many people believe that chewing tobacco or dipping snuff is safe because the product is not inhaled. Unfortunately, tobacco juice contains nicotine (the habit-forming substance found in cigarettes), many cancer-causing substances, and hundreds of other chemicals. In addition, most brands contain sweeteners which cause tooth decay, abrasives which wear down tooth surfaces, and salt which can contribute to high blood pressure and kidney disease.

Since smokeless tobacco is held in one area of the mouth for long periods of time, its use is associated with various oral hygiene problems and diseases. **Smokeless tobacco users have 50 times the rate of oral cancers, including cancer of the cheek, inner lip, pharynx, tongue, esophagus, palate, and larynx.** Inflammation and infection of the gums are common, and users are five times more likely to lose their teeth due to decay. Mouth wounds heal more slowly, and users have a lowered sense of taste and smell. Other social problems include brown stained teeth, a condition called black hairy tongue, and the unsanitary need to spit frequently.

TOBACCO AND THE FIRE SERVICE

If the national mortality averages hold true for the fire service, we lose almost 1,800 of our 1.1 million firefighters every year, or about five per day, to the hazards of smoking and other forms of tobacco abuse. Unfortunately, this data may actually understate the problem since many experts believe that a greater proportion of firefighters smoke than the general population.

Furthermore, most lung diseases are caused by substances that people breathe. Firefighters are exposed at work to a number of harmful products of combustion, including irritant gases, vapors, and particulates in smoke. As a result, studies suggest that firefighters are at increased risk of chronic lung disease and loss of lung function. According to the American Lung Association, cigarette smoking greatly increases these hazards.

A particular threat is carbon monoxide, a colorless, odorless gas that reduces the oxygen-carrying capacity of the blood. Its effects are first felt in tissues that are especially sensitive to a lack of oxygen—the brain and heart. Symptoms include headache, weakness, dizziness, dim vision, nausea, and vomiting. High concentrations can cause coma and death.

Smoking increases the levels of carbon monoxide in the blood, thus contributing to these symptoms and related dangers on the incident scene. Smoking also elevates blood pressure by constricting blood vessels and increasing heart rate. As a result, your heart has to work harder, potentially contributing to heart attack and stroke. Finally, smoking firefighters have a diminished sense of smell, and so have a reduced sensitivity to dangerous smoke and toxic gases.

In summary, smoking firefighters start with higher levels of carbon monoxide than non-smokers, and have reduced aerobic capacity. It is therefore reasonable to assume that smokers on average have reduced job performance and more injuries than non-smokers. Furthermore, data from several studies suggest an elevated risk for lung disease and coronary heart disease in smoking firefighters, but not in non-smoking firefighters.

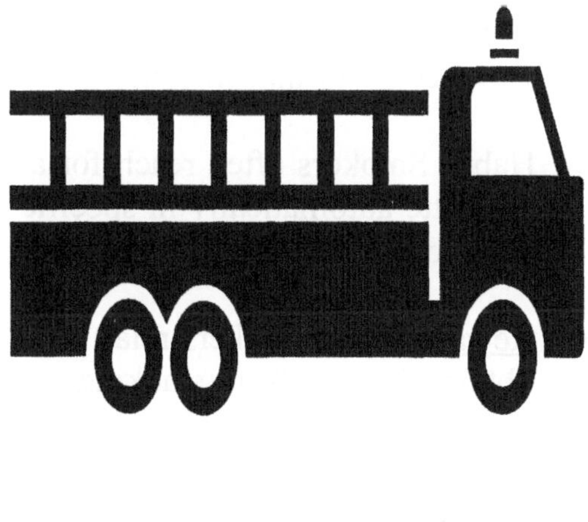

QUITTING SMOKING

The use of tobacco—like any form of chemical dependency—should be viewed as a disease that can be cured if dealt with effectively. About three million people quit smoking each year. In fact, nearly half of all adults who ever smoked have quit for life. Ninety percent of them did it on their own, without participation in a formal cessation program.

Besides the obvious health benefits, some other reasons smokers often give for quitting include:

- Feeling more in control of life
- Better smelling hair, breath, clothes, house, and car
- More stamina for work and leisure activities
- Less coughing, colds, and flu
- Reduced costs and inconvenience
- Consideration for family, friends, and others

However, as anyone who has ever tried knows, quitting smoking is not easy. Some of the challenges smokers must overcome to quit include:

- Habit: Smokers often reach for a cigarette automatically in specific situations every day.

- Reward: Most smokers relax or obtain pleasure from smoking.

- Stimulant: Some people feel smoking gives them more energy when they are tired.

- Weight gain: Some smokers gain weight after quitting.

- Social: Friends or relatives that smoke can be a negative influence.

- Time filler: Many people smoke when they are bored or have nothing to do.

- Coping: Smokers often light up when they feel worried, upset, sad, or angry.

In short, tobacco is perceived as serving a meaningful purpose in the smoker's everyday life. Moreover, most smokers are physically addicted to nicotine and will crave cigarettes when they stop. Withdrawal symptoms, which may last two to four weeks, can include dizziness, headaches, tiredness, coughing, tightness in the chest, trouble sleeping, constipation, hunger, and lack of concentration. Any plan to quit must take these factors into consideration.

Although quitting smoking can be done, the process is different for everyone. The appendix at the end of this chapter contains detailed suggestions from the Department of Health and Human Services on ways to quit smoking. If you use tobacco, you are strongly encouraged to read this material and find an approach that works for you. There's probably nothing else you can do that's more important for your health and well-being. Do it for yourself!

YOUR ROLE IN SUBSTANCE ABUSE

The basic rule of substance abuse is simple: prevention is far better and much easier than rehabilitation. Therefore, to maximize your health and wellness:

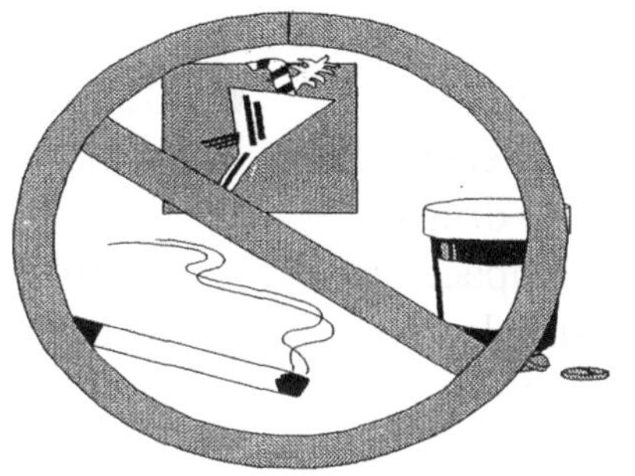

- Don't smoke or use smokeless tobacco.
- Don't drink alcohol or drink only in moderation.
- Don't use illegal drugs.
- Don't abuse legal medications.

As a member of the emergency services, you also have responsibilities to yourself, your co-workers, the department, and the public. These can be summarized as follows:

1. Take care of yourself. Eat well and participate in a fitness program to reduce stress and anxiety. Fit persons are less likely to need the psychological "crutches" offered by tobacco, alcohol, or drugs.

2. Be aware of the dangers. Learn the signs and symptoms of substance abuse, and watch for them in yourself and others.

3. Play it safe. Avoid people and situations that may lead to substance abuse. Foster a responsible environment at home and at work. Adopt stress management techniques that work for you (see Chapter 9 for suggestions.)

4. Help out others with a problem. Encourage and actively support your co-workers in their efforts to control the use of tobacco, alcohol, and drugs. You just might make a difference in someone's life!

5. Follow the rules. Learn and follow your department's policies and procedures on substance abuse.

If you even suspect you have a problem, seek help. Assistance is available through your department's EAP, government agencies, civic and church groups, health care institutions, private sector providers, etc. Local chapters of the American Lung Association, American Cancer Society, and American Heart Association can also help. Find out what your community has to offer, and take advantage of it. If you're in danger, don't wait until it's too late.

CHAPTER SUMMARY

In this chapter, you learned about the health impacts of substance abuse, the most important preventable health risk factor in the country. After defining substance abuse, you examined each of three major problems—alcohol, drugs, and tobacco—including their impact on the fire service. You used simple instruments to evaluate your own dependency on alcohol and drugs. Employee Assistance Programs and other possible sources of assistance were reviewed. You also thought about your own role in preventing and monitoring substance abuse, both on and off the job.

Having completed this chapter, you should now be able to:

- Define substance abuse and related terms.
- Identify health risks associated with alcohol, drug, and tobacco abuse.
- Assess your own dependency on alcohol and drugs.
- Discuss your role and the department's role in substance abuse prevention.
- Identify sources of information, counseling, and treatment.

BIBLIOGRAPHY

Baxter Healthcare Corporation, *The 1992 Baxter Survey of Health Habits* (conducted by Louis Harris and Associates), 1992.

Bell, Jerry, and Pat Bell, "Alcohol in the Workplace," *Professional Safety*, February 1989.

Center on Addiction and Substance Abuse at Columbia University, *The Cost of Substance Abuse to America's Health Care System*, 1993.

Department of Health and Human Services, *Nurses: Help Your Patients Stop Smoking*, National Institutes of Health, NIH Publication No. (ADM) 90-2962, October 1990.

Department of Health and Human Services, *What You Can Do About Drug Use in America*, DHHS Publication No. (ADM) 99-1572, 1988.

Estepp, M. H., and Elizabeth Redding, "Substance Abuse in the Fire Department," *The International Fire Chief*," June 1985.

Fitzgerald, S. T., S. C. Hammond, and K. A. Harder, "Role of the Employee Assistance Program in Helping the Troubled Worker, *Occupational Medicine*, 1989.

Health Communications, Inc., *Do You Know the Facts About Drugs?*, 1983.

International Association of Fire Fighters, *Developing Fire Service Labor/Employee Assistance Programs*, ISBN No. 0-942920-12-0, 1992.

McVernon, Father John, "Drugs, Drink and Duty," *Fire Engineering*, June 1984.

Meister, George R., *The Answer to Substance Abuse in the Fire Service: Identification and Rehabilitation*, National Fire Academy Executive Fire Officer Program, January 1990.

National Center for Health Statistics, *Health, United States, 1991*, Hyattsville, Maryland: Public Health Service, 1992.

National Institute on Alcohol Abuse and Alcoholism, *Facts About Alcohol and Alcoholism*, DHHS Publication No. (ADM) 80-31.

Stanford, Todd M., "The Hidden Disease," *Emergency*, September 1989.

United States Fire Administration, *Administrative Manual on Use of Drugs by Fire Department Members*, FA 77, May 1988.

APPENDIX: QUITTING SMOKING

QUITTING FOR KEEPS

Congratulations! You're ready to develop a new habit: not smoking. Like any other habit, it takes time to become a part of you; unlike most other habits, though, not smoking will take some conscious effort and practice. This material can be a big help. You'll find many techniques for developing the nonsmoking habit and holding on to it.

By reading this information carefully and reviewing it often, you'll become more aware of the places and situations that prompt the desire for a cigarette. You'll also learn many nonsmoking ways to deal with the urge to smoke. These are called coping skills. Finally, you'll learn what to do in case you do slip and give in to that urge.

Keep your guard up

The key to living as a nonsmoker is to avoid letting your urges or cravings for a cigarette lead you to smoke. Don't kid yourself: even though you've made a commitment not to smoke, you *will* sometimes be tempted. But instead of giving in to the urge, you can use it as a learning experience.

First, remind yourself that you've *quit* and you're a *non*smoker. Then, look closely at your urge to smoke and ask:

- Where was I when I got the urge?
- What was I doing at the time?
- Whom was I with?
- What was I thinking?

The urge to smoke after you've quit often hits at predictable times. The trick is to anticipate those times and find ways to cope with them without smoking. Naturally, it won't be easy at first. In fact, you may continue to want a cigarette at times. But remember, even if you slip, it doesn't mean an end to the nonsmoking you. It does mean that you should try to identify what triggered your slip, strengthen your commitment to quitting, and try again.

Look at the following list of typical triggers. Do any of them ring a bell with you? Check off those that might trigger an urge to smoke, and add any others you can think of:

- Working under pressure
- Feeling blue
- Talking on the telephone
- Having a drink or finishing a meal
- Watching television
- Driving your car
- Playing cards
- Drinking coffee
- Watching someone else smoke

If you're like so many new nonsmokers, the most difficult place to resist the urge to smoke is the most familiar: home. The activities most closely associated with smoking urges are eating, partying, and drinking. And, not surprisingly, most urges occur when a smoker is present.

How to dampen that urge

There are seven major coping skills to help you fight the urge to smoke. These tips are designed for you, the new nonsmoker, to help you nurture the nonsmoking habit.

1. Think about why you quit

Go back to your list of reasons for quitting. Look at this several times a day, especially when you're hit with an urge to smoke. The best reasons you could have for quitting are very personally yours, and these are also your best reasons for staying a nonsmoker.

2. Know when you're rationalizing

It's easy to rationalize yourself back into smoking. Don't talk yourself into smoking again. A new nonsmoker in a tense situation may think, "I'll just have one cigarette to calm myself down." If thoughts like this pop into your head, stop and think again! You know better ways to relax—nonsmoker's ways, such as taking a walk or doing breathing exercises.

Concern about gaining weight may also lead to rationalizations. Learn to counter thoughts such as "I'd rather be thin, even if it means smoking." Remember that a slight weight gain is not likely to endanger your health as much as smoking (cigarette smokers have about a 70 percent higher rate of premature death than nonsmokers). Develop a list of healthy, low-calorie snacks to help you combat hunger.

3. Anticipate triggers and prepare to avoid them

By now you know which situations, people, and feelings are likely to tempt you to smoke. Be prepared to meet these triggers head on and counteract them. Keep using the coping skills that helped you cut down and quit:

- Keep your hands busy: doodle, knit, type a letter.
- Avoid people who smoke; spend more time with nonsmoking friends.
- Find activities that make smoking difficult (gardening, washing the car, taking a shower). Exercise to help knock out the urge; it will help you feel and look good, too.
- Put something other than a cigarette in your mouth. Chew sugarless gum or nibble on a carrot or celery stick.
- Avoid places where smoking is permitted. Sit in the nonsmoking section in restaurants, trains, etc.

- Reduce your consumption of alcohol, which often stimulates the desire to smoke. Try to have no more than one or two drinks at a party. Better yet, have a glass of juice, soda, or mineral water with a celery stick to nibble on.

4. Reward yourself for not smoking

Congratulations are in order each time you get through the day without smoking. After a week, give yourself a pat on the back and a reward of some kind. Buy a new record or treat yourself to a movie or concert. No matter how you do it, make sure you reward yourself in some way. It helps to remind yourself that what you're doing is important.

5. Use positive thoughts

If self-defeating thoughts start to creep in, remind yourself again that you're a nonsmoker, that you don't want to smoke, and that you have good reasons for it. Putting yourself down and trying to hold out through willpower alone are not effective coping techniques. Mobilize the power of positive thinking!

6. Use relaxation techniques

Breathing exercises help to reduce tension. Instead of having a cigarette, take a long deep breath, count to 10, and release it. Repeat this five times. See how much more relaxed you feel?

7. Get social support

The commitment to remain a nonsmoker can be made easier by talking about it with friends and relatives. They can congratulate you as you check off another day, week, and month as a nonsmoker. Tell the people close to you that you might be tense for awhile, so they know what to expect. They'll be sympathetic when you have an urge to smoke and can be counted on to help you resist it. Remember to call on your friends when you're lonely or you feel an urge to smoke. A buddy system is a great technique.

Not smoking is habit-forming

Good for you! You've made the commitment not to smoke, and by using this information, you know what to do if you're tempted to forget that commitment. It's difficult to stay a nonsmoker once you've had a cigarette, so do everything possible to avoid it.

The following approaches include many of those most popular with ex-smokers. Remember that successful methods are as different as the people who use them. What may seem silly to others may be just what you need to quit, so don't be embarrassed to try something new. These methods can make your own personal efforts a little easier. Pick the ideas that make sense to you. And then follow through—you'll have a much better chance of success.

PREPARING YOURSELF FOR QUITTING

- Decide positively that you want to quit. Try to avoid negative thoughts about how difficult it might be.
- List all the reasons you want to quit. Every night before going to bed, repeat one of the reasons 10 times.
- Develop strong personal reasons in addition to your health and obligations to others. For example, think of all the time you waste taking cigarette breaks, rushing out to buy a pack, hunting for a light, etc.
- Begin to condition yourself physically: Start a modest exercise program; drink more fluids; get plenty of rest; and avoid fatigue.
- Set a target date for quitting, perhaps a special day such as your birthday, your anniversary, or the Great American Smokeout. If you smoke heavily at work, quit during your vacation so that you're already committed to quitting when you return. Make the date sacred, and don't let anything change it. This will make it easy for you to keep track of the day you became a nonsmoker and to celebrate that date every year.

KNOWING WHAT TO EXPECT

- Have realistic expectations; quitting isn't easy, but it's not impossible either. More than 3 million Americans quit every year.
- Understand that withdrawal symptoms are *temporary.* They usually last only 1-2 weeks.
- Know that most relapses occur in the first week after quitting, when withdrawal symptoms are strongest and your body is still dependent on nicotine. This will be your hardest time, so use all your personal resources—willpower, family, friends, and the tips in this material—to get you through this critical period successfully.
- Know that most other relapses occur in the first three months after quitting, when situational triggers—such as a particularly stressful event—unexpectedly occur. These are the times when people reach for cigarettes automatically, because they associate smoking with relaxing. It's hard to prepare yourself for this kind of situation, so it's important to recognize it if it *does* happen. Remember that smoking is a habit, but a habit you can break.
- Realize that most successful ex-smokers quit for good only after several attempts. You may be one of those who can quit your first try. But if you're not, *don't give up.* Try again.

INVOLVING SOMEONE ELSE

- Bet a friend you can quit on your target date. Put your cigarette money aside for every day, and forfeit it if you smoke. (But if you do smoke, *don't give up.* Simply strengthen your resolve and try again.)
- Ask your spouse or a friend to quit with you.
- Tell your family and friends that you're quitting and when. They can be an important source of support, both before and after you quit.

WAYS OF QUITTING

Switch Brands

- Switch to a brand you find distasteful.
- Change to a brand that's low in tar and nicotine a couple of weeks before your target date. This will help change your smoking behavior. However, *do not* smoke more cigarettes, inhale them more often or more deeply, or place your fingertips over the holes in the filters. All of these will increase your nicotine intake, and the idea is to get your body used to functioning without nicotine.

Cut down the number of cigarettes you smoke

- Smoke only half of each cigarette.
- Each day, postpone lighting your first cigarette one hour.
- Decide you'll smoke only during odd or even hours of the day.
- Decide beforehand how many cigarettes you'll smoke during the day. For each additional cigarette, give a dollar to your favorite charity.
- Change your eating habits to help you cut down. For example, drink milk, which many people consider incompatible with smoking. End meals or snacks with something that won't lead to a cigarette.
- Reach for a glass of juice instead of a cigarette for a "pick-me-up."
- Remember: Cutting down can help you quit, but it's not a substitute for quitting. If you're down to about seven cigarettes a day, it's time to set your target quit date and get ready to stick to it.

Don't smoke "automatically"

- Smoke only those cigarettes you *really* want. Catch yourself before you light up a cigarette out of pure habit.

- Don't empty your ashtrays. This will remind you of how many cigarettes you've smoked each day, and the sight and smell of stale butts will be very unpleasant.

- Make yourself aware of each cigarette by using the opposite hand or putting cigarettes in an unfamiliar location or different pocket to break the automatic reach.

- If you light up many times during the day without even thinking about it, try to look in a mirror each time you put a match to your cigarette—you may decide you don't need it.

Make smoking inconvenient

- Stop buying cigarettes by the carton. Finish one pack before you buy another.

- Stop carrying cigarettes with you at home and at work. Make them difficult to get to.

Make smoking unpleasant

- Smoke only under circumstances that aren't especially pleasurable for you. If you like to smoke with others, smoke alone. Turn your chair toward an empty corner and focus only on the cigarette and its many negative effects.

- Collect all your cigarette butts in one large glass container as a visual reminder of the filth smoking represents.

JUST BEFORE QUITTING

- Practice going without cigarettes.

- Don't think of *never* smoking again. Think of quitting in terms of one day at a time.

- Tell yourself you won't smoke today, and then don't.

- Clean your clothes to rid them of the cigarette smell, which can linger a long time.

ON THE DAY YOU QUIT

- Throw away all your cigarettes and matches. Hide your lighters and ashtrays.

- Visit the dentist and have your teeth cleaned to get rid of tobacco stains. Notice how nice they look, and resolve to keep them that way.

- Make a list of things you'd like to buy for yourself or someone else. Estimate the cost in terms of packs or cigarettes, and put the money aside to buy these presents.

- Keep very busy on the big day. Go to the movies, exercise, take walks, go bike riding.

- Remind your family and friends that this is your quit date, and ask them to help you over the rough spots of the first couple of days and weeks.

- Buy yourself a treat or do something special to celebrate.

IMMEDIATELY AFTER QUITTING

- Develop a clean, fresh, nonsmoking environment around yourself, at work and at home. Buy yourself flowers—you may be surprised how much you can enjoy their scent now.

- The first few days after you quit, spend as much free time as possible in places where smoking isn't allowed, such as libraries, museums, theaters, department stores, and churches.

- Drink large quantities of water and fruit juice (but avoid sodas that contain caffeine).

- Try to avoid alcohol, coffee, and other beverages that you associate with cigarette smoking.

- Strike up a conversation instead of a match for a cigarette.

- If you miss the sensation of having a cigarette in your hand, play with something else: a pencil, a paper clip, a marble.

- If you miss having something in your mouth, try toothpicks or a fake cigarette.

Avoid temptation

- Instead of smoking after meals, get up from the table and brush your teeth or go for a walk.

- If you always smoke while driving, listen to a particularly interesting radio program or your favorite music, or take public transportation for awhile, if you can.

- For the first 1-3 weeks, avoid situations you strongly associate with the pleasurable aspects of smoking, such as watching your favorite TV program, sitting in your favorite chair, or having a cocktail before dinner.

- Until you're confident of your ability to stay off cigarettes, limit your socializing to healthful, outdoor activities or situations where smoking isn't allowed.

- If you must be in a situation where you'll be tempted to smoke (such as a cocktail or dinner party), try to associate with the nonsmokers there.

- Try to analyze cigarette ads to understand how they attempt to "sell" you on individual brands.

Find new habits

- Change your habits to make smoking difficult, impossible, or unnecessary. For example, it's hard to smoke when you're swimming, jogging, or playing tennis or handball. When your desire for a cigarette is intense, wash your hands or the dishes, or try new recipes.
- Do things that require you to use your hands. Try crossword puzzles, needlework, gardening, or household chores. Go bike riding; take the dog for a walk; give yourself a manicure; write letters.
- Enjoy having a clean-mouth taste and maintain it by brushing your teeth frequently and using a mouthwash.
- Stretch a lot.
- Get plenty of rest.
- Pay attention to your appearance. Look and feel sharp.
- Try to find time for the activities that are the most meaningful, satisfying, and important to you.

When you get the crazies

- Keep oral substitutes handy. Try carrots, pickles, sunflower seeds, apples, celery, raisins, or sugarless gum instead of a cigarette.
- Take 10 deep breaths and hold the last one while lighting a match. Exhale slowly and blow out the match. Pretend it's a cigarette and crush it out in an ashtray.
- Take a shower or bath, if possible.
- Learn to relax quickly and deeply. Make yourself limp, visualize a soothing, pleasing situation, and get away from it all for a moment. Concentrate on that peaceful image and nothing else.
- Light incense or a candle instead of a cigarette.
- Never allow yourself to think that "one won't hurt"—it will.

ABOUT GAINING WEIGHT

Many people who are considering quitting are very concerned about gaining weight. If you're concerned about weight gain, keep these points in mind:

- Quitting doesn't mean you'll automatically gain weight. When people gain, most of the time it's because they eat more once they quit.
- The benefits of giving up cigarettes far outweigh the drawbacks of adding a few extra pounds. You'd have to gain a very large amount of weight to offset the many substantial health benefits that a normal smoker gains by quitting.

- Watch what you eat, and if you're concerned about gaining weight, consider the following tips:

  - Make sure you have a well-balanced diet, with the proper amounts of protein, carbohydrates, and fat.

  - Don't set a target date for a holiday, when the temptation of high-calorie food and drinks may be too hard to resist.

  - Drink a glass of water before your meals.

  - Weigh yourself weekly.

  - Chew sugarless gum when you want sweet foods.

  - Plan menus carefully, and count calories. Don't try to lose weight, just try to maintain your pre-quitting weight.

  - Have low-calorie foods on hand for nibbling. Choose foods that are both nutritious and low in calories. Some good choices are fresh fruits and vegetables, fruit and vegetable juices, low-fat cottage cheese, and air-popped popcorn without butter.

  - Take time for daily exercise, or join an organized exercise group.

IF YOU HAVE A RELAPSE

- Recognize that you've had a small setback. But your first cigarette or two didn't make you a smoker to start with, and a small setback doesn't make you a smoker again.

- Don't be too hard on yourself. One slip doesn't mean you're a failure or that you can't be a nonsmoker, but it is important to get back on the nonsmoking track *immediately.*

- Identify the trigger: exactly what was it that prompted you to smoke? Be aware of the trigger and decide *now* how you'll cope with it when it comes up again.

- Know and use the coping skills described above. People who know at least one coping skill are more likely to remain nonsmokers than those who don't know any.

- Sign a contract with yourself to remain a nonsmoker.

- If you think you need professional help, see your doctor. He or she can provide extra motivation for you to stop smoking. Your doctor also may prescribe nicotine gum as an alternative source of nicotine while you break the habit of smoking.

Adapted from: *Cleaning the Air: How to Quit Smoking...and Quit for Keeps*, U.S. Department of Health and Human Services, NIH Publication No. 92-1647, 1991.

COMPREHENSIVE WELLNESS FOR FIREFIGHTERS

Chapter 9

Managing Stress On and Off the Job

CHAPTER INTRODUCTION

For most people, stress is a normal part of everyday life. Surveys show that over 60% of the population experiences high levels of stress at least once a week, and almost one in five feels great stress every day. (Louis Harris 1992) These trends appear to be increasing at an alarming rate in today's ever-changing, fast-paced world.

We now know that stress is associated with many types of illnesses, including heart disease, gastrointestinal problems, backaches, and infections. In fact, **up to 80% of all non-traumatic deaths may really be due to stress**, according to the Surgeon General. Stress is also linked to homicides, suicides, accidents, substance abuse, crime, and many behavioral, interpersonal, and work-related problems.

In this chapter, you will learn what stress is and how it can affect you; the factors that contribute to stress and those that defend against it; and ways to manage stress in your own life.

LEARNING OBJECTIVES

After learning the information in this chapter, you will be able to:

- Define stress and its impact on health and personal well-being.
- Discuss the nature of stress in the fire service.
- Recognize sources and symptoms of stress in your own life.
- Identify ways to control stress on and off the job.
- Develop a personal strategy for stress management.

It is important to note that this material provides only a broad overview of a very complex subject. It is not intended as a substitute for psychotherapy, psychological treatment, individual counseling, or other forms of professional help that might be appropriate in certain situations. Moreover, further information and practice may be necessary to apply the stress reduction techniques described here. You are encouraged to get additional materials and assistance, as needed.

THE NATURE OF STRESS

WHAT IS STRESS?

When most people think of stress, they picture the pressures that people face in modern society—too much to do, oppressive time deadlines, competing priorities, financial worries, and so forth. Obviously, these factors place a strain on our lives, but all stress is not necessarily bad. Good stress, or ***eustress***, provides challenge and stimulation, contributing to the energy and enjoyment of life.

> "Stress has become one of the most serious health issues of the 20th century—a problem not just for individuals in terms of physical and mental disability, but for employers and governments who have started to assess the financial damage."
> International Labor Org.

Stress helps you recognize potential problems and opportunities, and motivates you to make positive changes in your life. It can even save your life in an emergency. But too much stress or stress that is particularly prolonged or frustrating—so called ***distress***—can be harmful to your health and well-being. It can lead to physical malfunction, disease, impaired job performance, and a broad range of psychological and social problems.

Stress is actually a normal and necessary response our bodies make to the environment in which we live. When a demand or threat is perceived, the body responds with a series of complex biochemical reactions that are designed to prepare it to act. These responses are pretty much the same no matter what causes the stress.

Stress then is "the body's nonspecific response to any demand placed on it, pleasant or unpleasant." (National Fire Academy) The demand can be physical, causing a direct effect on the body, or mental and emotional in nature.

STRESS IN SOCIETY

The negative effects of stress have become an epidemic in our country. In 1990, 41% of the adult population said that stress had at least some effect on their health, and 13% sought help in one form or another. (NCHS 1992) According to the American Institute of Stress, 75% to 90% of all visits to physicians involve stress-related complaints. Americans also resort to self-medication on a massive scale, taking tons of aspirins, sedatives, laxatives, and other forms of treatment every year in an effort to cope with the ravages of stress in their lives.

Governments and businesses also pay the price. The International Labor Organization, a United Nations agency, estimates that job stress costs employers about $200 billion a year in absenteeism, lower productivity, higher health insurance payments, turnover, increased accidents, and "burnout." In 1990, stress claims amounted to 15 percent of all worker compensation claims, a threefold increase in only 10 years.

For these reasons, the ability to manage stress is increasingly being recognized as a critical component of health and wellness. Individuals are learning how to recognize and control the signs and symptoms of stress in their lives. And more businesses and government agencies are taking steps to help their employees deal with stress-related problems. In 1985, over 60% of all worksites with 750 or more employees offered stress management programs. (NCHS 1992)

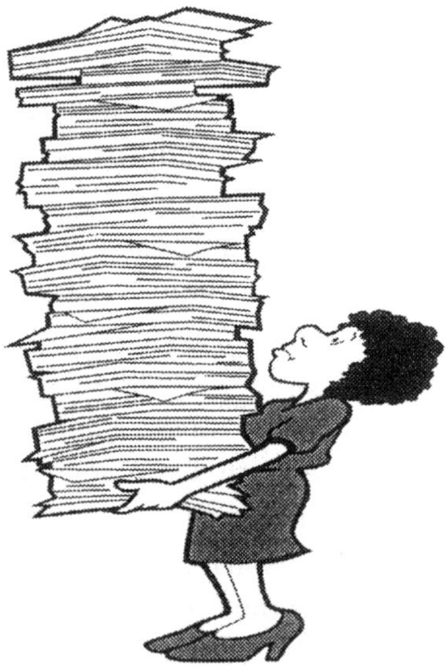

WHAT CAUSES STRESS?

Stress is caused by a vast array of factors in today's deadline-oriented, technological world. These **stressors** can be classified into several broad categories:

- **Environmental**—Many factors in the physical surroundings cause stress, including high noise levels, extremes of heat and cold, overcrowding, polluted air, and weather conditions. Continuous states of poverty and fear of violence can also be considered long-term environmental stressors.

- **Social/Interpersonal**—These factors relate to contact with other people, either on or off the job. Examples might include dysfunctional family relationships, abusive supervisors, arguments with fellow workers, group or peer pressures, conflicts with members of the public, lack of respect from young people, etc.

- **Work/Organizational**—Some jobs, such as emergency services worker, air traffic controller, and surgeon are inherently more stressful than others. Factors contributing to stress include responsibility for people's safety, personal danger, time urgency, work overload, boring or repetitive assignments, task ambiguity, unpleasant work conditions, lack of career opportunities, and other job-specific variables.

- **<u>Personality</u>**—These factors relate to traits of individuals—psychological makeup, beliefs, values, perceptions, goals, capabilities, etc. When a person's expectations or needs go unfulfilled, high levels of internal stress can result. Examples include guilt over perceived failings, anger at not being appreciated, a lack of assertiveness, extreme negativity or cynicism, etc.

- **<u>Life Change and Life Trauma</u>**—Events that cause a meaningful change or upheaval in a person's life or work situation, whether good or bad, are known to cause stress. Holmes and Rahe (1967) developed a scale to evaluate the stress associated with major life events, the top 30 of which are shown in Table 9-1.

Obviously, many different types of events and situations can cause stress. In fact, it has been said that <u>life is stress</u>—people responding, positively or negatively, to the world around them. The ability to control that response, therefore, largely determines the course and quality of each person's existence.

Table 9-1

Rank and Life Event	Mean Value
1. Death of spouse	100
2. Divorce	73
3. Marital separation	65
4. Jail term	63
5. Death of close family member	63
6. Personal injury or illness	53
7. Marriage	50
8. Fired at work	47
9. Marital reconciliation	45
10. Retirement	45
11. Health change—family member	44
12. Pregnancy	40
13. Sex difficulties	39
14. Gain of new family member	39
15. Business readjustment	39
16. Change in financial state	38
17. Death of close friend	37
18. Change in line of work	36
19. Change in arguments—spouse	35
20. Mortgage over $10,000	31
21. Foreclosure—mortgage or loan	30
22. Change—work responsibilities	29
23. Son or daughter leaving home	29
24. Trouble with in-laws	29
25. Great personal achievement	28
26. Spouse starting/stopping work	26
27. Beginning or ending school	26
28. Change in living conditions	25
29. Revision of personal habits	24
30. Trouble with boss	23

(Source: Holmes and Rahe 1967)

THE STRESS MECHANISM

The body's response to stress is a series of physical and emotional changes controlled by the brain and involving the nervous, endocrine (glandular), and musculoskeletal systems. The reaction is designed to prepare you to take positive protective action—to either combat or escape a perceived danger or challenge. This ***fight or flight*** response is absolutely normal and healthy; in fact, human beings could not have survived as a species without it.

The underlying biochemical processes are highly technical, but an overview is helpful for understanding your own reactions to stress (see Figure 9-1):

1. Information received by the senses is interpreted and analyzed in the cortex of the brain.

2. Depending on the brain's interpretation, strong emotions such as fear, anger, excitement, aggression, love, hostility, and disgust may be aroused.

3. If a significant threat or challenge is perceived, the brain communicates the need for a physical response to the rest of the body through the nervous and endocrine systems. Under the direction of the hypothalamus, the brain's "dispatch center," and the pituitary gland:

- The adrenal glands located on top or the kidneys produce powerful hormones, such as epinephrine (adrenalin), norepinephrine (noradrenaline), and a wide variety of corticoids.

- The voluntary nervous system, which controls intentional movements, sends messages preparing your muscles for action.

- The autonomic or involuntary nervous system sends extra blood to your muscles and slows down other bodily functions, such as digestion.

Figure 9-1 THE "FIGHT OR FLIGHT" RESPONSE

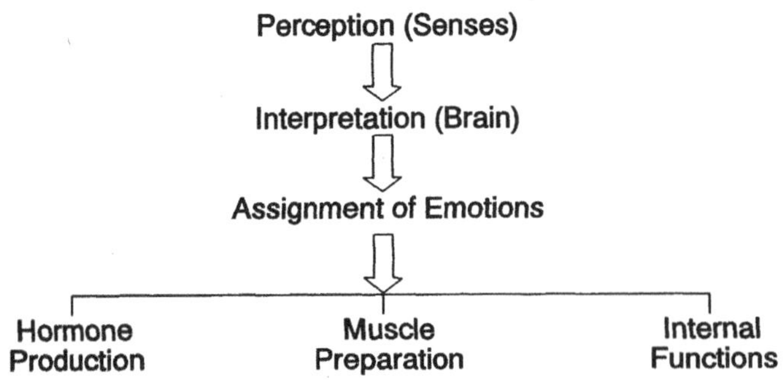

Physical Effects

The result of these changes is a heightened state of physical arousal and awareness. The effects, which are virtually the same no matter what causes the stress reaction, include increases in:

- Heart rate and blood pressure
- Oxygen consumption
- Dilation of coronary and deep muscle arteries
- Contraction of arteries close to the skin surface
- Metabolism and blood sugar levels
- Cholesterol and triglyceride levels
- Blood clotting capability
- Muscle tension and strength
- Dilation of pupils

These physical reactions cause the familiar sensations most people experience in times of stress—pounding heart, "clenched" stomach, cold and sweaty hands, muscle tremors, shortness of breath, and so forth. The effects may be brief or longer lasting, depending on the intensity and duration of the stressor and factors specific to the individual.

Cognitive and Emotional Effects

The stress response is also associated with a broad range of cognitive (thinking) and emotional reactions. Ideally, the result is a focused state of mind, useful for dealing with the stressor, whether it's responding to an incident, giving a speech, or coping with the sickness of a friend. Virtually the entire spectrum of human emotions—from fear, anger, and hostility to love, exhilaration, and compassion—may be involved. These emotions help people recognize and evaluate potential problems. They also motivate action and personal change.

However, when stress levels are excessive, a different type of cognitive and emotional response may occur. In effect, the mind tries to protect the person by shutting down "extraneous" mental processes, de-emphasizing other needs, or even mentally escaping the situation. Some possible symptoms include:

- Going on "auto-pilot"
- Difficulty concentrating and staying focused
- Reduced short-term memory
- Racing or obsessive thoughts
- Decreased mental flexibility
- Increased withdrawal and isolation
- Feelings of invulnerability
- Fantasies and wishful thinking

CONSEQUENCES OF STRESS

The stress reactions just described usually don't present a major problem if the body has an adequate opportunity to rest and recover after the experience. However, difficulties arise when fight or flight is an inappropriate or ineffective response to the situation. For example:

- When physical action is unsuitable or impossible—e.g., after being reprimanded by your supervisor or sitting in a traffic jam.
- When the cause of stress is continuous and beyond your control—e.g., long-term deadline pressures or unfair administrative policies.
- When stress levels are so high that they exceed the normal coping mechanisms available to the individual—e.g., major life changes or great pain (physical or emotional).

Types of Stress Reactions

Acute stress reactions are the result of a single powerful experience that overwhelms a person's ability to cope. Examples include some of the major life traumas discussed earlier, but even lesser events can have a significant impact. Most often, signs of stress appear immediately or within a relatively short period of time; in some circumstances, symptoms may not be apparent for weeks, months, or even years. This is referred to as **delayed stress**.

Stress reactions can also be caused by the combined effects of lower level stressors that occur over an extended period of time. In these situations, the body never has a chance to fully recover from the damaging effects of the stress reaction. If the stressor continues for long, the physical and psychological response can develop into a habit which becomes progressively harder to break. The individual may even adjust to the situation so that the unhealthy state seems normal.

Over time, this **chronic** or cumulative stress will damage the system to the point of malfunction or disease. Resistance to acute stress is also diminished. Symptoms may take years to develop and the interrelationships with other factors are often extremely complex. As a result, diagnosis and treatment may be very difficult.

The end result of chronic stress is sometimes referred to as "**burnout**," a state of mental, physical, and emotional exhaustion. As explained by experts in organizational behavior, "people with high aspirations and strong motivation to get things done are prime candidates for burnout under certain conditions. They are especially vulnerable when they find themselves in an organization that suppresses or limits their own initiative while constantly demanding that they serve the organization's own ends....The most likely effects of this are fatigue, frustration, and helplessness under the burden of overwhelming demands. The person literally exhausts his or her aspirations and motivation, much as a candle burns itself out." (Moorhead and Griffin 1989)

Physical/Medical Effects

As described above, stress produces a powerful total body reaction that affects all the body's organs and systems. Thus, it's not surprising that prolonged or unresolved stress can damage your health in many ways:

- Cardiovascular System—Excess production of hormones like epinephrine can lead to higher blood pressure, cardiac arrhythmia (eccentric heartbeat), athero-sclerosis, heart attacks, and stroke. Migraine headaches, caused by dilation of blood vessels in the scalp, may also be stress-related.

- Digestive System—Anxiety, another common stress symptom, affects the gastrointestinal system. Related problems can include nausea, ulcers, constipation, diarrhea, and ulcerative colitis, which can be life-threatening.

- Immune System—Stress can affect the body's ability to attack and destroy bacteria, viruses, and other foreign invaders. Lessened resistance leaves a person more vulnerable to common colds, infections, allergies, asthma, arthritis, and even cancer.

- Musculoskeletal System—People express their feelings through "body language." Repressed emotions and physical stress can contribute to unrelieved muscle tension and pain, fatigue, backache, headaches, and joint problems.

Behavioral Effects

Studies show that people experiencing high levels of stress are more likely to use drugs and tobacco and to drink too much alcohol. Other behavioral consequences include accident proneness, violence, and appetite disorders. For example, 20% of all fatal car accidents involve drivers who have suffered an upsetting experience within six hours before the crash, and one out of three accident victims was depressed. (McQuade 1993)

Of course, all of these stress-related effects influence performance on the job. Individuals coping with stress are more likely to call in sick or quit work. Decision-making ability and morale are affected, leading to declines in productivity and increases in accidents. Inappropriate coping behaviors can lead to conflicts with supervisors and co-workers. The results are damaging to the individual and disruptive to the organization.

Psychological and Social Effects

The health and behavioral consequences of excessive stress also take their toll on the victim's personal and family life. If left unchecked, these difficulties contribute to mental health problems and great personal pain. Symptoms may include depression, anxiety disorders, withdrawal and alienation, sleep disturbance, family discord and divorce, sexual dysfunction, personality changes, loss of self esteem, and burnout.

Activity 9-1

SIGNS AND SYMPTOMS OF STRESS

Excessive or prolonged stress can result in a vast array of possible signs and symptoms, depending on the individual, the cause of stress, and other variables. The ability to recognize these signals is the first step in learning how to deal with stress in a positive way.

During this activity, you will identify signs and symptoms of distress in your own life. The exercise will give you some insight into the principal ways you respond to stress. (Note: this activity is based on materials developed by Irwin, Mitchell and Bray, Navarre, and USFA.)

Instructions

1. In Parts A through D below and on the next page, place a check mark (√) next to the signs and symptoms of stress that you recognize in yourself. If you experience others that are not listed, list those as well in the blank spaces.

2. Review the lists you developed. Then place an asterisk (*) next to those signs and symptoms that you feel are your most important reactions to stress. If one of the categories (physical/medical, cognitive, emotional, or behavioral) is predominant, note that as well.

A. PHYSICAL/MEDICAL

_____ Headaches
_____ Muscle tension or aches
_____ Muscle tremors or shakes
_____ Chills or profuse sweating
_____ Weariness or fatigue
_____ Inability to sleep well
_____ Colds or allergies
_____ Weight change (up or down)
_____ Diarrhea, digestive upsets
_____ Changes in appetite

_____ Lowered sexual drive
_____ Skin rashes
_____ Pounding or racing heart
_____ High blood pressure
_____ Shortness of breath
_____ Rapid or shallow breathing
_____ Chest pain
_____ Ulcers
_____ ____________________
_____ ____________________

B. COGNITIVE

_____ Forgetfulness
_____ Inability to concentrate
_____ Reduced attention span
_____ Confusion
_____ Boredom
_____ Apathy or lethargy
_____ Low productivity
_____ Negative attitudes
_____ Racing thoughts
_____ Recurring images, flashbacks
_____ Nightmares, bad dreams
_____ Obsessive thoughts
_____ Going on "automatic pilot"
_____ Lack of creativity
_____ Reduced problem-solving, decision-making abilities
_____ ______________________
_____ ______________________

C. EMOTIONAL

_____ Anxiety or worrying
_____ Anger or irritability
_____ Feeling discouraged, frustrated
_____ Hopelessness or emptiness
_____ Loss of meaning or dirction
_____ Fear
_____ Guilt
_____ Depression ("the blues")
_____ Mood swings
_____ Crying spells
_____ Martyrdom, feelings of persecution
_____ Feeling that no one cares
_____ Self-doubt, low self-esteem
_____ Sense of isolation, separateness
_____ Inappropriate emotions
_____ Resistance to touching
_____ ______________________
_____ ______________________

D. BEHAVIORAL

_____ Excessive joking, "horseplay"
_____ Excessive "gallows humor"
_____ Teasing or belittling others
_____ Extreme or inappropriate cynicism
_____ Denying or repressing feelings
_____ Avoiding potentially stressful situations
_____ Ignoring the signs and symptoms of stress
_____ Pushing yourself too hard
_____ Ignoring safety precautions
_____ Taking it out on family members and friends
_____ Withdrawing from family and friends
_____ Not talking with people at work
_____ Using alcohol, drugs, or tobacco to "wind down"
_____ Sleeping more than usual
_____ Pacing or other nervous mannerisms
_____ Compulsive activity, inability to relax and "do nothing"
_____ Arguing or anger over insignificant matters
_____ Excessive complaining about supervisors, co-workers
_____ Excessive complaining about other aspects of the job
_____ Putting off work or decisions
_____ Blaming others for problems
_____ Taking unnecessary risks
_____ Difficulty accepting authority
_____ Increased rate of accidents
_____ ______________________
_____ ______________________

INDIVIDUAL DIFFERENCES

If stress is basically a predictable reaction of the body's nervous and endocrine systems, why do people respond so differently? Situations or events that cause one person stress—such as an upcoming performance test—may be viewed by another as an exciting challenge. Similarly, two people feeling the same stress may react differently—one becomes anxious and fearful, while the other turns angry and hostile.

The Mind-Body Connection

The reason people respond differently to stress is referred to as the mind-body connection, that complex process by which cognitive and emotional processes are translated into the activities of muscles and organs. In essence, **"stress isn't caused so much by external factors...as by the way we perceive them and cope with them."** (Stark 1992) As shown in Figure 9-2, there are two components of this system: 1) how your thoughts and feelings (not the situation or event itself) stimulate changes in the body, and 2) how your body's physical mechanism influences the way you think and feel.

Figure 9-2

THE MIND-BODY CONNECTION

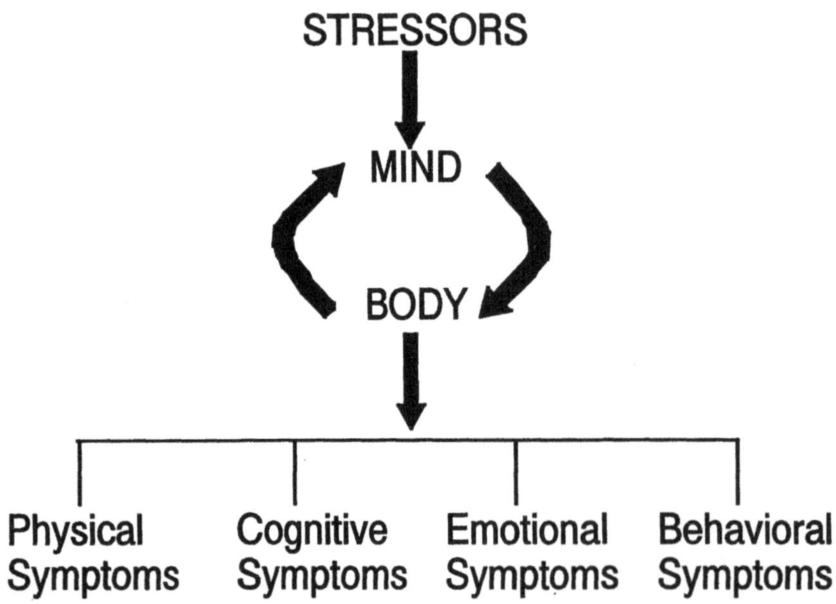

In this process, everyone is different because everyone has different thoughts, emotions, and physical equipment. Many factors are involved:

Genetics—Evidence indicates that some people are biologically more stress-resistant than others. Everyone's physical equipment varies, and sometimes the weakest link in the chain breaks first. People may also be genetically predisposed to respond to stress in certain ways. For example, women appear to be more likely to experience emotional reactions to stress, while men have more physical reactions. Similarly, one family may tend to experience gastrointestinal problems while another gets high blood pressure.

Culture—The beliefs and values transmitted by different cultures also influence how people perceive and react to life events. To some extent, people respond in ways that they are taught. For example, one study demonstrated that American executives may have less stress than those in similar positions in other countries.

Personality—Individual characteristics can make a difference. Traits linked to stress-related disease include low self-esteem, lack of assertiveness, inability to express anger, hostility or aggression in one's own defense, external loss of control, and feelings of helplessness. (USFA 1991) People who see themselves as complex may be better able to handle stress. The same may be true for thrill-seeking and risk-taking personalities.

Type A and Type B Personalities

Work done by Friedman and Rosenman in 1974 indicated that individual differences in temperament influence which people get heart disease. The result was the identification of so called "Type A" and "Type B" behavior patterns.

Type A personalities are characterized by intense drive, competitiveness, devotion to work, and a strong sense of time urgency for getting things done. They tend to be aggressive, ambitious, and impatient. Their behaviors reflect this basic nature: they usually move and talk rapidly, dominate conversations, feel guilty about relaxing, work on and think about several things at once, and seem preoccupied with their own thoughts.

Type B personalities, in contrast, have a more balanced and relaxed approach. They are not as driven or competitive; they even speak slower. Interestingly, Type B persons are not necessarily less successful at work. However, they are two to three times less likely to get coronary heart disease in middle age.

Most people are, of course, not purely one personality type or the other. It should also be noted that later research shows that Type A people who are enthusiastic and positive, who thoroughly enjoy their work, probably have no greater risk of heart disease. On the other hand, so called "hostile Type As" seem to have stronger stress reactions, a factor which contributes to future cardiovascular problems.

The checklist below will help you determine whether you possess some characteristic Type A personality traits. If many of the statements here are **often** true about you, you probably fall into the Type A personality category.

TYPE A CHARACTERISTICS

- √ Think about work when off duty
- √ Become impatient when events move slowly
- √ Feel vaguely guilty when relaxing or "doing nothing"
- √ Speak, eat, and walk at a rapid pace
- √ Set deadlines and work hard to meet them
- √ Do several things at the same time
- √ Feel compelled to compete against others
- √ Have hostile or aggressive feelings towards others
- √ Measure accomplishments against numerical goals
- √ Remain pre-occupied or unaware of surroundings
- √ Feel under continual time pressure
- √ Feel driven to advance from current position

RESISTANCE TO STRESS

Some research indicates that three personal qualities are important in determining a person's hardiness, or ability to resist stress. They are a sense of **control** over one's life, a strong **commitment** to important values and activities, and the ability to see change as a **challenge** rather than a threat.

These three qualities are reflected in the characteristics of men and women who deal well with stressful situations, as identified by Dr. Raymond Flannery of the Harvard University Medical School:

- ♦ Actively control their lives
- ♦ Look for active solutions to problems
- ♦ Committed to meaningful goals
- ♦ Use little nicotine and caffeine
- ♦ Relax at least 15 minutes a day
- ♦ Get regular aerobic exercise
- ♦ Actively involved with others

Promoting these qualities in your own life will help you control stress and stay healthy. More on stress management is presented later in this chapter.

> "The fact that the mind rules the body is, in spite of its neglect by biology and medicine, the most fundamental fact we know about the process of life."
> Franz Alexander

STRESS AND THE FIRE SERVICE

Every time the alarm goes off, firefighters and rescue workers are exposed to stress. Many incidents involve personal danger and life-or-death decisions. Physical demands are great, the stakes are high, and time is short. Sometimes, as soon as one incident is over, another one begins.

Back at the station, the situation may not seem much better. Work is unending, boring, or repetitive. Living and working conditions leave something to be desired. Conflicts with co-workers or dissatisfaction with management make the job a constant hassle. Sometimes, the rewards just don't seem worth it.

> "Stress is one of the most serious occupational hazards in the fire service, affecting health, job performance, career decision-making, morale, and family life. Emotional problems, as well as problems with alcohol and drugs, are becoming increasing evident. High rates of attrition, divorce, occupational disease and injury continue."
> U.S. Fire Administration

The National Fire Academy identifies some of the characteristics that makes firefighting stressful:

- High levels of uncertainty
- Limited control over the work environment
- Repeated emergency conditions
- Tensions between co-workers
- Exposure to human trauma
- Fear of death or injury

Research also shows that responsibility for the safety of others is a major stressor for emergency workers. As a result, supervisors, in particular, often experience high levels of stress.

Other organizational factors contributing to stress, as identified by Dr. Robert Hoffman, include poor supervision, lack of career opportunities, inadequate rewards, offensive policies, excessive paperwork, poor equipment, and lack of cooperation between jurisdictions. No wonder that firefighting and rescue work is considered one of the most stressful jobs in the world today!

Partially as a result of this stress, emergency responders may have higher rates of heart disease, cancer and other ailments than the general population. Divorce and substance abuse rates exceed the national average. It's also reasonable to assume that a disproportionate number of performance problems and injuries—both physical and psychological—result from stress on the job.

EMERGENCY SERVICES PERSONNEL

If firefighting and rescue work is so stressful, why do so many people choose, and even prefer, this line of work? Research indicates that a large number of emergency workers have in common certain personality traits that perhaps incline them to accept the risks and challenges of this occupation. According to Jeff Mitchell and Grady Bray (1990), experts in the field of emergency services stress, these traits can be summarized as follows:

- Need to be in control
- Obsessive (desire to do a perfect job)
- Compulsive (tend to repeat the same actions for similar events; traditional)
- Highly motivated by internal factors (e.g., job satisfaction)
- Action-oriented
- High need for stimulation
- Need for immediate gratification
- Easily bored
- Risk-takers
- Strong need to rescue and help people
- Highly dedicated
- Strong need to be needed

Understanding these characteristics is important for understanding emergency services stress. Remember, the way people think and feel—their personality—to a large extent determines how they respond under pressure.

Emergency services work requires immediate, decisive action, often under dangerous conditions. Established procedures must be followed precisely, and the primary reward is helping others. Therefore, most of the personality traits listed here would seem to match the typical emergency worker to the demands of the job. However, **these same traits may also make stress worse.** For example:

- Highly motivated personnel who try to do the "perfect" job are most vulnerable to burnout.

- The strong need to help people can lead to overwhelming frustration and guilt when victims are lost or the incident "goes bad."

- The inherent inability to predict or control emergency incidents can contribute to long-term anxiety.

- The lack of appreciation or other awards often causes frustration for emergency workers.

- An extreme sense of dedication may keep personnel on the job even when they are hurting themselves or their families.

The fire service culture can also contribute to the problem. In particular, some personnel continue to believe that stress is a sign of weakness. They silently endure stress or have trouble dealing with the problems of others. This emphasis on being "macho" can inhibit a member's ability to seek or give help, or even to recognize that a problem exists.

Activity 9-2

SOURCES OF FIRE SERVICE STRESS

Emergency services work presents a unique set of challenges that reflect the nature of the job and the people who fill it. This activity is designed to give you an opportunity to identify some of the stressors in your own work life.

A number of factors that studies show contribute to stress for fire and rescue personnel are listed below. Place a check mark (√) next to those that you feel personally cause you stress on the job. Add others, as appropriate. Then place an asterisk (*) next to those sources that cause you the <u>most</u> stress.

<u>Environmental Stressors</u>

_____ The sound of the alarm
_____ Long hours at work, at the incident scene
_____ Shift work, irregular schedules
_____ Lack of sleep or interrupted sleep on duty
_____ Noise, heat, and cold
_____ Toxic environments
_____ Overcrowding at the station
_____ Faulty or unsafe equipment
_____ ______________________________
_____ ______________________________
_____ ______________________________

<u>Social/Interpersonal Stressors</u>

_____ Lack of respect from government officials, the public
_____ Concern of family members for your safety
_____ Absence from the family when you are needed
_____ Working around chiefs, managers
_____ Personality conflicts with officers, co-workers
_____ Working with inexperienced, untrained personnel
_____ ______________________________
_____ ______________________________
_____ ______________________________

Activity 9-2 (Continued)

Work/Organizational Stressors

_____ Lack of feedback, encouragement, or appreciation
_____ Boredom or long inactive periods
_____ Ambiguous, inconsistent, or weak leadership
_____ Overall uncertainty, lack of control over work
_____ Lack of opportunities for advancement, development
_____ The need to make rapid decisions
_____ Responsibility for co-workers' safety
_____ Worry about layoffs, job security
_____ Concern about retirement, pensions, etc.
_____ ____
_____ ____
_____ ____

Personality Stressors

_____ Concern about making mistakes, harming others
_____ Criticism or "second guessing" after incidents
_____ Lack of job satisfaction, enjoyment
_____ Inability to do the best job possible
_____ Feelings of inadequacy, fear of failure
_____ Difficulty discussing problems or expressing feelings
_____ ____
_____ ____
_____ ____

Life Change and Life Trauma

_____ Encountering dead and injured victims
_____ Interactions with survivors and relatives of victims
_____ Death or injury of a co-worker
_____ Injury to self on the job
_____ Change of job responsibilities
_____ ____
_____ ____
_____ ____

CRITICAL INCIDENT STRESS

As part of their daily work, firefighters and rescue workers respond to incidents that trigger the fight or flight response—heart pounding, muscles primed, thoughts focused, etc. Although these "routine" incidents may contribute to cumulative stress, they usually are not powerful enough to cause a major stress reaction by themselves. The responders' basic resistance to stress and ability to recover are adequate to protect them.

However, certain events are so overwhelming that they can exceed an individual's capacity to cope. These so-called **critical incidents** can cause severe acute stress reactions, sometimes to virtually every person involved in the response. Examples of critical incidents include (Mitchell and Bray 1990):

- Death or serious injury to a fellow worker
- Incidents involving a relative or close friend
- Suicide of a fellow emergency worker
- A mass casualty or large-scale disaster
- Dealing with violent people at the incident scene
- Incidents with excessive media interest
- Contact with dead or severely injured children
- Death to a civilian caused by emergency operations

These types of incidents can produce extraordinary stress reactions, even years after the event. Potential consequences include all the physical, cognitive, emotional, and behavioral effects discussed earlier. In severe cases, victims suffer from recurring and obtrusive images (obsessive thoughts about the incident, flashbacks, daydreams, and nightmares); a deepening sense of withdrawal and isolation; a deterioration of thinking processes; and feelings of guilt, hopelessness, intense grief, loss of emotional control, and depression.

According to Mitchell, "recent studies indicate that better than 85 percent of emergency personnel have experienced acute stress reactions after working at one or more critical incidents similar to those presented above. Fortunately, the majority of emergency personnel experience only temporary stress reactions and recover within a few weeks. Others take several months to overcome fully the effects of critical incidents, and a small number (two to four percent) may experience such profound effects that their jobs, families, health, and happiness are permanently impaired."

This latter condition, referred to as **Post-Traumatic Stress Disorder** (PTSD), is a potentially serious psychological condition that can cause severe malfunction and distress. It is not considered a normal stress reaction. Diagnosis and treatment should be left to trained medical and mental health professionals.

CRITICAL INCIDENT STRESS DEBRIEFING TEAMS

> "The fire department shall adopt a written policy that establishes a program designed to relieve the stress generated by an incident that could adversely affect the psychological and physical well-being of fire department members."
>
> NFPA 1500, 9-1.5

Managing critical incident stress in fire services organizations requires special knowledge, skills, and procedures. To cope with this challenge, a growing number of jurisdictions around the country have established **Critical Incident Stress Debriefing (CISD) Teams**, a concept initially researched and developed by Dr. Mitchell.

The CISD Team is a comprehensive programmatic approach for dealing with the special needs and personalities of emergency services personnel. It includes activities designed to help responders prepare for stressful events, as well as those during and after the incident that minimize or control negative effects.

The CISD Team includes health care professionals, emergency services personnel, and sometimes representatives of the clergy. Members receive special training in the CISD process and related disciplines. Typically, the team provides services to all emergency response agencies and personnel—fire, police, EMS, hospital, volunteer, etc.—within a given jurisdiction or region. Over 200 such teams currently operate in the United States.

CISD Team Services

The services provided by the CISD Team are designed to keep healthy members healthy and on the job. They are not generally intended as psychological treatment or individual care for persons with severe problems. The services typically include:

- Training—CISD Teams sponsor and conduct training for all emergency services personnel within the jurisdiction. Training covers the causes and consequences of critical incident stress, methods of stress reduction and control, and sources of assistance.

- On-Scene Support Services—During an incident, peer support personnel may offer limited assistance to *obviously distressed* co-workers. They may also provide advice to command staff and support for victims and their families.

- Demobilization Services—After large-scale or prolonged incidents, a demobilization center may be established to help facilitate the transition back to "normal" working conditions. A limited amount of stress-related information is usually provided at this time, often in the form of handouts. Emergency workers also get a chance to eat and relax, hear announcements, and, if desired, share their reactions and feelings on an individual or group basis.

- Defusings—This small-group process focuses on the needs of more seriously affected workers. It is conducted within a few hours of the incident, usually by one of the department's command officers. Defusings provide a relatively informal and unstructured setting for members to express their reactions and feelings without fear of criticism or critique. Stress-related information may be disseminated.

- Critical Incident Stress Debriefing—The formal CISD is a structured group process conducted between one and three days after the incident. The meeting is directed by a mental health professional, with help from other team members. Typically, all personnel involved in the incident attend. The CISD, which usually lasts about three hours, provides an opportunity for personnel to discuss what happened during the incident in a supportive environment and to "ventilate" their thoughts and feelings. CISD Team members also provide stress reduction education and information, emphasizing that physical and emotional symptoms are normal reactions to abnormal events.

- Follow-Up Services—Based on needs identified during the formal CISD, team members provide additional services over the next few days, weeks, months, or even years. These may include follow-up meetings, individual contacts, referrals, advice to command staff, spousal debriefings, family education and support programs, general information dissemination, and so forth.

According to Mitchell, over 9,000 debriefings have been held since 1983, the vast majority for one or two victims of critical incident stress. Affected personnel are encouraged but not forced to actively participate in all phases of the process. Strict confidentiality is maintained.

MANAGING LIFE AND WORK STRESS

While it may be impossible to live completely without stress, there are ways to avoid it, control it, or minimize its impact. According to the United States Fire Administration, **stress management is "the systematic application of one or more therapeutic, educational, and common-sense techniques that aim to reduce or eliminate excessive stress."** An emphasis is placed on practical, preventive measures you can take everyday to stay healthy and productive.

Stress management should be viewed as a normal part of life in today's hectic, pressure-packed environment. It just makes common sense for everyone, especially emergency responders, to prepare as well as they can for the potentially destructive stressors they face on and off the job. Stress management, therefore, does not imply weakness, mental illness, or the inability to "take it." In fact, it implies just the opposite.

THE STRESS MANAGEMENT PROCESS

As described previously, the stress reaction is a complex series of perceptual, cognitive, emotional, and physical responses of the mind-body system to outside stressors. When stress levels are excessive or prolonged, they can result in a wide variety of symptoms and problems that vary according to the situation and the person.

The goal of stress management is to interrupt this sequence of events before damage can be done. As depicted graphically in Figure 9-3, there are four basic strategies:

- Minimizing Stressors—Proactive steps to avoid, eliminate, or reduce the stressors in life.
- Changing Perceptions—Techniques to alter the way problems are perceived or to channel stress more productively.
- Relaxation—Methods to influence the mind and control the body.
- Building Physical Resistance—Ways to increase the body's ability to resist and recover from stress.

Each of these four methods will be discussed in more detail. However, it should be noted that this chapter provides just a very brief overview of these complex topics. Readers wishing to learn these skills may need additional assistance or instruction.

Figure 9-3

The Stress Management Process

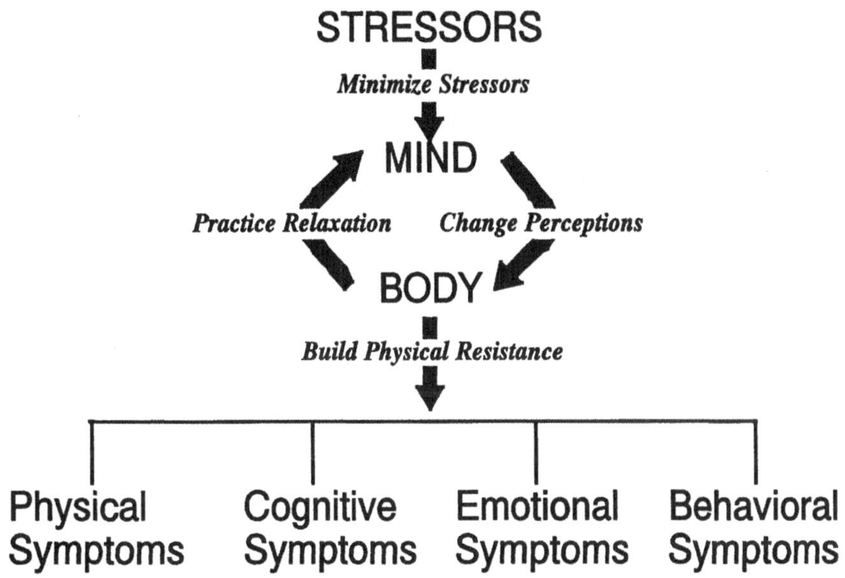

MINIMIZING STRESSORS

When it comes to stress, **prevention is always better than treatment**, and the best way to prevent problems is often to attack the source. Methods for reducing outside stressors include several basic lifestyle strategies, such as leading a balanced life, fostering support groups, and promoting personal and professional growth. In addition, you can implement proactive measures to "take charge" of specific stressors in your life.

Leading a Balanced Life

A life in balance includes a wide variety of interests and pursuits: family, friends, work, hobbies, entertainment, exercise, spirituality, leisure activities, and education. Diverse interests help people limit their exposure to stress from any one source, enabling them to keep problems in perspective. A well-rounded life also provides sources of support and a range of outlets when pressures mount.

Because of the stressful nature of emergency services work, firefighters and rescue workers need to develop and maintain interests outside the job. For many people, this means active planning—mapping out leisure time in advance, setting priorities, promoting personal relationships, etc. The process may take some extra effort, but the benefits—less stress, a greater sense of control, and a fuller life—are worth it.

Support Groups

For most people, it helps to talk to someone about their concerns and problems. Research indicates that simply discussing difficult issues with sympathetic listeners actually reduces stress chemicals in the body. The process also helps people put problems in perspective, identify possible solutions, and reduce feelings of isolation or uniqueness.

Support groups provide the psychological backup everyone needs at different times in their lives. This role is often played by family, friends, and co-workers. Some people join special interest organizations, discussion groups, or social clubs to meet like-minded people. The role may also be played by concerned outsiders, including CISD Team members, clergy, and mental health professionals.

Unfortunately, communicating about personal matters is particularly difficult for many fire service members. Others have no one to turn to who is both willing to listen and who understands the unique problems that emergency workers face. These people lack a valuable resource in the battle against stress. Thus, **the ability to talk about personal issues and to build strong networks of supporters should be viewed as stress management <u>skills</u> that all personnel need to develop.**

Personal and Professional Growth

The one constant in life is that things change—relationships, responsibilities, roles, technologies, surroundings, etc. What's worse, things seem to get more and more complex all the time. The need to constantly adapt to this dynamic environment is a major source of stress in modern life.

The best way to increase your ability to deal with change and complexity is to take advantage of opportunities for personal and professional growth. Formal education and other experiences that increase your knowledge and skills provide you with a sense of competence and control over what you do. This confidence, in turn, helps you to view new situations as a challenge rather than a threat.

For fire service supervisors, especially those who come up through the ranks, professional growth may mean additional training in the administrative, management, and "people" skills needed for their new responsibilities. For emergency responders, it means active participation in technical training, drills, exercises, and critiques. For everyone, it means a positive attitude and a desire to learn. The result will be improved individual and team performance—in short, less work-related stress.

Managing the Environment

In addition to basic lifestyle strategies, everyone has to deal with specific events or situations that cause stress in their lives. Sometimes, the easiest way is simply to avoid or remove the stressor. However, this option isn't always available or appropriate in the social and work situations most people face every day.

Several important methods for minimizing the major sources of chronic stress in many people's lives—interpersonal conflicts and occupational responsibilities—are briefly described below. These and others are basically just different approaches for "taking charge" of the situation and directing it towards a positive end.

Time Management—Time management provides techniques to help people organize their internal resources and use them more effectively. Related skills include task analysis, value and goal setting, pacing, and delegating responsibility. Sometimes, the process can be as simple a making a list of everything you need to do, ranking them in order of importance, and establishing a simple "game plan."

Role Management—Everyone fills a variety of roles in life (spouse, parent, family member, friend, etc.) and at work (supervisor, subordinate, peer, leader, etc.). Sometimes, people adopt unrealistic expectations about doing a "perfect" job in each of these roles, contributing to overload. At other times, roles may be unclear or actually conflict with one another. Role management includes techniques for analyzing an individual's varied roles and taking proactive steps to eliminate problems.

Conflict Resolution—Conflict occurs when an individual or organization feels that its goals are being blocked by another. (This same situation usually produces healthy competition when behavior is regulated by rules and procedures that are perceived to be fair.) Conflict can be a catalyst for creativity and positive change, but too much produces stress. Strategies for resolving conflict include methods that promote common goals, clarification of roles, coordination, and communication.

Assertiveness Training—Some people have trouble expressing themselves appropriately or effectively. Others are uncomfortable with interpersonal confrontation and conflict. The result can be a source of constant disappointment or anger, leading to frustrated goals, social problems, and loss of self-esteem. Assertiveness training provides the confidence and skills people need to deal with the relationships in their lives. Techniques include active listening, dealing with aggressive people, speaking honestly and diplomatically, giving and receiving feedback, etc. Sometimes, the solution is as simple as learning to say "no" to unreasonable demands.

CHANGING PERCEPTIONS

Minimizing stressors can help reduce problems, but this option is not always available. Often, the situations or events that cause stress are outside your ability to control. At other times, stress is caused more by the way a stressor is *perceived* than by the stressor itself. In other words, **what you think determines how you feel.**

Internal Dialogue

Let's take an example. On the highway, another motorist cuts you off, almost causing an accident. The incident makes you so angry that you are still upset two hours later. In this case, you might believe that the other motorist caused you to be angry, but an important element is missing here—how you "talked to yourself" about the event.

This internal dialogue goes on within everyone almost all the time. Two examples of self-talk in this case might be:

- "There is absolutely no way he should have done that. That guy's a jerk."
- "There are a lot of crazy drivers out here. I'm lucky to be alive."

Obviously, these different internal responses to the same event will result in very different stress reactions, both emotionally and physically. The first leads to hostility and anger, maybe even causing you to drive aggressively and unsafely. The second might bring a feeling of relief and a resolve to "drive defensively." Over time, each of these thought patterns becomes a habit that largely determines how you respond to traffic situations.

Cognitive Restructuring

Contrary to what many people believe, **you can change the way you think and feel**. Many types of psychotherapy and counseling help people see problems from a different perspective. In stress management, a technique called cognitive restructuring focuses on identifying irrational or dysfunctional thought patterns. Harmful stressors are reexamined in a way that produces a more positive effect. As summarized by USFA, steps in this process are as follows:

1. **Confront the Stressor**—carefully describe the situation and its effects, including your emotions.

2. **Analyze Your Reaction**—rationally examine your thought patterns and responses during and immediately following the event.

3. **Rethink the Situation**—Generate other ways to view the event that are more positive and helpful.

4. **Select an Alternative**—pick one from your list that will reduce stress and improve the situation.

5. **Try It Out**—Deliberately adopt the new interpretation and assess its effects.

It's important to note that this type of rational self-analysis and mental rehearsal is not self-deception or denial. Any interpretation you select must be well-thought out and acceptable to you. Cognitive restructuring merely provides a way to think through your values, beliefs, goals, and habits in a certain area. Then, in effect, you "try on" others to see how they fit. The approach allows you to adjust your mental attitude, perhaps by redefining problems, setting new priorities, positive thinking, or viewing situations with humor.

RELAXATION

Another way to control your response to stress is through relaxation exercises, both mental and physical. In this context, relaxation does not refer to vacations, leisure activities, or sleep. It is a purposeful and active process used to increase awareness and energy while quieting the mind and body. Many different approaches and variations exist.

Deep Breathing

Rapid and shallow breathing may be both a symptom and a cause of stress. Controlling your breathing pattern affects the fight or flight mechanism (perhaps by regulating oxygen and carbon dioxide levels in the blood) and contributes to relaxation and stress reduction. Most techniques emphasize slow and deep breaths, making sure to "belly breathe" from the diaphragm (i.e., your abdomen should expand more than your chest). Inhale through your nose, pause slightly, and then exhale long and forcefully, while focusing on the awareness of relaxation.

Progressive Muscle Relaxation

Flexing and then releasing tense muscles can help burn up stress chemicals and trigger a relaxation response in the body. These exercises can be performed sequentially for all muscle groups or just for particularly tight areas. The procedure typically involves isometrically contracting the muscles for 5-10 seconds, then consciously releasing the tension, all the while focusing on the sensations being experienced. The process should never produce pain or discomfort.

Mental Techniques

A variety of mental techniques can be used to achieve a relaxed state of mind. Examples include meditation, in which you free your mind of thoughts while remaining quiet and still; autogenic training, which uses verbal clues and concentration on sensations such as heaviness and warmth in the body; visualization, where you picture yourself in enjoyable and relaxing scenes; and guided imagery, which involves directed imaginings. Typically, these activities require dedication, self-control, practice, and an environment with minimal distractions.

Yoga

The increasingly popular practice of yoga includes physical poses, breathing techniques, and exacting, deliberate movements that are designed to reduce stress and improve strength, endurance, flexibility, and awareness. Some versions, which combine yoga and aerobics, even provide a cardiovascular workout. The various positions, which stretch and strengthen opposing muscle groups, may be held for long or short periods of time. Some schools of yoga also include mental aspects like meditation and chanting.

Biofeedback

Biofeedback is a treatment technique in which you learn to improve your health by being aware of signals from your own body. Sophisticated biofeedback machines are used to monitor your internal functions, providing information that can then be used to direct treatment. The principle is the same as when you take your temperature to decide whether you are well enough to get out of bed. Through biofeedback, you learn how to recognize harmful stress and control the mind-body connection to achieve a relaxed state, thus changing habitual reactions to stress. When these skills become second nature, the biofeedback machines are no longer needed.

Using Relaxation Techniques

Some of these relaxation exercises take time to learn and special conditions (quiet, darkness, equipment) to implement. As a result, they may seem to be less useful for emergency responders. However, with practice, many people learn to trigger the relaxation response almost immediately under a wide variety of conditions. The resulting calming effect can lead to improved confidence and performance, while protecting the mind and body from excessive stress.

The key is finding out what works best for you. For example, action-oriented people often experience muscle tension as a symptom of stress; they may find passive activities like meditation frustrating, but benefit by progressive muscle relaxation. Yoga is particularly suitable for internally directed and physically oriented people. Visualization techniques help many people deal with anxiety. Others can relax simply by listening to music, taking a bath, or going for a walk.

BUILDING PHYSICAL RESISTANCE

This final category describes lifestyle strategies for maximizing the body's ability to resist and recover from stress. The approaches discussed here—physical exercise, diet and nutrition, substance abuse prevention, and getting enough sleep—are perhaps the most basic and effective stress management techniques. They are particularly important for firefighters and rescue workers, who need both physical fitness and stress control to function effectively on the job.

Physical Exercise

The entire stress reaction is designed to prepare your heart, lungs, and muscles for physical activity. It's not surprising, then, that exercise helps to dissipate the physical and emotional arousal caused by stress. In fact, "regular, vigorous physical exercise is probably the single most beneficial way of dealing with stress and tension." (USFA 1991)

The health promoting benefits of physical fitness are well-known: reduced heart attacks, lower blood pressure, improved cholesterol levels, weight loss, less injuries on the incident scene, etc. Other advantages of exercise in the battle against stress include:

- Lower levels of toxic stress chemicals in the blood
- Enhanced ability to recover from stress' harmful effects
- Reduced muscular tension
- Increased confidence, optimism, self-esteem
- Positive outlet for aggression and hostility
- Improved performance, competence on the job, sense of control
- Improved physical appearance and sleep patterns

Aerobic exercise is particularly beneficial. Ideally, workouts should be vigorous enough to improve your level of cardiovascular fitness—i.e., moderate to high intensity activities sustained for a minimum of 20 minutes at least three times a week. Other forms of physical recreation can also be helpful, provided you stay active and enjoy what you are doing. Highly competitive sports, however, can increase stress for some people.

Diet and Nutrition

Excess weight is both a cause of stress and a result of it. On one hand, obesity places the body under physical strain, leads to various health problems, and contributes to low self-esteem. Certain foods also escalate the stress reaction or deplete the body of needed vitamins and minerals. On the other hand, many people react to stress by overeating. The resulting body fat compounds other problems and leads to dieting, another source of physical and psychological stress.

Proper diet and nutrition will improve the overall health of firefighters and minimize related stressors. Basic guidelines can be summarized as follows:

1. Limit caffeine, which stimulates the central nervous system and mimics the stress reaction.

2. Avoid excessive consumption of refined sugar, which adds calories, depletes B-complex vitamins, and leads to low levels of blood glucose (hypoglycemia).

3. Limit the use of salt, which can promote high blood pressure, excessive fluid retention, and a build-up of pressure in the central nervous system.

4. Restrict the intake of saturated fat and cholesterol, which contribute to atherosclerosis and heart disease.

5. Eat more complex carbohydrates, fruits, and vegetables to get the vitamins, minerals, and fiber you need for good health.

6. Balance the calories you eat with those burned in physical activity to maintain an appropriate body weight.

7. Consider taking a multi-vitamin supplement during times of high stress.

Substance Abuse Prevention

The use of alcohol, drugs, and tobacco is a major cause of stress in modern society. Substance abuse is a primary factor in most leading causes of death and disease. Related problems include accidents and injuries, interpersonal difficulties, poor work performance, physical and psychological dependency, and mental illness. The resulting costs to both the individual and the community are staggering.

Substance abuse also leaves people more vulnerable to stress reactions. Alcohol is a depressant and irritant which affects the nervous, endocrine, and immune systems. Tobacco contains nicotine, a powerful chemical which stimulates the stress response in the body and depletes needed vitamins. Drugs can alter the functioning of the mind-body connection in many ways, depending on the type, amount consumed, and means of ingestion.

Sometimes, these products seem to offer a temporary solution or escape in times of stress. In actuality, they limit your ability to handle the underlying problems, and they add a whole range of new ones. The best way to deal with the issue is obvious:

- Drink alcohol moderately or not at all
- Never use alcohol while on duty
- Don't start smoking, or quit immediately
- Don't abuse legal or illegal drugs

Getting Enough Sleep

Difficulty sleeping is a common symptom of stress. Individual needs vary, but most people should get between seven and nine hours sleep per night. Unfortunately, about one third of the population suffers from insomnia, and 15 percent sleep 6½ hours or less. The problem appears to be getting worse—the proportion of Americans sleeping the recommended amount has dropped from 64% in 1983 to 58% in 1992. (Louis Harris 1992)

Although a link between sleep deprivation and illness has not been proven, other negative effects are well known. Inadequate sleep results in a general feeling of fatigue which can affect mental performance, concentration, and memory capabilities. Consequences often include irritability and negative moods, decreased work performance, increased accidents, and difficulties in social relationships. The symptoms get worse the longer the problem persists.

Getting enough sleep can be a particular concern for emergency personnel whose biological clock is upset by frequent disruptions and shift work. (It takes about a week to reset the body's natural rhythms controlling sleep.) Since people have a tendency to adapt to their work situation, many don't even realize a problem exists.

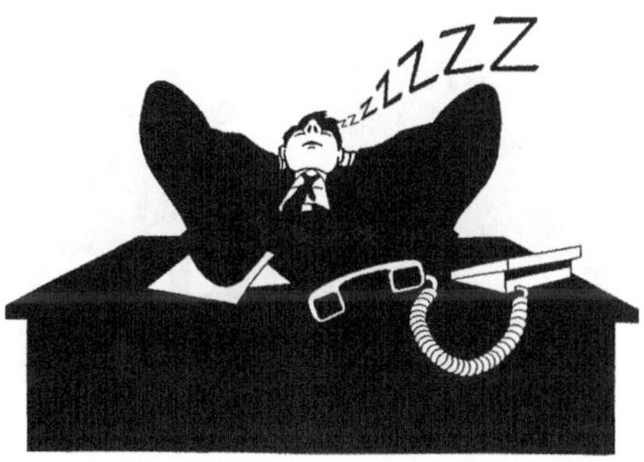

Most sleep problems are the result of medical or mental health problems that can be successfully treated by a professional. General tips for people with occasional difficulty sleeping include:

- Establish a regular sleep pattern, going to bed and getting up at the same time each day. Eliminate naps. Get regular exercise, especially in the late afternoon or early evening.

- Relax for about an hour before going to bed. Read, take a warm bath, listen to music, etc., but avoid vigorous physical or mental activities. Don't work or watch television in bed.

- Cut out caffeine and tobacco before bedtime. Alcohol can help you drop off, but sleep will frequently be light or disrupted.

- If your diet can handle it, try a late night snack of carbohydrates and milk (hot or cold). Limit other liquids to avoid midnight trips to the bathroom.

- Use deep breathing or mental relaxation techniques to help you fall asleep. If nothing happens within about 20 minutes, get up and do something until you are sleepy. Then try again.

PROFESSIONAL HELP

Sometimes, stress can become overwhelming in spite of measures you take to control it. In these situations, it is critical to avoid delays or an over-reliance on self-help or amateur psychology. Human emotions and stress reactions are highly complex, and inadequate or inappropriate treatment can make matters worse. **If you suffer from severe or prolonged symptoms like those described in Activity 9-1, you are strongly encouraged to get the professional assistance you need.**

Mental Health Professionals

Many different types of mental health professionals and services are available in most communities. These services are usually very specialized, depending on the practitioner's level of training and area of interest. Examples include psychotherapy, treatment with drugs, psychological testing, hypnosis, biofeedback, family or job counseling, and so forth.

Choosing the right professional is extremely important. First, learn something about the various sources of assistance within your department and the community. Then obtain some general information about the individual practitioner's qualifications, experience, methods, costs, etc. If possible, get references from trusted friends or other sources. Finally, call and ask questions to make sure the service is right for you.

Fire Department Services

An increasing number of fire and emergency medical departments now provide resources to help their members cope with work and life stress. Often, this support is administered through the department's Employee Assistance Program (EAP), which has been established to aid members and their families (see Chapter 8). Each department is different in the resources and services available. It is critical that you understand your department's policies and programs so you can participate effectively if the need arises.

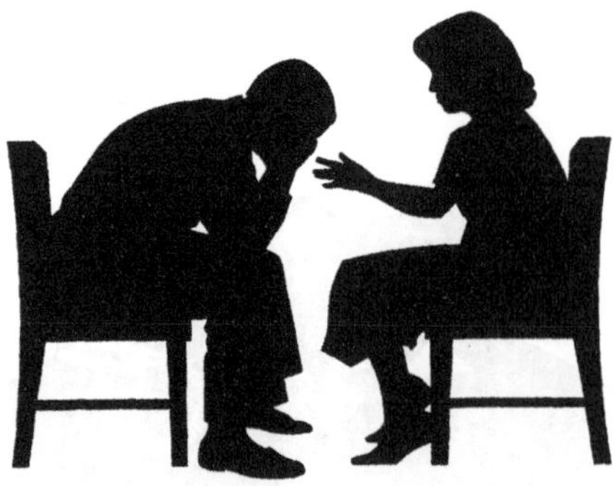

Activity 9-3

DEVELOPING A PERSONAL PLAN

When it comes to stress management, everyone is different. What works for one person or situation may not work for another. Therefore, everyone needs to analyze their own needs in order to select strategies that make sense for them.

This activity gives you an opportunity to think through a major source of stress in your life and develop a simple action plan to address it. The method used here can be helpful for any type of stress, but it's best suited for situations or events that are complex and somewhat predictable.

The approach is basically an organized way of thinking—breaking problems down into smaller components that are easier to analyze. You actually go through similar thought processes all the time, but formally writing down the steps can be helpful for complex issues. Remember: if the problem was simple, you probably would have already found a solution.

INSTRUCTIONS

Using the following worksheets, complete the steps below to prepare a stress management action plan.

Worksheet 1

1. **Define the Stressor**—Select an important source of stress in your life. (If desired, refer back to Activity 9-2.) Define it clearly and succinctly in one or two sentences.

2. **Describe the Stressor**—Think about the stressor and describe how and why it affects you. In particular, clarify:

   - When/where/how it occurs (specific circumstances or conditions)
   - How it upsets you (signs and symptoms—refer to Activity 9-1, if desired)
   - Why it upsets you (this is the hard part—be honest!)

3. **Determine Your Goals**—Write down how you would like the stressor and/or your response to change. Be as specific as you can, listing measurable objectives, if possible.

Worksheet 2

4. **Brainstorm Strategies**—Generate a list of options you could pursue to reach your goals, anything from specific action steps to learning new stress management skills. Don't worry about evaluating the options now; just list as many as come to mind. Try to identify several in each of the following categories:

    - Minimizing the Stressor—ways to avoid or change the stressor itself.
    - Changing Your Perceptions—ways to change the way you view the situation.
    - Relaxation Techniques—ways to control your physical and emotional state.
    - Building Physical Resistance—ways to increase your physical threshold for stress.
    - Getting Help—sources of assistance (personal or professional) you could recruit in your plan.

5. **Evaluate the Alternatives**—From your list, select several strategies that seem to have the best chance of success. Then evaluate those options by ranking them (high, medium, or low) according to the following criteria:

    - Time and effort needed
    - Emotional and financial costs
    - Tradeoffs—related problems, issues, etc.

Worksheet 3

6. **Develop the Plan**—Based on your analysis, select several action steps that you are willing and able to implement short-term (within 3 months) and long-term (over 3 months). Where appropriate, assign completion dates.

Revise your plan until you are satisfied. Then sign and date it. In the future, review the plan at regular intervals, fine-tuning until you reach your goals. With practice, the steps you take will become easier, and you will be able to apply your new skills to other areas of your life.

Activity 9-3 (Continued)

WORKSHEET 1

1. **DEFINE THE STRESSOR**:

____

____

____

2. **DESCRIBE THE STRESSOR**:

   Where/when/how it occurs: ______________________

____

____

____

   How it upsets you: ______________________

____

____

____

   Why it upsets you: ______________________

____

____

____

3. **DETERMINE YOUR GOALS**:

____

____

____

____

Activity 9-3 (Continued)
WORKSHEET 2

4. BRAINSTORM STRATEGIES	5. EVALUATE OPTIONS		
Minimizing the Stressor	T/E*	E/FC*	OT*
♦ ________________	____	____	____
♦ ________________	____	____	____
♦ ________________	____	____	____
♦ ________________	____	____	____
Changing Your Perceptions			
♦ ________________	____	____	____
♦ ________________	____	____	____
♦ ________________	____	____	____
♦ ________________	____	____	____
Relaxation Techniques			
♦ ________________	____	____	____
♦ ________________	____	____	____
♦ ________________	____	____	____
♦ ________________	____	____	____
Building Physical Resistance			
♦ ________________	____	____	____
♦ ________________	____	____	____
♦ ________________	____	____	____
♦ ________________	____	____	____
Getting Help			
♦ ________________	____	____	____
♦ ________________	____	____	____
♦ ________________	____	____	____
♦ ________________	____	____	____

* T/E = Time & Effort; E/FC = Emotional/Financial Costs; OT = Other Tradeoffs

Activity 9-3 (Continued)
WORKSHEET 3

6. DEVELOP THE PLAN

Short-Term Plan **Date**

- ♦ ____________________
- ♦ ____________________
- ♦ ____________________
- ♦ ____________________
- ♦ ____________________
- ♦ ____________________

Long-Term Plan **Date**

- ♦ ____________________
- ♦ ____________________
- ♦ ____________________
- ♦ ____________________
- ♦ ____________________
- ♦ ____________________

Plan Review Date: ____________________

Signature/Date: ____________________

CHAPTER SUMMARY

Stress is a normal reaction to extraordinary events and difficult situations. When managed appropriately, it contributes to the richness of life. When levels exceed the ability to cope, it can destroy health, emotional stability, performance, and personal relationships. This is particularly true for firefighters and rescue personnel, who face unique dangers and challenges as a normal part of their occupation.

In this chapter, you learned about the nature of stress: what causes it and how it affects individuals and society. You also examined the unique characteristics of fire and rescue work that contribute to stress, with a particular emphasis on critical incident stress and related departmental services. You identified symptoms and causes of stress in your own life. Then you looked at ways to minimize or control the negative effects of too much stress. Finally, you practiced a method to analyze and plan for major sources of stress on or off the job.

Having completed this chapter, you should now be able to:

- Define stress and its impact on health and personal well-being.
- Discuss the nature of stress in the fire service.
- Recognize sources and symptoms of stress in your own life.
- Identify ways to control stress on and off the job.
- Develop a personal strategy for stress management.

BIBLIOGRAPHY

Flannery, David R., "Managing Job-Related Stress," *Fire Chief*, February 1991.

Holmes, Thomas H., and Richard H. Rahe, "The Social Adjustment Rating Scale," *J. Psychosomatic Research*, 11:213-218, 1967.

Irwin, Terrence M., *Everyday Stress in the Fire Department*, Executive Fire Officer Program: National Fire Academy, August 1989.

Louis Harris and Associates, Inc., *The Baxter Survey of American Health Habits*, Study No. 923009, December 1992.

McQuade, Walter, and Ann Aikman, *Stress: What It Is, What It Can Do to Your Health, How to Handle It*, New York: Signet, 1993.

Mitchell, Jeff, Ph.D., and Grady Bray, Ph.D., *Emergency Services Stress: Guidelines for Preserving the Health and Careers of Emergency Services Personnel*, Englewood Cliffs, N.J.: Prentice Hall, Inc., 1990.

Moorhead, Gregory, and Ricky W. Griffin, Chapter 7: "Work Stress," *Organizational Behavior*, Boston: Houghton Mifflin Company, 1989.

National Center for Health Statistics, *Health, United States, 1991*, Hyattsville, Maryland: Public Health Service, 1992.

National Fire Academy, Unit 5: "Stress," *Firefighter Health and Safety: Program Implementation and Management*, Student Manual and Instructor Guide.

Navarre, Raymond J., *Stress and Firefighters*, Ph.D. Dissertation: University of Toledo, December 1993.

Public Health Service, *Plain Talk About...Handling Stress*, DHHS Publication No. (ADM) 91-502, Reprinted 1991.

Shearer, Robert W., "Occupational Stress in the Fire Service," *Professional Safety*, April 1989.

Stark, Elizabeth, "Stress: It's All Relative...and Relatively Easy to Manage," American Health, December 1992.

United States Fire Administration, *Stress Management: Model Program for Maintaining Firefighter Well-Being*, FA-100, February 1991.

Chapter 10

Maintaining Wellness Through Lifestyle Management

CHAPTER INTRODUCTION

Previous chapters examined different aspects of wellness, such as physical fitness, nutrition, and substance abuse. You learned exercises designed to improve flexibility, aerobic conditioning, and muscular fitness. Hopefully, you also began to look at other elements of your lifestyle—diet, stress, use of alcohol and tobacco, etc.—that could affect your risk for injury or disease.

This concept of lifestyle management is critical for improving your health. **Wellness must be viewed as a long-term commitment that can only be implemented by adopting daily patterns that promote fitness and health.** This does not mean that you have to live your life by a set of inflexible rules or always be deprived of things you want. But for most of us, it involves some changes in habits and attitudes that we have learned over the course of a lifetime.

This final chapter attempts to bring together the various components of wellness, both as a refresher of what you already learned and as a foundation for future personal growth. After discussing major health risks and wellness trends in the United States, you take a look at your own lifestyle. Making and (more importantly) maintaining lifestyle changes is discussed next. Finally, you examine your own wellness interests and long-term goals.

LEARNING OBJECTIVES

After learning the information in this chapter, you will be able to:

- Identify major health risks in the United States.
- Identify major wellness trends in the United States.
- Examine your own wellness behaviors to determine possible areas for improvement.
- Discuss guidelines for making and maintaining personal lifestyle changes.
- Prepare a personal wellness plan that takes into account your own health needs and goals.

HEALTH RISKS IN THE UNITED STATES

STATISTICAL OVERVIEW OF MAJOR HEALTH RISKS

The 10 leading causes of death in the United States in 1989 are shown in Table 10-1 and Figure 10-1. Heart disease and cancers of various kinds are by far the leading killers, accounting for about 1.25 million deaths per year. In fact, heart disease and cancers take the lives of well over twice as many people as the next eight leading causes combined. (Note: The primary source of data for this section is the National Center for Health Statistics.)

Table 10-1

		Deaths
1.	Heart Disease	733,867
2.	Cancers	496,152
3.	Strokes	145,551
4.	Accidents	95,028
5.	Chronic Lung Diseases	84,344
6.	Pneumonia and Influenza	76,550
7.	Diabetes Mellitus	46,833
8.	Suicide	30,232
9.	Chronic Liver Diseases	26,694
10.	Homicide	22,909

Source: NCHS 1992

Figure 10-1

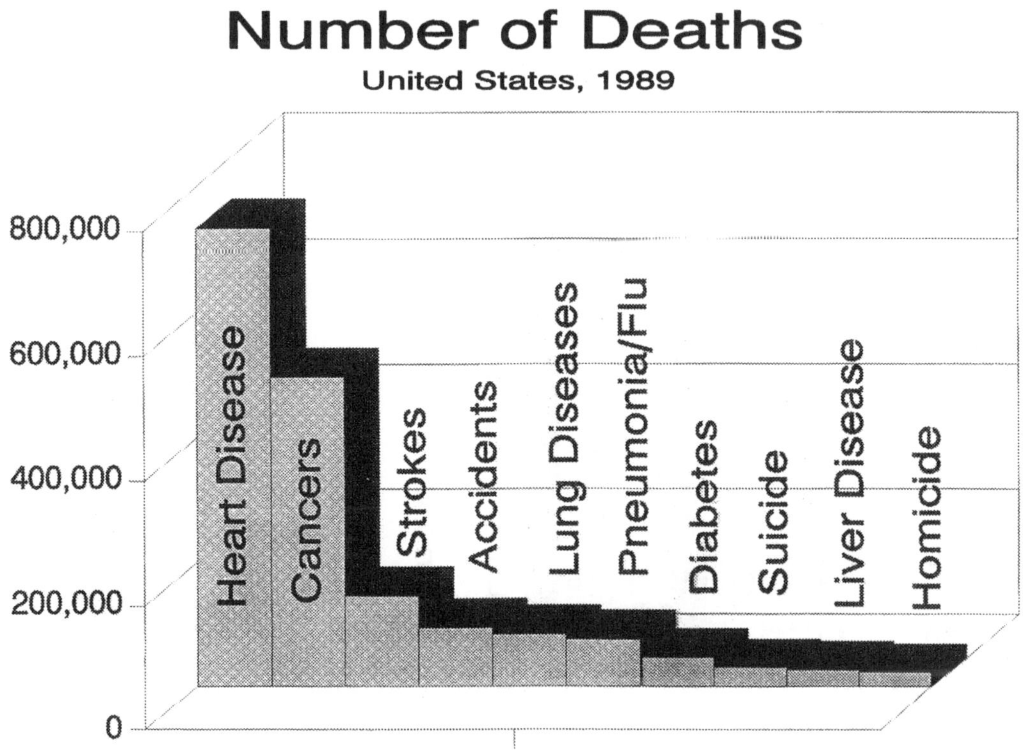

Premature Mortality

Another way of viewing the "Big 10" health risks in this country considers years of potential life lost before age 65 (see Table 10-2 and Figure 10-2, below). This measure of **premature mortality** takes into account the age of victims, so causes of death for younger people are weighed more heavily. Using this measure, the toll of accidents, homicides, and suicides takes on even greater importance because they cause a disproportionate loss of productive years of life and, presumedly, greater suffering.

Table 10-2

		Years*
1.	Heart Disease	649.7
2.	Cancers	843.3
3.	Strokes	109.5
4.	Accidents	1028.9
5.	Chronic Lung Diseases	62.4
6.	Pneumonia and Influenza	84.9
7.	Diabetes Mellitus	67.0
8.	Suicide	307.1
9.	Chronic Liver Diseases	107.5
10.	Homicide	338.5

* Per 100,000 population

Source: NCHS 1992

Figure 10-2

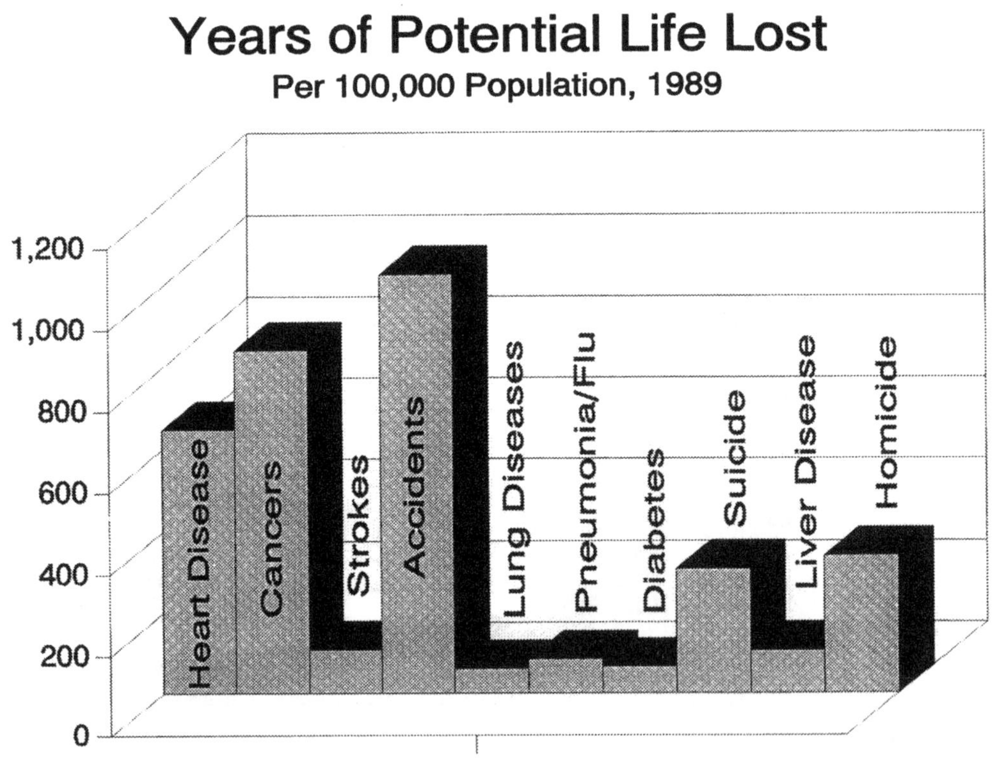

Risk by Age Category

The impact of these health risks varies for different populations. Table 10-3 below lists the leading causes of death by age category. These data show that death by various forms of violence is more likely among younger groups. As people get older, the incidence of heart disease and stroke increase, reflecting the cumulative nature of atherosclerosis. Related statistics include the following:

- Between 1988 and 1989, the death rate for human immunodeficiency virus (HIV) infection increased by 32 percent to become the 11th leading cause of death. Its rate among women doubled between 1984 and 1990.
- Suicide rates are particularly high among the young and old. The rate of suicide has doubled since 1968 among persons aged 15-19.
- In 1989, drug-related deaths stood at 4.3 per 100,000 population, up from 2.7 in 1978. Nationwide, about 10 percent of all homicides are drug-related, although rates are much higher in many cities.
- Between 1980 and 1989, the death rate for lung cancer increased by 42 percent for white women and 30 percent for black women, while staying fairly stable for men of both races.

In reviewing these figures, it should be noted that for virtually all health risks, members of certain races and ethnic groups, people with low income, and people with disabilities have a higher risk of premature death, disease, and disability. For example, premature mortality is almost twice as high for blacks as for whites, and twice as high for males as for females of both races. Socioeconomic status is also linked to the incidence of heart disease.

Table 10-3

RISK OF DEATH BY AGE CATEGORY

#	15-24	25-44	45-64	65 and Over
1.	Accidents	Accidents	Cancer	Heart Disease
2.	Homicide	Cancer	Heart Disease	Cancer
3.	Suicide	HIV Infection	Stroke	Stroke
4.		Heart Disease	Accidents	Lung Diseases
5.		Suicide	Lung Diseases	Pneumonia/Flu

Source: NCHS 1992

TRENDS IN WELLNESS

In some ways, recent trends in wellness seem to be going in the right direction. Overall, life expectancy (in years) at birth has increased from 47.4 in 1900 to 75.3 in 1989 (71.8 for men and 78.6 for women). Over a 10-year period, chances for surviving the effects of cancer have improved from 41% to 47% for men while staying virtually the same for women at 57%.

The death rate for adults has declined 30% between 1977 and 1989. This positive result is due primarily to reduced rates of cigarette smoking, lower mean blood cholesterol, and increased control of high blood pressure, which have, in turn, led to declines in mortality from heart disease and stroke. (NCHS 1992)

The agency continues, "in the same period, mortality from motor vehicle crashes also declined substantially. Lower rates of alcohol use, increased seat belt use, and changes in speed limits have contributed to this reduction." Another positive factor has been increased use of smoke detectors.

Figure 10-3 shows changes in death rates for the five leading causes of death. Of particular note, heart disease rates declined between 1970 and 1989 by 39%, and those for strokes went down by 58%. Death rates from accidents also declined significantly, while those for chronic lung diseases have gone way up. (NCHS 1992)

Figure 10-3

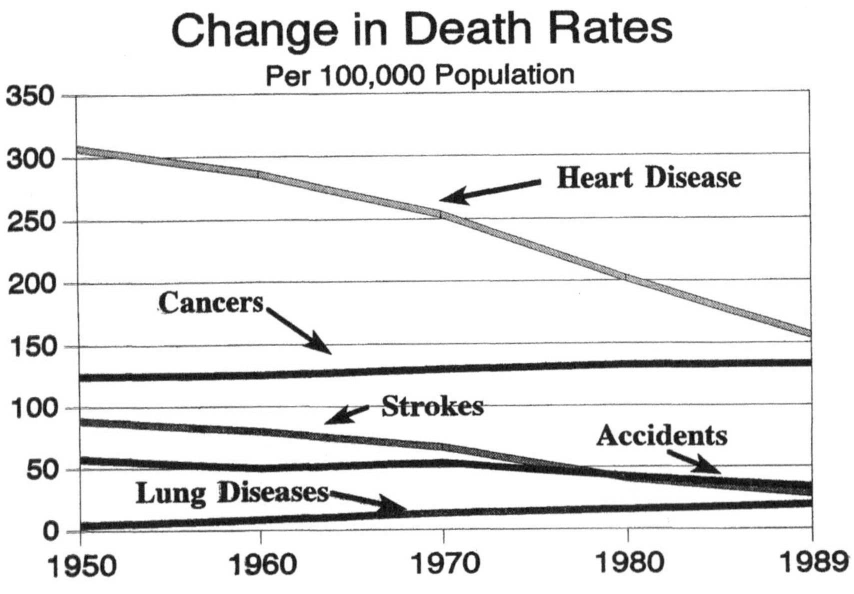

Recent Trends

Unfortunately, some of the positive trends of the past two decades seem to have leveled off or actually even started to reverse themselves. The amount people exercise has stabilized, and they're eating less well. Stress levels have soared. Too many people still smoke and drink excessively. In fact, "the most significant improvements made over the past several years have been in areas where healthful behavior is mandated by law." (Louis Harris 1992)

> "For the third straight year, Americans failed to improve their health behavior, and in a number of cases we sacrificed the gains of the early- and mid-1980s. For example, we're sleeping less and eating less carefully than we did a decade ago, and we're exercising about the same as in 1983 (and less than we did a year ago)."
> (Louis Harris 1992)

Several trends, both related to nutrition, are of special note:

- The mortality rate of cancer is 8% higher today than in 1971. Death rates may exceed those for heart disease within a matter of years.

- The number of people who weigh at least 20% more than their ideal body weight has increased a remarkable 8% in only 11 years.

Still, most Americans described their overall health in 1990 as good to excellent. Among persons 15-44 years of age, only about 5% said their health was fair or poor; the corresponding figure for those aged 45-64 was roughly 16%. As might be expected, people who are elderly, black, who live in poverty, or have little education are far more likely to describe their health as fair or poor than those who do not fall into those categories.

The table on the next page summarizes the practice of key preventive behaviors in the United States, according to the *1992 Baxter Survey of American Health Habits*. Important categories are examined in more detail on the following pages. (Note: self-reported health data are particularly susceptible to various sources of statistical error.)

Table 10-4

PERCENTAGE OF POPULATION PRACTICING PREVENTIVE BEHAVIORS (1992)

	Total %
Exercise and Body Composition	
Get strenuous exercise three or more days a week	33
Are not overweight	34
Diet and Nutrition—Try a lot to:	
Eat enough fiber	53
Avoid eating too much fat	51
Avoid eating too much salt	46
Avoid eating too many high-cholesterol foods	44
Eat vegetables in the cabbage family	57
Substance Abuse	
Do not smoke cigarettes	76
Drink alcohol moderately or not at all	88
Never use illegal drugs	95
Control of Stress	
Do not feel under great stress frequently	67
Get seven or eight hours of sleep most nights	58
Socialize with others at least once a week	82
Periodic Examinations and Tests	
Blood pressure reading at least once a year	84
Cholesterol check at least once a year	56
Dental checkup at least once a year	73
Safety Precautions	
Have a home smoke detector	90
Always drive at or below speed limit	49
Never drive after drinking	83
Always wear seat belts when in front seat of car	70

Source: Louis Harris 1992

Activity 10-1

CW-F WELLNESS QUIZ

This wellness quiz is designed primarily as a self-education tool and a review of the information in previous chapters. It asks you to rate yourself on behaviors that are part of any healthy lifestyle. It may help you identify goals for change in your own life, or determine priorities among different goals.

The quiz is divided into five parts. Each part focuses on a specific wellness component:

Part A:	Physical Fitness—Exercise and Body Composition
Part B:	Diet and Nutrition
Part C:	Substance Abuse and Health
Part D:	Stress Management
Part E:	Personal Safety and Medical Examinations

For most people, making the changes needed for a healthy lifestyle takes time. This wellness quiz can serve as a baseline as you go through the process, just like the physical fitness assessment you completed in Chapter 2. For this reason, you may want to take the quiz every three or six months to help you monitor your progress and stay focused on your goals.

Instructions

1. Each section of the quiz begins with a review of current trends related to the specific wellness area. (Note: the materials summarize research covered in depth in previous chapters.)

2. Then you will have an opportunity to evaluate yourself. Think about the behaviors listed in the quiz. For each behavior, assign yourself a score, using the following scale:

2 points	This healthy behavior is a <u>regular</u> part of my lifestyle.
1 point	This healthy behavior is <u>often</u> part of my lifestyle.
0 points	This healthy behavior is <u>sometimes</u> part of my lifestyle.
-1 point	This healthy behavior is <u>rarely or never</u> part of my lifestyle.

3. Total your scores for each section of the questionnaire. Then transfer the scores to the summary worksheet which follows.

PART A: PHYSICAL FITNESS–EXERCISE AND BODY COMPOSITION

Exercise

Inactive people have a higher risk of heart disease and a lower chance of post-heart-attack recovery. A sedentary lifestyle also contributes to unhealthy levels of blood cholesterol. Regular physical exercise provides many other benefits, including improved stamina and strength, better performance on and off the job, reduced injuries, and improved self-esteem.

While over three quarters of the public claim to get regular exercise, only about one-third exercise strenuously three or more times a week, a slight decline from recent years. About one in five people say they never exercise at all. Younger adults, men, Westerners, and people who say they are in excellent health are more likely to get strenuous exercise.

Body Composition

Excess weight is associated with high blood pressure, elevated blood cholesterol, diabetes, heart disease, stroke, some cancers, and gall bladder disease. It also may be a factor in osteoarthritis of the weight-bearing joints. Approximately one quarter of all adults, or about 34 million people, are overweight; half of them are trying to lose weight.

Using a different measure based on standard height-weight tables, the Baxter survey found that fully two-thirds of the population (66%) is overweight. This measure has been increasing steadily over the last decade, probably due more to decreased physical activity than eating more calories. The proportion of underweight people has stayed fairly constant; those within the recommended weight range has declined 6% since 1983.

Figure 10-4

FREQUENCY OF STRENUOUS EXERCISE

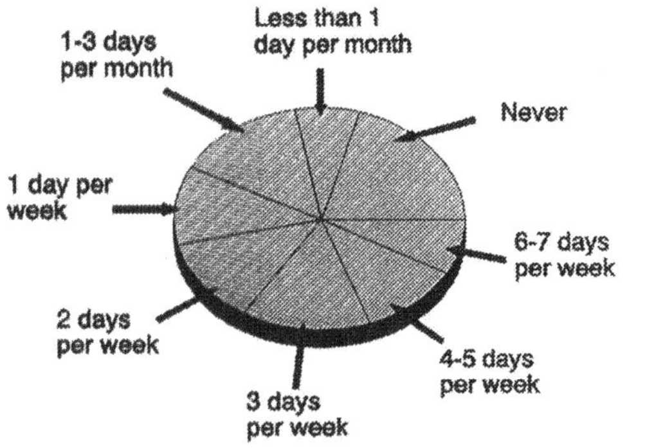

Figure 10-5

ADULT WEIGHT RANGES

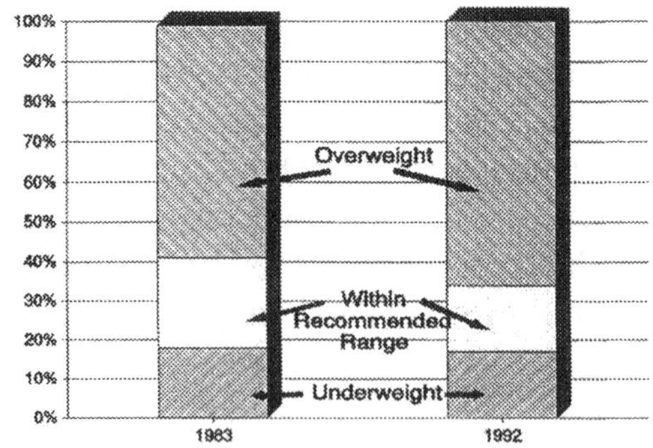

Activity 10-1 (Continued)

CW-F WELLNESS QUIZ: PART A

PHYSICAL FITNESS— EXERCISE AND BODY COMPOSITION	SCORE (-1 to 2)
1. Regularly perform static stretches to improve flexibility in all major muscle groups.	
2. Engage in strenuous aerobic activity for at least 20 minutes three or more times per week.	
3. Participate in a regular program of strength training at least 2-3 times per week.	
4. Conduct an adequate warm-up and cool-down with each exercise activity.	
5. Exercise at moderate levels of intensity, appropriate for my level of physical conditioning.	
6. Do not engage in competitive recreational sports without adequate conditioning.	
7. Maintain a healthy level of body fat (under 19% for men and 25% for women).	
8. Avoid rapid weight loss and gain.	
9. Occasionally review personal eating behaviors and assess their impact on my weight and health.	
10. Balance eating schedules and amounts of food with daily energy needs.	

TOTAL SCORE ________

Key: 2 points This healthy behavior is a regular part of my lifestyle.

1 point This healthy behavior is often part of my lifestyle.

0 points This healthy behavior is sometimes part of my lifestyle.

-1 point This healthy behavior is rarely or never part of my lifestyle.

PART B: DIET AND NUTRITION

Diet and nutrition is implicated in one-third of all cancer deaths, a large proportion of heart attacks, stroke, diabetes, liver disease, and atherosclerosis. It is a factor in high blood pressure, which affects about 30 percent of American adults, and blood cholesterol levels, a problem for over 50 percent of adults. Other related health problems include osteoporosis, gallstones, and tooth decay. As a result, poor nutrition is considered by many experts to be second in importance only to smoking as a controllable health risk.

"In 1992, Americans appear to be putting less effort into following good diet and nutrition principles. Attention to nearly every area measured has fallen, both since last year and since 1983. The largest decreases in the past year occurred in the much-hyped areas of avoiding too much fat and too much cholesterol, both falling by a sizable six points since 1991." (Louis Harris 1992)

About one-half of the population appears to be making a concerted effort to eat well. In particular, Americans try hardest to eat vegetables in the cabbage family (57%), to eat enough fiber (53%), and to avoid eating too much fat (51%). Nutrition habits seem to improve with age.

Figure 10-6

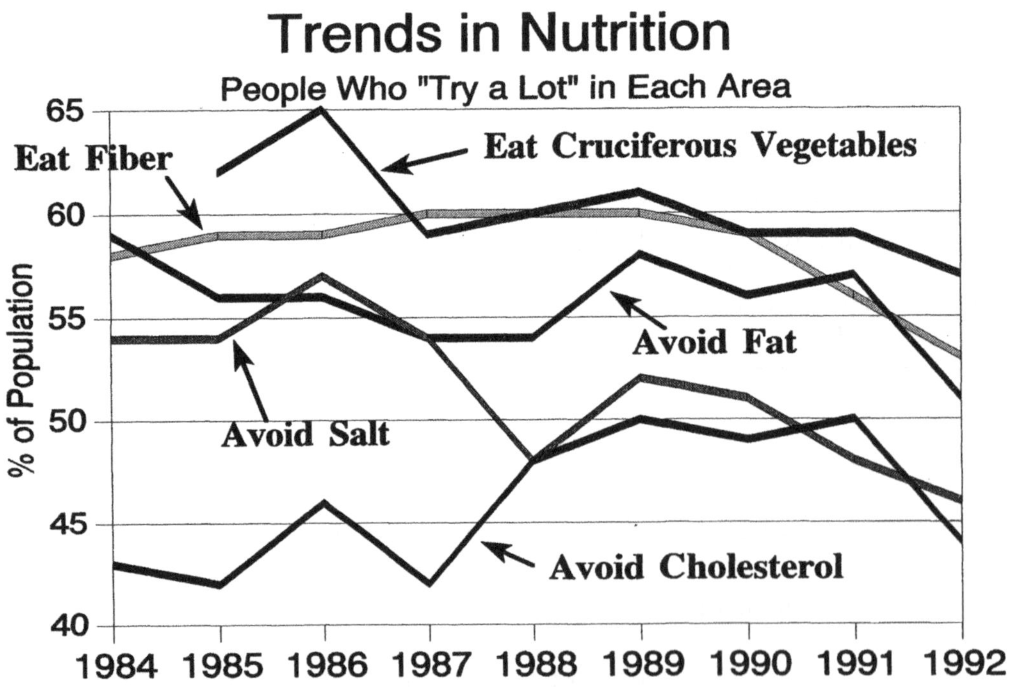

Activity 10-1 (Continued)

CW-F WELLNESS QUIZ: PART B

DIET AND NUTRITION	SCORE (-1 to 2)
1. Avoid eating too much fat, especially saturated fat.	
2. Avoid eating too many high-cholesterol foods, particularly egg yolks and organ meats (like liver).	
3. Eat plenty of fruits and vegetables (five or more servings daily).	
4. Eat plenty of carbohydrates—rice, pasta, bread, potatoes, beans, etc. (six or more servings daily).	
5. Avoid eating too much salt or sodium (more than 6 grams daily).	
6. Regularly eat vegetables in the cabbage family (cauliflower, broccoli, brussels sprouts, kale, etc.).	
7. Eat a wide variety of foods.	
8. Limit consumption of meat to six ounces per day or less.	
9. Regularly read food labels and monitor amounts of food eaten.	
10. Take steps to learn more about nutrition and healthful eating alternatives.	

TOTAL SCORE __________

Key: 2 points This healthy behavior is a regular part of my lifestyle.

1 point This healthy behavior is often part of my lifestyle.

0 points This healthy behavior is sometimes part of my lifestyle.

-1 point This healthy behavior is rarely or never part of my lifestyle.

PART C: SUBSTANCE ABUSE AND HEALTH

Tobacco

According to the Department of Health and Human Resources, "cigarette smoking has been identified as the largest risk factor for mortality in the United States. Over 400,000 lives are lost each year from smoking, primarily from lung cancer, cardiovascular disease, and chronic obstructive lung disease. The adverse effects of cigarette smoking on pregnancy and infant health are also well documented." A recent American Cancer Society study found that at least one-third of all smokers will die of smoking related causes. People who smoke are also more likely to adopt other risky behaviors, such as excessive drinking, illegal drug use, and many others. (Louis Harris 1992)

About 24% of the adult population smoked in 1992, a reduction of about 2% in just the last two years. This drop continues the steady decline in smoking over the last two decades, possibly due to public education campaigns aimed at smokers, more restrictive laws in public places, and social pressures. However, the proportion of women who smoke has increased rapidly in recent years, a major factor in their increased rates of lung cancer.

In addition to cigarette smoking, about 2% of the public smoke a cigar, 3% smoke a pipe, and 4% use chewing tobacco. Use of smokeless tobacco, which causes oral cancer and other diseases, may actually be increasing, particularly among young men.

Figure 10-7

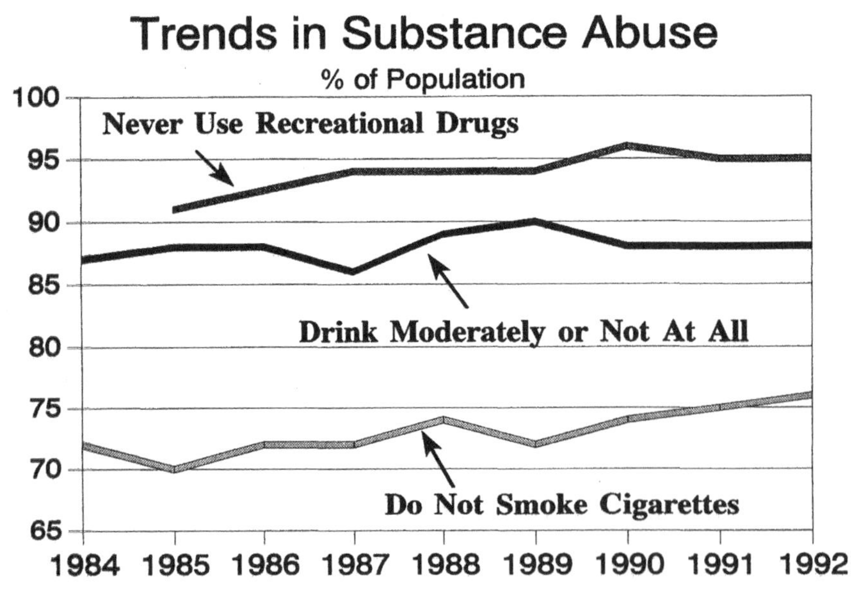

Alcohol

Alcohol is an addictive and dangerous drug associated with various forms of cancer, heart disease, cirrhosis of the liver, damage to the brain and other organs, birth defects, and a wide variety of other health problems. In addition, alcohol is a factor in motor vehicle and other types of accidents, violent crimes, and suicide. Alcohol-related problems were estimated to cost over $42 billion in 1975, including medical expenses and lost productivity (e.g., increased employee absenteeism).

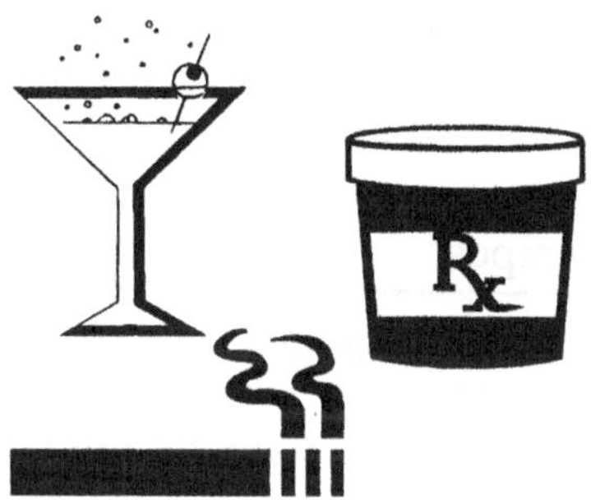

The proportion of problem drinkers—roughly 10 percent—has remained fairly stable over the last decade. According to the National Institute on Alcohol Abuse and Alcoholism, there were about 9.5 million alcoholics in the United States in 1985. However, the proportion of people who drink moderately (1-3 drinks on a day when they drink) has declined 6% between 1983 and 1992. Furthermore, about 40% of Americans say they never drink alcohol, up from 34% over the same period. Women and older people are more likely to drink moderately or to abstain than men and younger adults.

Legal and Illegal Drugs

Health effects associated with drug abuse differ depending on the substance chosen and the method of intake. However, in general, drug use can lead to physical and psychological addiction and a vast array of physical, mental, and social problems. Furthermore, abuse of drugs is a factor in accidents, injuries, and lost productivity, both on and off the job.

Marijuana is the most common illicit drug, used by about 5% of the population in 1990. After marijuana, cocaine use ranked second, with other drugs in the 0.5-1.5% range. In 1992, rates appear to be relatively unchanged, with 95% of the population reporting that they never use recreational drugs. Of particular note, the proportion of younger adults (aged 18-29) abstaining from drug use has increased from 79% from 1984 to 91% in 1992. However, some recent reports indicate that this trend may be reversing somewhat lately for certain drugs like LSD.

Activity 10-1 (Continued)

CW-F WELLNESS QUIZ: PART C

SUBSTANCE ABUSE AND HEALTH	SCORE (-1 to 2)
1. Do not smoke cigarettes.	
2. Do not smoke cigars or pipes.	
3. Do not use smokeless tobacco products.	
4. Avoid smoky environments and sources of secondary smoke whenever possible.	
5. Drink alcohol moderately or not at all on a daily basis.	
6. Never engage in binge drinking (five or more drinks on any one occasion).	
7. Never drink while at work or on duty.	
8. Never use illegal drugs (marijuana, cocaine, LSD, etc.)	
9. Never take legal medications except as prescribed by a doctor.	
10. Never become physically or psychologically addicted to any substance.	

TOTAL SCORE ________

Key: 2 points This healthy behavior is a regular part of my lifestyle.

1 point This healthy behavior is often part of my lifestyle.

0 points This healthy behavior is sometimes part of my lifestyle.

-1 point This healthy behavior is rarely or never part of my lifestyle.

PART D: STRESS MANAGEMENT

Stress is associated with homicides, suicides, injuries and deaths to children inflicted by abusing parents, mental illness, alcoholism, drug use, divorce, and criminal behavior. It contributes to many illnesses, including heart disease. Stress is also linked with behavioral and interpersonal problems, such as disturbed sleep, impatience, lack of motivation, decreased productivity, and many others. For these reasons, stress may be responsible for up to $20 billion in losses to the American economy.

In 1990, 41% of the population 18 years of age and over indicated that stress had at least some effect on their health; 13% had sought help from family, friends, professionals, or self-help groups. The corresponding percentages for 1985 were 44% and 11%, respectively. (National Health Interview Survey.)

This trend seems to be increasing, as more people report feeling under great stress. In 1992, 63% of the public reported they felt great stress at least once a week, versus 55% in 1983. A total of 18% say they feel great stress every day. In addition, the proportion of Americans reporting getting the recommended 7-8 hours sleep a night has dropped from 64% in 1983 to 58% in 1992.

Figure 10-8

FREQUENCY OF GREAT STRESS

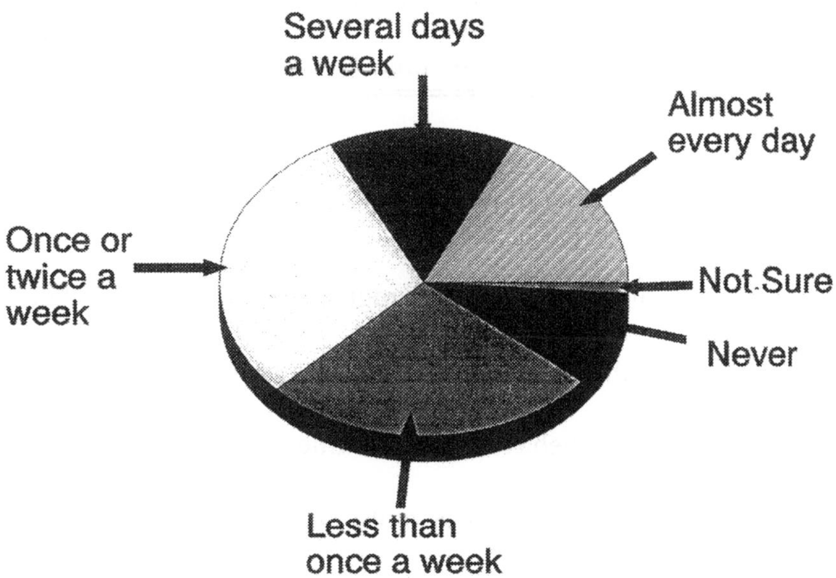

Activity 10-1 (Continued)

CW-F WELLNESS QUIZ: PART D

STRESS MANAGEMENT	SCORE (-1 to 2)
1. Avoid situations that cause undue stress whenever possible.	
2. Get seven or eight hours of sleep on most nights.	
3. Socialize with others at least once a week.	
4. Practice personal relaxation techniques (e.g., meditation, systematic relaxation, biofeedback, yoga, etc.) during periods of anxiety.	
5. Maintain hobbies and personal interests outside of the job and other responsibilities.	
6. Engage in regular exercise and/or other physical activity.	
7. Take advantage of support systems and other sources of assistance in times of need.	
8. Recognize and look out for signs of stress in myself and others.	
9. Look for ways to make my job challenging and enjoyable.	
10. Practice communicating my real feelings to family and friends.	

TOTAL SCORE __________

Key:	2 points	This healthy behavior is a regular part of my lifestyle.
	1 point	This healthy behavior is often part of my lifestyle.
	0 points	This healthy behavior is sometimes part of my lifestyle.
	-1 point	This healthy behavior is rarely or never part of my lifestyle.

PART E: PERSONAL SAFETY AND MEDICAL EXAMINATIONS

Personal Safety

Accidents and their adverse effects are the fourth leading cause of death and the leading cause of premature mortality in the country. By themselves, motor vehicle crashes, about half of them alcohol-related, rank as the sixth leading cause of death. Among young people (25 and under), alcohol-related traffic accidents are the leading cause of death and spinal cord injury. Other areas of concern include home accidents, falls, drownings, residential fires, and accidents with firearms.

Over the last decade, death rates from most types of accidents have declined. The following chart shows trends for car crashes, children's home accidents, falls, and drownings. In addition, residential fire deaths have declined about 17%, unintentional deaths from firearms are also down 17%, and tap water scald injuries requiring hospital care have been reduced about 26%.

Trends in personal safety behaviors are mixed, with some improving and some not. Many more homes are equipped with smoke detectors (up 22% since 1983), but the proportion of households with someone who smokes in bed has stayed about the same. More Americans are wearing seat belts every year, but driving at or below the speed limit has declined. Perhaps most hopefully, the proportion of drivers who say they drive after drinking continues to fall sharply, down to 17% in 1992 from 32% in 1983.

Figure 10-9

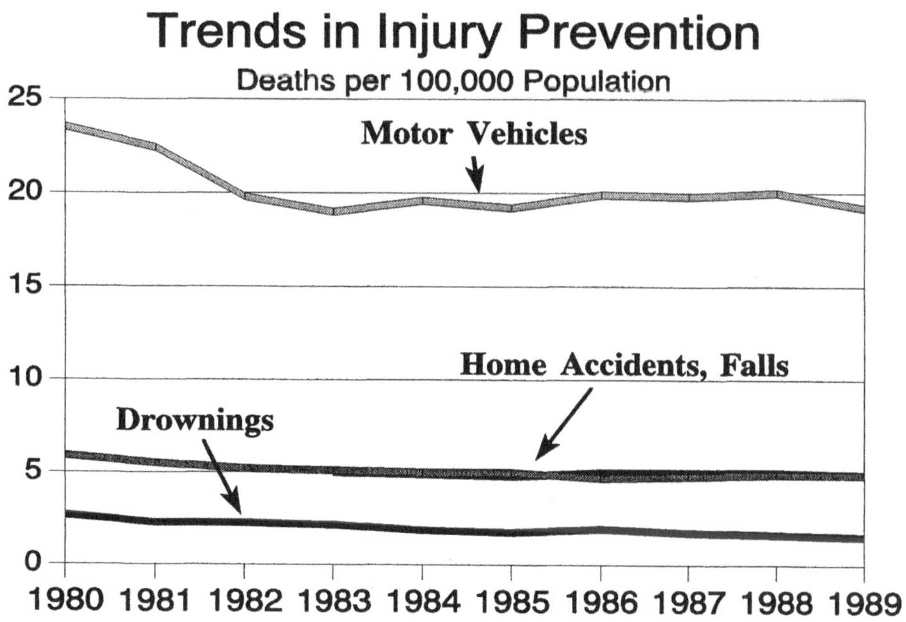

According to the Coalition for Consumer Health and Safety, the 10 most avoidable hazards (not ranked by risk) are rollover crashes in sport and utility vehicles; crash injuries from not using seat belts; falls from playground equipment; falls and burns from unsupervised use of baby walkers; breathing problems from secondhand tobacco smoke; infant drownings in five-gallon buckets; accidents and disease caused by excessive drinking; sexually transmitted diseases from improper contraceptive use; head injuries from not wearing bicycle helmets; and illness from improperly cooked foods.

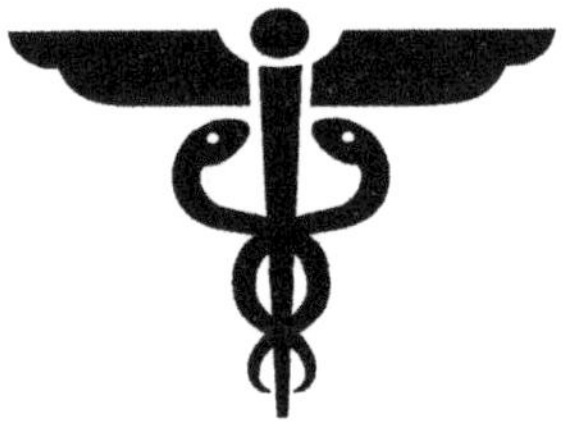

Medical Examinations

Health promotion includes activities, such as certain medical examinations and tests, to help identify potential problems early and to take appropriate action. Important areas include regular physical examinations, blood pressure readings, blood cholesterol tests, and immunization. Surveillance of infectious diseases—such as hepatitis B, HIV, tuberculosis, pneumonia, and meningitis—is of special concern to firefighters and emergency care providers. For women, breast examinations, mammograms, and pap tests should be a regular part of prevention.

Most Americans are willing to visit their health care providers for preventive exams and tests. Review of behaviors in this area reveals the following:

- A substantial portion of the public (84%) have a blood pressure reading at least once a year, about the same as 10 years ago.
- More people have their blood cholesterol checked at least annually—56% in 1992, up 8% since 1985.
- About three quarters (73%) of the population goes to the dentist for treatment or a check-up at least once a year, up marginally over the past decade.
- Approximately half (49%) of adult women examine their breasts once a month to detect cancer, an increase of 12% since 1983.
- About two thirds of women aged 40 and over report having a mammogram at least every two years, a 3% drop since the previous year.
- Eight in ten adult women say they have a Pap smear at least every two years, an increase of 5% since 1983.

Activity 10-1 (Continued)

CW-F WELLNESS QUIZ: PART E

PERSONAL SAFETY AND MEDICAL EXAMINATIONS	SCORE (-1 to 2)
1. Always wear seat belts when traveling in a passenger vehicle.	
2. Always drive at or below the legal speed limit.	
3. Never drive under the influence of alcohol or drugs.	
4. Avoid potentially violent situations where someone could be seriously injured.	
5. Always practice proper techniques for lifting and carrying objects.	
6. Have blood pressure checked at least once a year.	
7. Get a cholesterol screening at least once a year.	
8. Get a dental check-up at least once a year.	
9. Take immediate steps to address health problems that develop.	
10. Avoid exposure to infectious diseases through immunizations, personal protective equipment, safe sexual practices, etc.	

TOTAL SCORE ________

Key: 2 points This healthy behavior is a regular part of my lifestyle.

1 point This healthy behavior is often part of my lifestyle.

0 points This healthy behavior is sometimes part of my lifestyle.

-1 point This healthy behavior is rarely or never part of my lifestyle.

Activity 10-1 (Continued)

SUMMARY WORKSHEET

Transfer your total score from each of the five separate sections of the CW-F Wellness Quiz to the worksheet below. Then total your scores and compare the result with the key below.

WELLNESS CATEGORIES	SCORE (-10 to 20)
A. Physical Fitness—Exercise and Body Composition	
B. Diet and Nutrition	
C. Substance Abuse and Health	
D. Stress Management	
E. Personal Safety and Medical Examinations	

GRAND TOTAL SCORE _________

Key: 80-100 You take very good care of yourself. Congratulations!

60-79 You take good care of yourself, but could improve in certain areas.

40-59 You take reasonable care of yourself, but should do better.

20-39 Your lifestyle needs significant improvement.

Below 20 Your lifestyle may be hazardous to your health.

LIFESTYLE AND PERSONAL CHANGE

In the last section, you learned about health trends in this country and what Americans are doing to prevent or minimize their risk of death, disease, and injury. This information emphasizes the relationship between lifestyle—an individual's patterns of everyday living—and health. In short, **you can completely control many risk factors by maintaining a healthy lifestyle**.

Most people—about 9 out of 10 adults—already know that high blood pressure, cigarette smoking, high cholesterol levels, obesity, and a high fat diet are risk factors for heart disease. Most adults are also familiar with at least some of the basic lifestyle guidelines for health. As a result, the incidence of heart disease and stroke in this country has declined dramatically over the past twenty years. There have been improvements in other areas as well.

However, many people continue to follow unhealthful lifestyle patterns, even though they know better. Why does this happen? The answer seems to lie in the psychology of change, a subject of critical importance in any health and wellness program.

MAKING LIFESTYLE CHANGES

If change is "making something different," then lifestyle changes involve making *ourselves* different. For most people, adopting new habits and patterns is very difficult, and the process seems to get harder as we get older. However, some people are more comfortable with change, and others even enjoy it.

Resistance to change, even small changes, is normal. In fact, a constructive resistance to change is actually healthy. Often, "old ways" were adopted because they worked; doing things a new way sometimes leads to unexpected problems. Imagine making drastic changes in your life every time a new idea comes along!

However, everyone has room for improvement in some aspect of their lives, and most people want to steer their lives in a positive direction. Therefore, each of us has to deal with the psychology of change. The capacity for change can literally determine the outcome of our lives.

Some reasons why individuals resist beneficial change include:

- Lack of awareness—Individuals must first recognize that change is beneficial; then they need enough information to follow through.
- Habit—Often it's just easier to do things the way we learned to do them in the past.
- Security—Some people feel uncomfortable or insecure doing things a new way—fear of the unknown.
- Cultural blocks—Personal background and learned values strongly affect the change process.
- Social factors—Peer pressure, job requirements, and other situational variables can make change harder (or easier).

The capacity for change is rooted in basic human characteristics—needs, perceptions, beliefs, and values. As a result, **making lifestyle changes is complex, and the process is different for everyone**. Although some genetic factors may contribute, the major forces that shape our personal approach to change result from a combination of life experience and environmental factors.

In short:

Personality
+ Life Experience
+ Environment
Capacity for Change

Each of these factors is discussed in more detail below.

Personality

Adults can be grouped into three general categories based on their openness or resistance to change:

- A small percentage thrive on change and seek different ways of doing things "just for the sake of change."
- The great majority are not actively looking for change but are willing to change for the right reason (i.e., with adequate motivation).
- A small percentage actively dislike almost any type of change and go out of their way to avoid it.

Figure 10-10

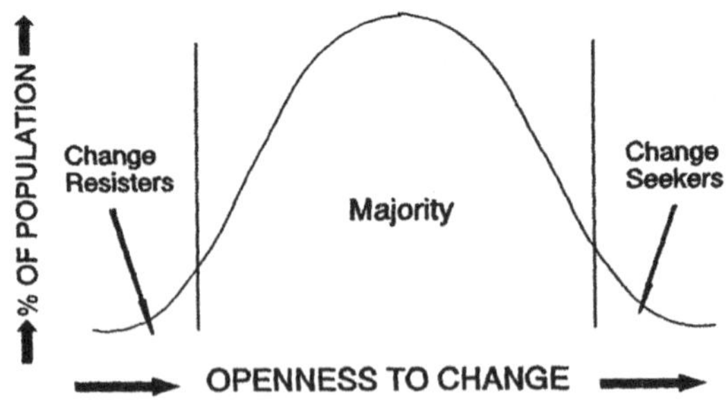

Life Experience

Life experience from the time you were a child affects your attitude about change. Every time you tried to make changes in your life, there were consequences. If these consequences were usually good, you probably became more open to change. If the consequences were negative, you learned through the years that change was painful—something to avoid as much as possible.

Environment

Outside factors—family, friends, co-workers, job situations, social interactions, etc.—strongly influence most people's desire for personal change, as well as their ability to make and maintain changes over time. If family members at home (primary environment) or co-workers at the fire department (secondary environment) are open to change and supportive, their attitudes may directly or indirectly "tip the scale" in favor of constructive change. Unfortunately, the opposite is also true.

Fire and rescue personnel spend more time on the job, and they function more like a family, than most other professions. Therefore, it is imperative that they encourage and support each other in making positive lifestyle changes. It is often particularly helpful to have a buddy or a team at work trying to accomplish important goals together.

Personal Capacity for Change

Lifestyle is critical to health and wellness, and all of us have room to improve. Furthermore, our bodies and situations change as we get older, whether we like it or not. Therefore, each of us needs to address lifestyle changes at various times throughout our lives.

To get a very broad indicator of your capacity or tendency to make and maintain personal lifestyle changes, take the simple quiz on the next page (Activity 10-2). No matter what the results, remember that anyone can change his or her habits and daily patterns if they want to enough.

The general guidelines that follow can be remembered by the acronym ***CHANGE***. These "rules of thumb" have been shown to be useful for people wishing to initiate and maintain a personal behavioral change, like losing weight or quitting smoking. Although the focus here is on lifestyle change to promote health and fitness, the guidelines are equally appropriate in other areas.

The bottom line is that everyone has to figure out what works best for him or her. The process becomes easier the more you practice it and learn about yourself.

Activity 10-2

PERSONAL CAPACITY FOR CHANGE

For each question, circle the number that most closely corresponds with your answer. Then total the results and compare with the score key.

	Strongly Disagree				Strongly Agree
1. **Personality**: In general, I enjoy new experiences and actively look for opportunities to improve myself.	1	2	3	4	5
2. **Life Experience**: In the past, I have usually been successful in attempts to make important changes in my life.	1	2	3	4	5
3. **Environment**: Typically, my family, friends, and co-workers support me in making positive changes in my life.	1	2	3	4	5

Key: Capacity for Change

TOTAL SCORE _____

12-15	High
7-11	Medium
3-6	Low

CHANGE™: GUIDELINES FOR PERSONAL GROWTH

C = **CONVICTION AND COMMITMENT**. The hardest part is often believing you can change and deciding you want to change—i.e., committing yourself to the process. To help establish this psychological foundation, actively foster beliefs and values that support the change you want to make, particularly:

- The end result of change is worth the effort.
- The process of change is within my control.
- The responsibility for change is mine and I accept it.

Techniques that help you visualize the outcome and benefits of the proposed change, and that strengthen your resolve, contribute to personal power.

H = **HELPS AND HINDRANCES**. Know yourself: what supports you and what serves as an obstacle, distraction, or temptation. Promote those things that help you; avoid people or situations that don't. Why make the process any harder than necessary?

A = **ATTITUDE AND APPROACH**. Take a long-term, proactive approach: start with a positive attitude, analyze the situation, and "plan to succeed." Cultivate a positive outlook by finding out what "carrots" and "sticks" work for you. Identify the best road to your destination and travel it in your mind. Plan for potholes and stormy weather.

N = **NATURAL AND NECESSARY**. There is usually a variety of methods to achieve any given outcome. Determine what you need and what you want, and think through the requirements of different options. Whenever possible, pick ones that feel right for you—that fit your personality, interests, and responsibilities.

G = **GOALS AND GRADUALISM**. Make sure you get what you want and want what you get. Think of the process as a journey—if you're not sure where you're going, you won't know how to get there or when you've arrived. Take one step at a time:

- Define realistic, long-term goals that you are willing to commit to.
- Identify specific short-term objectives you can complete in 2-3 months at most.
- Select a limited number of objectives that you know you can achieve.
- Monitor progress and update objectives until your long-term goals are met.

E = **EXPECTATIONS AND ENJOYMENT**. Change is a process, not an event. Find ways to motivate yourself over the long haul (rewards, challenges, games, etc.). Be realistic in your expectations—if one approach doesn't work, try another. Make sure you enjoy the process as well as the results or you may not stick with it.

Activity 10-3

INDIVIDUAL WELLNESS PLANNING

THE CHANGE PROCESS

As noted previously, making and, more importantly, maintaining lifestyle changes involves many factors, and it's a highly personal process. **Only you can decide what works best for you in different situations**. However, behavioral scientists know that many attempts fail because people don't take the time to think through what they want and what they will have to do to get it.

This analytical process is not difficult—in fact, you do it informally all the time whether you realize it or not. But it is sometimes helpful to use a more systematic approach, particularly for important or difficult goals you want to accomplish.

Steps in this simplified change process can be equated to the phases of emergency operations, as shown in Table 10-5:

Table 10-5

COMPARISON OF PLANNING STEPS

EMERGENCY RESPONSE	PERSONAL CHANGE
1. Respond to the alarm	1. Recognize the need for change
2. Establish incident priorities	2. Set personal goals
3. Conduct size-up	3. Analyze the situation
4. Develop strategy and tactics	4. Select objectives and methods
5. Develop an action plan	5. Develop an action plan
6. Implement the plan: incident operations	6. Implement the plan: behavioral change
7. Conduct a post-incident critique/debriefing	7. Evaluate your progress and modify the plan

PURPOSE OF ACTIVITY

This activity defines the steps of a simple personal planning process. You are encouraged to go through the steps, using a lifestyle goal of your own choosing. The exercise will give you an opportunity to think about some of the factors that affect your own personal change style. Although details of the process may vary in different situations, the basic approach is equally appropriate for any type of personal goal—health and fitness, career, social, educational, etc.

<u>**Instructions**</u>

1. Select a broad long-term **goal**—an area in your life in which you would like to make a lifestyle change. Define your goal in one or two sentences.

2. List the **benefits** you will receive when you accomplish this goal—why it will be worth the effort. Try to envision how you will feel when you are successful. Make sure you clarify your <u>real</u> motivations for making the change.

3. Brainstorm a variety of smaller steps, or **objectives**, you could take to help reach your goal. For example, to lose weight, you could give up dessert, quit drinking soda, stop snacking between meals, eat more vegetables, etc. List as many as possible. Then go back and select a few to work on over the next 2-3 months.

4. Identify the **helps** and **hindrances** you will face—possible sources of support and obstacles that could make the change more difficult. Be sure to include your own strengths and weaknesses on the list.

5. Select several specific action steps you will take over the next 2-3 months. Include ways to maximize the "helps" and minimize the "hindrances." Add dates and other details as appropriate. Most importantly, be realistic—don't plan more than you are actually willing to do. Set yourself up for success!

6. Look over the plan and revise it until you're satisfied. Then select a date, perhaps 1-2 months from now, when you will review and update the plan. Finally, commit yourself to carrying it out by signing it at the bottom.

PERSONAL WELLNESS PLAN

A. Goal / Reason(s): ___

___

___

___

B. Benefits: ___

___

___

___

___

___

___

___

C. Objectives ___

___

___

___

___

___

___

___

___

___

___

___

___

D. Helps: ___

___

___

___

___

___

___

___

___

Hindrances: ___

___

___

___

___

___

___

___

___

___

___

E. Action Steps/Dates ___

___

___

___

___

___

___

___

___

___

___

___

___

___

___

F. Personal Commitment:

Plan Review Date ___

___

Signature

Consolidating Your Plan

During this activity, you prepared an action plan for one wellness goal. Since wellness looks at many different facets of life, you may have more than one goal (e.g., to lose weight, quit smoking, and reduce stress). To develop a comprehensive wellness plan, simply prepare separate action plans for each goal. When you are done, you may want to integrate the separate plans into one document for convenience. A form like the one on the next page may be useful for this purpose.

ACTIVITY SUMMARY

This activity provided practice in using a simple model for personal planning, whether for wellness or any other area of your life. Other approaches may be equally as effective. The key is to approach the process systematically and to find a method that works for you.

Whether you choose this method or another, remember the goal is to analyze the situation as clearly as possible and develop a plan that maximizes your chance of success. Writing it down just helps to structure your thinking process. In short:

- **Self-analysis and planning are the keys to success in making any type of personal change.**
- **The ability to make and sustain personal change is the key to controlling your lifestyle.**
- **Lifestyle is the key to health and wellness.**

However, no approach works if you don't believe you can change or if you don't want to. Change is a process that becomes easier the more you practice it and learn about yourself. Stick with it and you will become the person you want to be.

CONSOLIDATED WELLNESS PLAN

Goal	Action Step/Date
1.	■ /
	■ /
	■ /
	■ /
2.	■ /
	■ /
	■ /
	■ /
3.	■ /
	■ /
	■ /
	■ /
4.	■ /
	■ /
	■ /
	■ /
5.	■ /
	■ /
	■ /
	■ /

CHAPTER SUMMARY

Wellness can be defined as a comprehensive philosophy or approach to improve the quality of life and to promote lifetime health and well-being. In this chapter, you took a broad look at some of the different components of wellness, including physical fitness and exercise, diet and nutrition, control of dangerous substances, stress management, personal safety, and periodic medical examinations.

After discussing health risks and wellness trends in the United States, you used a self-assessment instrument to identify areas in your own lifestyle that could be improved. Tips for making and maintaining lifestyle changes were discussed next. Finally, you practiced using a simple model for personal planning.

Having completed this chapter, you should now be able to:

- ♦ Identify major health risks in the United States.
- ♦ Identify major wellness trends in the United States.
- ♦ Examine your own wellness behaviors to determine possible areas for improvement.
- ♦ Discuss guidelines for making and maintaining personal lifestyle changes.
- ♦ Prepare a personal wellness plan that takes into account your own health needs and goals.

BIBLIOGRAPHY

Centers for Disease Control, "Behavioral Risk Factor Surveillance, 1986-1990," *Morbidity and Mortality Weekly Report*, Vol. 40/No. SS-4, December 1991.

Louis Harris and Associates, Inc., *The Baxter Survey of American Health Habits*, Study No. 923009, December 1992.

National Center for Health Statistics, *Health, United States, 1991*, Hyattsville, Maryland: Public Health Service, 1992.

National Fire Academy, "Module II: Firefighter Health and Physical Fitness," *Firefighter Safety and Survival: The Company Officer's Responsibility*, 1988.

Pollock, Michael L., Jack H. Wilmore, and Samuel M. Fox III, *Health and Fitness Through Physical Activity*, New York: John Wiley & Sons, 1978.

Squires, Sally, "More Americans Are Too Fat, Study Shows," *The Washington Post*, July 20, 1994.

United States Fire Administration, *Administrative Manual on Use of Drugs by Fire Department Members*, FA 77, May 1988.

United States Fire Administration, *Physical Fitness Coordinator's Manual for Fire Departments*, 1990.

United States Fire Administration, *Stress Management: Model Program for Maintaining Firefighter Well-Being*, FA-100, February 1991.

University of California, Berkeley, *The Wellness Encyclopedia: The Comprehensive Family Resource for Safeguarding Health and Preventing Illness*, Boston: Houghton Mifflin Company, 1991.

INDEX

Printed and bound by CPI Group (UK) Ltd, Croydon, CR0 4YY
16/09/2026
14963450-0001